ALLERGY AND IMMUNOLOGY SECRETS

ALLERGY AND IMMUNOLOGY SECRETS

Stanley M. Naguwa, M.D.

Clinical Professor
Division of Rheumatology/Allergy and Clinical Immunology
Department of Internal Medicine
University of California, Davis, School of Medicine
Davis, California
Staff Rheumatologist
Veterans Affairs Northern California Healthcare System
Mather, California

M. Eric Gershwin, M.D.

The Jack and Donald Chia Professor of Medicine
Chief, Division of Rheumatology/Allergy and Clinical Immunology
Department of Internal Medicine
University of California, Davis, School of Medicine
Davis, California

HANLEY & BELFUS, INC./Philadelphia

Publisher: HANLEY & BELFUS, INC.
                  Medical Publishers
                  210 South 13th Street
                  Philadelphia, PA 19107
                  (215) 546-7293; 800-962-1892
                  FAX (215) 790-9330
                  Web site: http://www.hanleyandbelfus.com

Note to the reader: Although the information in this book has been carefully reviewed for correctness of dosage and indications, neither the authors nor the editors nor the publisher can accept any legal responsibility for any errors or omissions that may be made. Neither the publisher nor the editors make any warranty, espressed or implied, with respect to the material contained herein. Before prescribing any drug, the reader must review the manufacturer's current product information (package inserts) for accepted indications, absolute dosage recommendations, and other information pertinent to the safe and effective use of the product described. This is especially important when drugs are given in combination or as an adjunct to other forms of therapy.

Library of Congress Cataloging-in-Publication Data

Allergy and immunology secrets / edited by Stanley M. Naguwa, M. Eric Gershwin.
        p. ; cm.—(Secrets Series®)
    Includes bibliographical references and index.
    ISBN 1-56053-414-1 (alk. paper)
        1. Allergy—Miscellanea. II. Immunology—Miscellanea. I. Naguwa, Stanley M., 1945–
II. Gershwin, M. Eric, 1946– III. Series.
        [DNLM: 1. Allergy and Immunology—Examination Questions.   2.
Hypersensitivity—Examination Questions. QW 18.2 A434 2001]
    RC585.A4454 2001
    616.97—dc21

                                                        00-065443

ALLERGY AND IMMUNOLOGY SECRETS   ISBN 1-56053-414-1

Last digit is the print number: 9   8   7   6   5   4   3   2   1

CONTENTS

CONTRIBUTORS

Rahmat Afrasiabi, M.D.
Assistant Clinical Professor, Department of Internal Medicine, University of California, Davis, School of Medicine, Davis, California; University of California, Davis, Medical Center, Sacramento, California; Enloe Hospital, Chico, California

Christopher Chang, M.D., Ph.D.
Associate Professor, Department of Internal Medicine, University of California, Davis, School of Medicine, Davis, California; University of California, Davis, Medical Center, Sacramento, California

Richard S. DeMera, M.D.
Division of Rheumatology/Allergy and Clinical Immunology, Department of Internal Medicine, University of California, Davis, School of Medicine, Davis, California; University of California, Davis, Medical Center, Sacramento, California

Gordon Garcia, M.D.
Assistant Clinical Professor, Department of Pediatrics, University of California, Davis, School of Medicine, Davis, California; Kaiser Foundation Hospital, Sacramento, California

M. Eric Gershwin, M.D.
The Jack and Donald Chia Professor of Medicine and Chief, Division of Rheumatology/Allergy and Clinical Immunology, Department of Internal Medicine, University of California, Davis, School of Medicine, Davis, California

Katherine E. Gundling, M.D., FACP
Associate Adjunct Professor, Department of Dermatology, University of California, Davis, School of Medicine, Davis, California; University of California, Davis, Medical Center, Sacramento, California

Rosemary L. Hallett, M.D.
Division of Rheumatology/Allergy and Clinical Immunology, Department of Internal Medicine, University of California, Davis, School of Medicine, Davis, California

Maurice E. Hamilton, M.D.
Clinical Professor, Division of Rheumatology/Allergy and Clinical Immunology, Department of Internal Medicine, University of California, Davis, School of Medicine, Davis, California

Russell J. Hopp, D.O.
Professor, Department of Pediatrics, Creighton University School of Medicine; St. Joseph Hospital, Omaha, Nebraska

Joshua S. Jacobs, M.D.
Assistant Clinical Professor, Department of Internal Medicine, University of California, Davis, School of Medicine, Davis, California; Staff Allergist, John Muir Medical Center, Walnut Creek, California

Nicholas J. Kenyon, M.D.
Division of Pulmonary and Critical Care Medicine, Department of Internal Medicine, University of California, Davis, School of Medicine, Davis, California

Sarah Kuhl, M.D., Ph.D.
Division of Rheumatology/Allergy and Clinical Immunology, Department of Internal Medicine, University of California, Davis, School of Medicine, Davis, California; Sacramento Veterans Affairs Medical Center, Mather, California

James C. Leek, M.D.
Clinical Professor of Medicine, Division of Rheumatology/Allergy and Clinical Immunology, Department of Internal Medicine, University of California, Davis, School of Medicine, Davis, California

Samuel Louie, M.D.
Professor, Division of Pulmonary and Critical Care Medicine, Department of Internal Medicine, University of California, Davis, School of Medicine, Davis, California

Massoud Mahmoudi, D.O., Ph.D.
Clinical Assistant Professor, Department of Internal Medicine, College of Osteopathic Medicine, University of Medicine and Dentistry of New Jersey, Stratford, New Jersey; California Pacific Medical Center, San Francisco, California

Stanley M. Naguwa, M.D.
Clinical Professor, Division of Rheumatology/Allergy and Clinical Immunology, Department of Internal Medicine, University of California, Davis, School of Medicine, Davis, California; Staff Rheumatologist, Veterans Affairs Northern California Healthcare System, Mather, California

Kristina Hoffman Philpott, M.D.
Allergy and Immunology Department, Palo Alto Medical Foundation; Stanford University Hospital, Palo Alto, California

Bruce T. Ryhal, M.D.
Associate Clinical Professor, Department of Internal Medicine, University of California, Davis, School of Medicine, Davis, California; Senior Physician, Department of Allergy, Kaiser-Permanente Medical Center, Roseville, California

Arif M. Seyal, M.D.
Associate Clinical Professor, Division of Allergy and Clinical Immunology, Department of Internal Medicine, University of California, Davis, School of Medicine, Davis, California; Chief, Department of Allergy and Clinical Immunology, Permanente Medical Group, Roseville, California

E. Bradley Strong, M.D.
Assistant Professor, Department of Otolaryngology-Head and Neck Surgery, University of California, Davis, School of Medicine, Davis, California; University of California, Davis, Medical Center, Sacramento, California

Suzanne S. Teuber, M.D.
Associate Professor, Division of Rheumatology/Allergy and Clinical Immunology, Department of Internal Medicine, University of California, Davis, School of Medicine, Davis, California

Robert D. Watson, Ph.D., M.D.
Allergy Department, MedClinic, CHW Medical Foundation; Mercy General Hospital, Sacramento, California

Mark J. Zlotlow, M.D.
Assistant Clinical Professor, Department of Pediatrics, University of California, Davis, School of Medicine, Davis, California; Assistant Chief, Allergy Department, North Valley CSA, Permanente Medical Group, Roseville, California

PREFACE

Allergies are among the most common chronic problems of childhood and the most frequent complaints of adults. Several national studies have demonstrated that up to 20% of people in the United States suffer from allergic rhinitis and up to 10% suffer from asthma. More than 90% of patients with allergies require some form of intermittent drug therapy. These overwhelming statistics, as well as the chronic and sometimes restrictive nature of allergies, result in significant stress for patients and families. However, despite the widespread nature of asthma and allergies and the fact that they have been well characterized throughout reported medical history, the basic disease process is only now being defined. Indeed, there are large numbers of etiologies that interact in the common pathways of allergic disease.

Because of the ubiquitous nature of allergies, physicians in many disciplines are called upon to treat allergic patients. Although the majority of research on allergy occurs at large university medical centers, the bulk of medical care is delivered throughout the community by primary care physicians. At the University of California, we have emphasized the need for continued and intensive education of our housestaff in order to improve the care of people who suffer from allergic disease. The specialization of allergy and immunology, one of the most exciting disciplines in medicine, attracts students from both pediatrics and internal medicine. In addition, with the growing numbers of adult-onset allergy, even gerontologists need to be kept abreast of advances in the management of immunologic problems. In this volume, our goal has been to bring together important issues for housestaff and for primary care physicians of all backgrounds. We have provided readers with useful materials to help them in their board examinations and perhaps even stimulate a career in allergy and immunology. Most importantly, we hope it improves the care of patients.

Stanley M. Naguwa, MD
M. Eric Gershwin, MD

1. GENETICS AND EPIDEMIOLOGY OF ALLERGIC DISEASE

Russell J. Hopp, D.O.

EPIDEMIOLOGY OF ALLERGIC DISEASES IN THE UNITED STATES

1. What is the current prevalence of atopic dermatitis in the United States?

An international study of the prevalence of symptoms of allergies and asthma (International Study of Asthma and Allergies in Childhood–ISAAC) evaluated the current prevalence of atopic eczema with the question "ever had an itchy rash which was coming and going for at least six months?" In the sole United States site, Seattle, the 12-month prevalence was 9.4% for adolescents age 13 to 14 years. There was a lifetime prevalence of 19.4%.

The worldwide literature on atopic dermatitis was reviewed as of 1992. The conclusions in a study by Schultz-Larsen were that the prevalence rates for atopic dermatitis were 10–12%, and that less than 15% maintain their disease after puberty.

2. What is the prevalence of allergic rhinoconjunctivitis in the United States?

ISAAC evaluated the current prevalence of allergic rhinoconjunctivitis with the questions, "In the past 12 months have you had a problem with sneezing, or a runny, or blocked nose when you DID NOT have a cold? Or the flu?," and (if yes), "In the past 12 months, has this nose problem been accompanied by itchy-watery eyes?" In the United States, two sites in Chicago and a site in Seattle, asked these questions of more than 7,000 children age 13–14 years. The 12-month prevalence ranged from 12% to 22%.

The third National Health and Nutrition Examination Survey, 1988–94 (NHANES III), collected data on seasonal and perennial allergic rhinoconjunctivitis. Based on survey data, the prevalence of allergic rhinitis is: 19.9%, 26.8%, and 29.6% in the age groups 6–11 years, 12–17 years, and 18 years and older, respectively. Of the 71 million people with allergic rhinitis, based on the current US population, 13.6 million have continuous symptoms.

3. What percent of the US population has positive allergy skin tests?

A survey of allergy skin test reactivity in the United States through the auspices of the National Health and Nutrition Examination Survey, 1976–80 (NHANES II), showed that the rates of skin test response to one or more common allergens was greatest in adolescents and young adults. Males were more often positive than females, and blacks were more often positive than whites. In the age group 6–11 years, 18% of whites and 28% of blacks were positive. In the age group 12–17 years, 23% of whites and 36% of blacks were positive, with similar rates for subjects in the age group 18–24 years. Rates were lower in subjects older than 25 years for both racial groups.

4. What is the current prevalence of asthma in children in the United States?

The Centers for Disease Control and Prevention (CDC) has surveyed and summarized asthma statistics in the United States. Since 1979, the Ninth International Classification of Diseases (ICD-9) has been used for defining asthma for mortality analysis, using codes 493 to 493.9.

The CDC released a comprehensive report in 1998, documenting a 75% increase in self-reported asthma from 1980 to 1994. This increase crossed all races, both genders, and all age groups. Children demonstrated remarkable increases: 160% in those 0–4 years of age and 74% for those 5–14 years of age.

Using data generated by 1995 state-specific estimates of asthma, the CDC estimated that in 1998 there were 17 million people in the United States with asthma. Asthma was defined as having been physician diagnosed and symptomatic within the past 12 months. State-specific rates ranged from 5.8% to 7.2%.

NHANES III collected data on the prevalence of asthma in the United States. Prevalence was determined by a physician diagnosis at any time, but with symptoms in the past year. In ages 6–11 years, the prevalence was 6.6%; prevalence was 9.6% for those 12–17 years of age.

5. What is the prevalence of adult-onset asthma?

Adult-onset asthma has not gained a national or international sense of urgency, as has pediatric-onset asthma. The available data, however, suggests increasing trends. The United States National Health Interview Survey from 1980 through 1994 reported the average annual rate of self-reported asthma. Per 1,000 individuals, rates were given for ages 15–34, 35–64 and ≥ 65 years. The results are presented below.

AGE	1980	1981–83	1983–86	1987–89	1990–92	1993–94
15–34	27.7%	30.2%	35.1%	40.1%	41.7%	51.8%
35–64	28.1%	33.1%	32.0%	36.8%	42.3%	44.6%
≥ 65	30.7%	34.4%	38.9%	42.1%	36.4%	44.6%

The cumulative prevalence of asthma in US adults was ascertained by the Second National Health and Nutrition Examination Survey, 1976–80. Defined as ever being told by a physician that he/she had asthma, and/or frequent problems with wheezing in the past 12 months, the rates were 9.9% for ages 12–44 years, 11.8% for ages 45–64 years, and 12.4% for ages 65–74 years.

NHANES III collected data on the prevalence of asthma in the United States. Prevalence was determined by a physician diagnosis at any time, but with symptoms in the past year. In ages 18 years or older, the prevalence was 5.9%.

In the United States, deaths with asthma as the underlying cause have increased in the adult population from 1960 through 1995. Using the results from ICD-9, 1979 and following, the number of deaths of adults 65 years of age or greater has increased from 1,481 in 1979 to 2,972 in 1995, a 200% increase. In adults ages 34–65 years, an increase of 186% in asthma-associated deaths occurred during the same years, although the total number of deaths is about 60% of the older adults.

EPIDEMIOLOGY OF ALLERGIC DISEASES OUTSIDE
OF THE UNITED STATES

6. What is the current prevalence of atopic dermatitis?

ISAAC evaluated the current prevalence of atopic eczema with the question, "ever had an itchy rash which was coming and going for at least six months?" The 12-month prevalence results for children ages 13–14 years ranged from virtually nonexistent in China and Albania, to between 15% and 20% in Nigeria, the United Kingdom, Finland, and Sweden.

In other studies using doctor diagnosis, the prevalence of atopic eczema in German children 6 years old was 15.7% in East Germany and 12.9% in West Germany. In Danish children ages 5–16 years, the prevalence was 7%. A lifetime rate, based on questionnaire, of 24% was found in Norwegian children, ages 7–12 years. In children ages 3–11 years in the United Kingdom, the current prevalence was 11.5%, with a lifetime rate of 20%, based on clinic chart data.

7. What is the prevalence of allergic rhinoconjunctivitis?

ISAAC evaluated the current prevalence of allergic rhinoconjunctivitis with the questions, "In the past 12 months have you had a problem with sneezing, or a runny, or blocked nose when you DID NOT have a cold? Or the flu?," and (if yes), "In the past 12 months, has this nose problem been accompanied by itchy-watery eyes?" The 12-month prevalence data ranged from less than 5% in several former Soviet bloc nations to well over 25% in Nigeria, Paraguay, and Hong Kong, and near 25% in Argentina, Canada, and Australia. The United Kingdom was similar to the United States at 12–22%, depending on the site.

8. What is the current prevalence of asthma in children?

ISAAC evaluated the prevalence of asthma and asthma symptoms in children ages 6–7 years and ages 13–14 years throughout the world in the mid-1990s. For children ages 6–7 years, the question to their parents of "Ever had asthma?" resulted in a prevalence of 10.2% globally, with the Oceanic area of New Zealand and Australia having a prevalence of 26.8%, at the high end, and the eastern and northern European regions being the lowest at 3.2%. Rates in children ages 13–14 years, for the question "Ever had asthma?" revealed rates of 26% in the Oceanic region and 4.4% for the eastern and northern European regions. Rates in the United Kingdom were the highest for all Western European regional countries, over 19% for the UK, and 13.0% for all Western European countries, inclusive of the UK.

9. What is the prevalence of adult-onset asthma?

The European Commission Respiratory Health Study, a multicenter survey of the prevalence and determinants of asthma in adults 20–44 years of age, is probably the most recent comprehensive study of the disease symptoms in young adults. In the 45 centers reporting data, the median 12-month prevalence of asthma attacks was 3.1%, treatment for asthma was 3.5%, the maximum prevalence in any center was 9.7% for attacks, and 9.8% for treatment.

INTERRELATIONSHIP OF THE ATOPIC DISEASES

10. What are the known relationships between the common allergic diseases?
Atopic dermatitis, the most usual early presenting atopic disease, is a herald for the development of allergic rhinitis and/or asthma. Nearly 50% of children with atopic dermatitis will develop either rhinitis and/or asthma.

NHANES III collected data on the prevalence of asthma in the United States. Prevalence was determined by a physician diagnosis at any time and with symptoms in the past year. In children ages 6–11 years, the prevalence was 6.6%; in adolescents ages 12–17 years, it was 9.6%; for those age 18 years or older, the prevalence was 5.9%. Further analysis based on reports of allergic symptoms and/or atopy that was determined by positive skin tests, revealed that 80% of children ages 6–11 years, 86% of adolescents ages 12–17 years, and 93% of adults age 18 years or older with asthma also had concomitant atopic or allergic manifestations.

ISAAC evaluated the prevalence of asthma and asthma symptoms, allergic conjunctivitis and atopic dermatitis in children ages 6–7 years and 13–14 years throughout the world in the mid-1990s. The symptoms of asthma (A), allergic rhino-conjunctivits (AR), and atopic eczema (AE) for the previous 12 months were compared by regression analysis.

COMPARISON	REGRESSION COEFFICIENT	SIGNIFICANCE
A versus AR	0.75	$p < 0.0001$
A versus AE	0.74	$p < 0.0001$
AR versus AE	0.71	$p < 0.0001$

FACTORS INFLUENCING THE DEVELOPMENT OF ATOPIC DISEASES

11. Are there differences in the risk factors for the different atopic diseases?
Despite the close relationship between the atopic diseases, there are risk factors differences that could account for the development of these diseases. Asthma, in particular, has both allergic and nonallergic factors that have been casually associated with its development. In contrast, allergic rhinitis is, by definition, due totally to atopy, and the biggest risk factor, beyond a genetic predisposition, are allergen exposure. Atopic dermatitis is probably more similar to asthma, but the biggest risk factor is atopy.

In addition, it is possible to have factors that reduce the development of an allergic disease. Breast-feeding is a classic example.

12. What is an odds ratio?
Epidemiologic data is commonly expressed as a relative risk or odds ratio. A relative risk is used with cohort studies, and odds ratio are used with case-control studies. A ratio of 1.0 indicates no effect, a ratio > 1.0 indicates an effect, and a ratio < 1 indicates the studied "risk" factor is actually of benefit to the individual.

13. How are atopy, allergy, and allergic rhinitis defined in epidemiologic studies.

Being atopic or allergic is generally defined as having evidence for specific IgE, regardless of any specific clinical diagnosis. This is defined, in various reports, as having a positive immediate skin test with a typical wheal and flare, having a positive RAST, or having an IgE level greater than two standard deviations above the mean. The last criterion is generally less useful.

Allergic rhinitis is a clinical diagnosis, which in most epidemiologic studies is either self- or parental reported, or termed "allergic rhinitis" if symptoms compatible with allergic rhinitis are reported. It is uncommon to see both atopy and self-reported allergic rhinitis used together to define allergic rhinitis.

14. What are the risk factors for being atopic?

The most common reason for being atopic is parental presence of atopy. The risk for being atopic is 1.4 if only the mother is atopic, and the same if only the father is atopic. If both parents are atopic, the odds ratio (risk) is 2.8. Other studies show that 90% of atopic children have at least one atopic parent; that 66% of children were atopic when one parent was atopic; and that 75% of children were atopic if both parents were atopic. That children with two atopic parents can be found to be nonatopic (at the time of testing) suggests that environment factors necessary for sensitization must also exist!

15. What risk factors are conducive to the development of asthma? What is the level of risk for these factors?

CAUSATIVE FACTOR	RELATIVE RISK OR ODDS RATIO (SINGLE REPORT UNLESS OTHERWISE NOTED)
Specific allergen-positive skin tests	*Alternaria* was 5.0 House dust was 2.9
Passive smoke exposure	Pooled odds ratio from the analysis of 60 studies was 1.21
Prematurity	Birthweight < 1,500 grams was 1.61; respiratory distress syndrome was 2.95; prematurity was 1.34
Familial factors: Adoption	Adoptive mother atopic was 3.2; adoptive father atopic was 1.9
Weight	Highest quintile for weight was boys 2.3; girls 1.5
Antibiotics	Use of antibiotics was 2.74; use of antibiotics before age 1 year was 4.05

16. What other factors influence the development of asthma, but with a less quantifiable risk?

CAUSATIVE FACTOR	SUBJECTIVE RISK (AUTHOR'S OPINION)
Gender: boys before age 10 years; girls after puberty	Well-documented
Bronchial hyperresponsiveness	Rarely measured before developing asthma, but its presence in an atopic person is a moderate risk
Atopic dermatitis in infancy or early childhood	Moderate risk

(Table continued on next page.)

CAUSATIVE FACTOR	SUBJECTIVE RISK (AUTHOR'S OPINION)
Atopy	Moderate risk
Racial/ethnic	In the United States, it is closely associated with socio-economic factors; African-Americans and Puerto Ricans are at a higher risk
Socioeconomic factors	Higher risk in lower income families
Air pollution	Small risk, if any
Attendance at day care	Small risk
Cockroach exposure	Moderate risk
Alum-containing vaccinations	Questionable, but theoretically increases TH2 responses
Respiratory syncytial virus infection	With a serious RSV infection, the risk is very high

17. If a parent has asthma, what are the risk factors that may enhance the development of asthma in the offspring?

A study from the National Jewish Center for Immunology and Respiratory Medicine prospectively studied this issue. One hundred fifty asthmatic pregnant women were recruited. Twenty-eight fathers were also asthmatic. At age 3 years, the child's asthma status was identified, and the risk factors for the development of asthma assessed. The risk factors were compared individually and in combination.

FACTORS	PROBABILITY OF ASTHMA AT AGE 3 YEARS (%)
No risk factors	2
Psychosocial stressers	6
IgE > 10 IU at age 6 months	7
Frequent illness (> 8)	7
Frequent illness and IgE > 10 IU	22
Frequent illnesses, IgE >10 IU at age 6 months, and excessive psychosocial factors	55

18. Are there any factors that reduce asthma risk?

The pooled odds ratio for the effect of breast-feeding for more than 3 months on the development of asthma is 0.80. Breast-feeding has numerous beneficial effects for infants, and should remain the choice for nutrition for newborns. Its benefit as an asthma prophylaxis appears conservative, but could be significant if breast-feeding could be increased.

An increased ingestion of 3-omega fatty acids, common in a diet rich in fish, may have a modest effect in reducing asthma prevalence.

19. What risk factors are conducive to the development of allergic rhinitis and what are their levels of risk? What factors may reduce allergic rhinitis development?

RISK FACTORS FOR ALLERGIC RHINITIS	RISK (QUALITATIVE OR QUANTITATIVE) FOR ALLERGIC RHINITIS DIAGNOSIS OR SYMPTOMS
Month of birth	May be a factor for regions with high seasonal pollens counts.
Western life style	Increased
Parental allergy/atopy	Increased
Lower birth order	Increased
Multiple gestation	Increased
Younger birth mother	Increased
Food allergy (atopy)	Increased
Traffic related air pollution	Increased
Not breast-feeding	Increased
Atopy (+ allergy skin tests)	Increased
Childhood farm environment	Decreased
Breast-feeding	Decreased

20. What risk factors are conducive to the development of atopic dermatitis and what are their levels of risk? What factors may reduce atopic dermatitis development?

RISK FACTORS FOR ATOPIC DERMATITIS	RISK (QUALITATIVE OR QUANTITATIVE) FOR ATOPIC DERMATITIS
Parental atopic dermatitis	Increased
Parental allergy	Increased
No siblings	Increased
Animals exposure in bedroom	Increased
Heavy traffic exposure	Increased
Higher socioeconomic advantages	Increased
High newborn eosinophilia	Increased
Low breast-milk IgA	Increased
Strict maternal dietary restrictions and breast feeding	May reduce or postpone
Domestic hard water	Increases

21. Can the "hygiene hypothesis" explain the increased incidence of asthma and allergy?

It has been proposed that living in a highly developed country might be detrimental risk factor for development of asthma and/or atopy. This is, in part, supported by studies showing a larger family size, and even an indoor pet, having a protective effect on the development of atopic diseases. Results from studies of this nature focus on the concept of TH1 and TH2 CD4+ T-cells. TH1 cells are responsible for

thwarting serious infectious agents, while TH2 cells are seemingly involved with atopic responses. If children are more vigorously using their TH1 T-cells, less stimulation of TH2 occurs.

If the hygiene hypothesis has merit, it probably has more validity in highly developed nations, although it may play a role in rural versus urban differences in developing nations.

22. Describe the role of air pollution in the development of an allergic disease.

Because air pollution, increased diesel particulates, and ozone are all common urban air pollution problems, it has been suggested that the increase in asthma incidence could be associated with these pollutants. The most convincing argument against this, however, is the data coming from surveys of asthma and allergy in reunified Germany. In several studies, the incidence of childhood asthma was not greater in East Germany, the more industrialized and polluted country, and atopy was more common in West Germany.

The direct role of ozone, NO_2, and diesel particulates, and the increase in asthma in industrialized nations, has not been adequately answered, and continued evaluations on their role(s) should continue.

GENETIC FACTORS IN ATOPIC DISEASE

23. Why should segregation analysis be used?

This method of analysis suggests the pattern of inheritance of a disorder or phenotype by observing how it is distributed with families. The absence or presence of asthma, atopy, or a serum IgE level, can be used as the variable of interest. Segregation analysis compares the affected phenotype in the families with the expected phenotype using various statistical models. The analysis can provide a suggestion for the mode of inheritance and whether a single gene or multiple genes are responsible.

24. What are candidate gene studies?

The most commonly performed genetic studies of asthma focus on nuclear families, sib pairs, or large extended families. In these evaluations, surrogate representation of the asthmatic condition is used to define the disease. The most important concern is to "correctly" pick the surrogate(s) that best "equate(s)" to the clinical state. In most studies a combination of factors is used to identify the proband (index subject) as "asthmatic."

A candidate gene study is an a priori approach. In essence, the search for the "asthma" gene is preselected, based on known biologic information about asthma. This method of genetic analysis identifies whether the "asthmatic" proband, or surrogate, has a statistical association with polymorphisms (simple repeat-sequence loci) occurring with the candidate gene or regions of specific chromosomes. If there is a significant association between the surrogate (i.e., a positive methacholine challenge) and a known marker on a specific chromosome, by inference, the "gene" for the asthma condition or the surrogate marker for the asthma condition may be on that chromosome and near that repeat-sequence loci. By using other loci on the same chromosome, the closeness or distance from known candidate genes can be determined.

ATOPY-RELATED SURROGATES	ASTHMA-RELATED SURROGATES
Serum IgE at a specific "elevated" level	+ Methacholine challenge
+ Skin test(s) to standardized allergens	+ Histamine challenge
+ RAST test(s)	Clinical diagnosis of asthma
	Reversibility to a beta-agonist
	Combinations of Column A and Column B

25. Describe the genome search approach for the genes for asthma or allergy.

The genome search approach takes an unbiased stance, relative to asthma biology, and allows unsuspected genes to be identified. The Collaborative Study on the Genetics of Asthma (CSGA) has detected a number of potential candidate gene areas for further research. Using the entire genome, linkages to specific marker areas are sought. Further evaluations using other markers on these "new" candidate genes can then be used to establish potential linkage, and unique biologic reasons for the biology of asthma.

26. How can studies of structural gene variations assist in the genetics of asthma?

If a candidate gene is the cause of asthma, a reasonable approach to elucidating the etiology of asthma is to study the various forms (polymorphisms) of a specific gene. For example, differences in the IL-4 alpha subunit, the beta-chain of the high-affinity receptor for IgE, and the beta-adrenergic receptor have been found. The question is whether these structural differences account for the disease itself or for different phenotypes or severity of the disease.

27. What have been the results of genetic studies of serum IgE levels?

Segregation analysis has been the predominant method in the attempt to determine the inheritance of IgE levels. A critical issue has been uncovered, in that the basal IgE level may be controlled by a gene(s) separate from the gene(s) responsible for the IgE response to specific allergens. This is evident by the fact that IgE *is* detectable in most humans, but specific IgE is *not* detected in all humans

The major studies of serum IgE levels to date, using segregation analysis, have generally supported an heritable model, but with varying genetic models, including major gene, either recessive or codominant. Other authors have shown polygenic, genetic heterogeneity, and no genetic effect.

A suggestion has been made that a recessive gene may be responsible for basal IgE levels, and is supported by the analysis of random families, while a dominant gene may be involved in high IgE levels, as ascertained through asthma families.

28. Which cytokines are responsible for IgE production? What is known about the genetics of these cytokines?

Genetic linkage has been identified between total serum IgE and a region on chromosome 5q31-33. This region codes for a variety of cytokines genes that have critical importance in understanding atopy. These include IL-3, IL-4, IL-5, IL-9, and IL-13. Most importantly, IL-4 and IL-13 are known to participate in IgE synthesis by influencing class switching to IgE by human B cells. The genes for these two cytokines are closely localized to 5q31 chromosome. The most recent studies suggest that IL-13 is the more critical cytokine for IgE production.

Linkage studies for atopy, either elevated IgE levels or positive skin tests, show statistical association with, initially, the locus for IL-4, but more convincingly with the locus for IL-13. There is a suggestion that the "basal" level of IgE might be regulated by the gene(s) for IL-13.

29. List the chromosomes that have been linked by using the candidate gene approach to factors associated with IgE or atopy.

To date, IgE levels and/or atopy have been linked to 5q; serum IgE levels to 12q, atopy to 11q, and 14q for specific IgE responses. These data also support the variability seen in segregation analysis of serum IgE levels.

30. What is the HLA system?

Human leukocyte antigen (HLA), is the major histocompatibility complex in humans. The genetic control for the HLA system is on chromosome 6. These genes encode proteins of three different types: Classes I, II, and III. Class III proteins are complement proteins. There are three Class I loci: HLA-A, HLA-B, and HLA-C, and each has multiple alleles. The Class I alleles are specific to the individual codes for HLAs that resides on nucleated cells. These antigens can be tissue typed.

Class II molecules are encoded by the DR, DP, and DQ regions of the HLA complex. The Class II molecules are mostly limited to cells responsible for immunity. There are different loci for each of the three Class II regions, and these alleles code for the specific Class II molecules that reside on T and B lymphocytes.

Because Class I and Class II molecules are encoded by genes, they can be used as markers for determining the likelihood of inheriting other genetic traits, such as highly specific IgE responses.

31. Describe allergenic epitopes.

The antigenic location on a large allergen that the human IgE antibody recognizes is the allergenic epitope. Each allergen has one or more major epitopes. These epitopes can be identified by a positive allergic skin-test reaction. Peanut, for example, expresses three major epitopes, Ara h 1–3. Because these proteins are available for skin testing, it is possible to "fingerprint" each atopic patient to their exact epitope profile. A patient's specific epitope IgE response can then be compared to his or her HLA characteristics and statistical associations between HLA type and specific epitope antigen-IgE response. Examples are shown below.

ALLERGEN	HLA	ETHNIC GROUP
Der p 1 (House dust mite)	HLA-DPB1	
Bet v I (Birch)	HLA-DR3	Caucasian
Amb a V (Ragweed)	HLA-DR2	Caucasian
Lol p I-III (Rye grass)	HLA-DR3	Caucasian

BIBLIOGRAPHY

1. Bodner C, Godden D, Seaton A: Family size, childhood infections and atopic diseases. The Aberdeen WHEASE Group. Thorax 53:28–32, 1998.
2. Borish L: Genetics of allergy and asthma. Ann Allergy Asthma Immunol 82:413–424, 1999.

3. Ernst P, Cormier Y: Relative scarcity of asthma and atopy among rural adolescents raised on a farm. Am J Respir Crit Care Med 161:1563–1566, 2000.
4. Forecasted state-specific estimates of self-reported asthma prevalence—United States, 1998. MMWR Morb Mortal Wkly Rep 47(47):1022–1025, 1998.
5. Gergen PJ, Turkeltaub PC, Kovar MG: The prevalence of allergic skin test reactivity to eight common aeroallergens in the U.S. population: Results from the second National Health and Nutrition Examination Survey. J Allergy Clin Immunol 80:669–679, 1997.
6. Graves PE, Kabesch M, Halones M et al: A cluster of seven tightly linked polymorphisms in the IL-13 gene is associated with total serum IgE levels in three populations of white children. J Allergy Clin Immunol 105:506–513, 2000.
7. Gray L, Peat JK, Belousova E, Xuan W, Woolcock AJ: Family patterns of asthma, atopy and airway hyperresponsiveness: An epidemiological study. Clin Exp Allergy 30:393–399, 2000.
8. Hall IP: Genetics and pulmonary medicine 8:Asthma. Thorax 54:65–69, 1999.
9. International Study of Asthma and Allergies in Childhood (ISAAC): Worldwide variations in the prevalence of asthma symptoms. Eur Respir J 12:315–335, 1998.
10. International Study of Asthma and Allergies in Childhood (ISAAC): Worldwide variation in prevalence of symptoms of asthma, allergic conjunctivitis, and atopic eczema. Lancet 351:1225–1232, 1998.
11. Peat JK, Li J: Reversing the trend: Reducing the prevalence of asthma. J Allergy Clin Immunol 103:1–10, 1999.
12. Peterson B, Saxon A: Global increases in allergic respiratory disease: The possible role of diesel exhaust particulates. Ann Allergy Asthma Immunol 77:263–270, 1996.
13. Mrazek DA, Klinnert M, Mrazek PJ et al: Prediction of early-onset asthma in genetically at-risk children. Pediatr Pulmonol 27:85–94, 1999.
14. Postma DS, Bleecker ER, Amelung PJet al: Genetic susceptibility to asthma—bronchial hyperresponsiveness coinherited with a major gene for atopy. N Engl J Med 333:894–900, 1995.
15. Rona RJ, Duran-Tauleria E, Chinn S: Family size, atopic disorders in parents, asthma in children, and ethnicity. J Allergy Clin Immunol 99:454–60, 1997.
16. Rosenstreich DL, Eggleston P, Kattan M et al: The role of cockroach allergy and exposure to cockroach allergen in causing morbidity among inner-city children with asthma. N Engl J Med 336:1356–1363, 1997.
17. Schultz-Larsen F: The epidemiology of atopic dermatitis. Monogr Allergy 31:9–28, 1993.
18. Schwartz J, Gold D, Dockery DW, Weiss ST, Speizer FE: Predictors of asthma and persistent wheeze in a national sample of children in the United States. Association with social class, perinatal events, and race. Am Rev Respir Dis 142:555–562, 1990.
19. Shirakawa T, Enomoto T, Shimazu S, Hopkin JM: The inverse association between tuberculin responses and atopic disorder. Science 275:77–79, 1997.
20. Sigurs N, Bjarnson R, Sigurbergsson F, Kjellman B: Respiratory syncytial virus bronchiolitis in infancy is an important risk factor for asthma and allergy at age 7. Am J Respir Crit Care Med 161:1501–1507, 2000.
21. Sporik R, Holgate ST, Platts-Mills TA, Cogswell JJ: Exposure to house-dust mite allergen (Der p I) and the development of asthma in childhood. A prospective study. N Engl J Med 323:502–507, 1990.
22. Surveillance for asthma—United States, 1960-1995. MMWR Morb Mortal Wkly Rep 47(No. SS-1):1–27, 1998.
23. The Collaborative Study on the Genetics of Asthma (CSGA): A genome-wide search for asthma susceptibility loci in ethnically diverse populations. Nat Genet 15:389–392, 1997.
24. Thomas NS, Wilkinson J, Holgate ST: The candidate region approach to the genetics of asthma and allergy Am J Respir Crit Care Med 156(4 Pt 2):S144–451, 1997.
25. Variations in the prevalence of respiratory symptoms, self-reported asthma attacks, and use of asthma medication in the European Community Respiratory Health Survey (ECRHS). Eur Respir J 9:687–695, 1996.
26. von Mutius E, Martinez FD, Fritzsch C, Nicolai T, Roell G, Thiemann HH: Prevalence of asthma and atopy in two areas of West and East Germany. Am J Respir Crit Care Med 149:358–364, 1994.
27. Weitzman M, Gortmaker S, Sobol A: Racial, social, and environmental risks for childhood asthma. Am J Dis Child 144:1189–94, 1990.
28. Wickens K, Pearce N, Crane J, Beasley R: Antibiotic use in early childhood and the development of asthma. Clin Exp Allergy 29:766–771, 1999.
29. Wuthrich B: Clinical aspects, epidemiology, and prognosis of atopic dermatitis. Ann Allergy Asthma Immunol 83:464–470, 1999.
30. Xu J, Wiesch DG, Meyers DA: Genetics of complex human diseases: Genome screening, association studies and fine mapping. Clin Exp Allergy 28(Suppl 5):1–5, 1998.

2. IMMUNOLOGY AND PATHOPHYSIOLOGY OF ALLERGIC DISEASE

Maurice E. Hamilton, M.D.

1. Describe the physical properties of immunoglobulins.

Immunoglobulins comprise a heterogeneous group of glycoproteins that constitute about 20% of total serum proteins and migrate with gamma- and, to a lesser extent, beta-globulins during protein electrophoresis.

All immunoglobulins are composed of two identical heavy (H) chains and two identical light (L) chains covalently linked by disulfide bonds between cysteine residues. Each chain contains an aminoterminal sequence characterized by significant diversity in the amino acid residues, the variable (V) region, and a carboxyterminal sequence with less variability, the constant (C) region.

Within each chain are globular regions known as domains: the domains in the light chains are termed V_L and C_L, whereas those in the heavy chains are named V_H, C_H1, C_H2, C_H3, and C_H4. The segment of heavy chains between the first two constant domains, C_H1 and C_H2, constitutes the hinge region.

2. What are the products of enzymatic digestion of immunoglobulins by papain and pepsin?

Digestion of immunoglobulins by papain splits the molecule on the aminoterminal side of the disulfide bonds joining the heavy chains and yields two antigen-binding fragments, Fab. Each Fab contains an entire light chain, the V_H and C_H1 domains of a heavy chain, and a crystallizable fragment, Fc, that is composed of the carboxyterminal halves of the heavy chains.

Pepsin cleaves the heavy chains on the carboxyterminal side of the disulfide bonds linking these chains to produce a divalent antigen-binding fragment, $F(ab')_2$, which is composed of two Fab regions and the hinge region with intact disulfide bonds, in addition to small peptides.

3. Characterize the antigen-binding site and its relationship to antibody function.

Amino acids within the variable regions of the heavy and light chains form the antigen-binding site, which is closely associated with segments that display significant diversity, the hypervariable regions.

Binding of antigen to immunoglobulin induces conformational changes in the constant regions of the heavy chains. These changes permit the carboxyterminal portion to bind to Fc receptors on the surface of lymphocytes and macrophages and to the first component of complement, C1q.

4. How do immunoglobulin allotypes differ from idiotypes?

Allotypes represent minor polymorphic or allelic variations in the amino acid sequences (usually a single amino acid substitution) in the constant regions of heavy

13

and light chains that segregate according to Mendelian genetics. They usually do not alter function. Gm allotypes are associated with γ chains, Am allotypes with α chains, and Inv allotypes with κ light chains.

Idiotypes refer to antigenic determinants within the variable regions of heavy and light chains that may encompass the antigen-binding sites, particularly the hypervariable regions. Shared idiotypes on structurally different immunoglobulins are termed public- or cross-reactive idiotypes, whereas idiotypes expressed on only a limited number of closely related antibodies are called individual or private idiotypes.

5. Discuss the relationship between antiidiotypic antibodies and antigens.

Some antiidiotypic antibodies are believed to resemble the structure of the original antigen that induced antibody formation. Thus, if the antigen-binding site represents a negative image or "cast" of the antigen, then an antiidiotypic antibody directed against the antigen-binding site may resemble a negative image of the antigen-binding site, or the original antigen itself. Antiidiotypic antibodies may modulate immune function and do form immune complexes that may be pathogenic.

6. How are light chains classified?

Light chains are subdivided based on antigenic differences in the constant regions into λ (lambda) and κ (kappa) types. In humans, the proportion of kappa to lambda chains is about 2:1.

7. What is the structural basis for the classification of immunoglobulins?

Immunoglobulins are classified on the basis of structural differences in the constant regions of the heavy chains into five classes or isotypes—IgG, IgA, IgM, IgD, and IgE—which correspond to the heavy chains γ (gamma), α (alpha), μ (mu), δ (delta), and ε (epsilon), respectively. IgG, IgA, and IgM may be further categorized into subclasses based on antigenic differences in the structure of the C_H regions (e.g., IgG1–IgG4, IgA1, and IgA2).

8. Describe the structural differences between the immunoglobulin classes.

Mu and epsilon chains consist of five domains (V_H, C_H1, C_H2, C_H3, and C_H4), whereas gamma and alpha chains are composed of four domains (V_H, C_H1, C_H2, and C_H3).

IgG, IgE, and IgD exist only as the basic immunoglobulin unit consisting of two heavy chains and two light chains, whereas IgA and IgM also exist as polymers. In the circulation, IgA exists in both monomeric and dimeric forms. IgA in secretions exists as a dimer and includes a J chain and a secretory piece synthesized by epithelial cells. IgM is secreted as a pentamer composed of five immunoglobulin units joined by disulfide bonds and a J chain. Although the J chain is present in all polymeric immunoglobulin molecules with more than two basic units, the secretory component is uniquely associated with IgA.

9. What is the proportion of each immunoglobulin class in the circulation?

In normal humans, IgG comprises about 75% of total serum immunoglobulins, IgA 15%, IgM 10%, IgD 0.2%, and IgE 0.004%.

10. Characterize the function of each immunoglobulin class.

IgG represents the predominant antibody in the secondary immune response. It is the only immunoglobulin capable of crossing the placenta. IgG activates complement via the classical pathway. The ability of the IgG subclasses to bind complement varies, being greatest for IgG3 and IgG1. IgG2 is a poor activator of complement and IgG4 is unable to bind complement. The C1q binding site on IgG appears to be located in the C_H2 domain.

IgG Fc receptors (FcγR) on cells such as macrophages bind IgG1 and IgG3 via the C_H3 domain of the Fc region, mediating phagocytosis and antibody-dependent cell-mediated cytotoxicity (ADCC) following binding of specific antigen. Fcγ receptors have also been identified on B cells, neutrophils, basophils, eosinophils, and platelets.

IgM is the predominant antibody in the early immune response, the initial immunoglobulin expressed on the surface of B cells, and the most efficient complement-fixing antibody (requiring binding of antigen to only one antibody molecule).

IgA is the primary immunoglobulin class in secretions, including tears, saliva, and mucus, providing the primary defense against local pathogens.

IgD, like IgM, functions as a membrane-bound antigen receptor on the surface of B lymphocytes. Some data indicate that binding of antigen to surface IgD may stimulate B cell maturation. In addition, surface IgD may inhibit the induction of B-cell tolerance.

IgE, a monomeric antibody with a molecular weight of 190,000 daltons, binds to effector cells via its Fc portion and plays a key role in mediating allergic reactions and cytotoxicity to parasites following binding of specific antigen.

11. Describe the location and kinetics of IgE production.

IgE-producing plasma cells are distributed primarily in lymphoid tissue adjacent to the respiratory and gastrointestinal tracts. The highest concentrations are found in the tonsils and adenoids. The half-life of IgE is only 2 to 3 days in the circulation vs. about 14 days in human skin.

12. Which cytokines regulate IgE synthesis?

Interleukin-4 (IL-4) and IL-13 are the only cytokines capable of inducing IgE synthesis. IL-4 induces isotype switching from IgM to IgG4 and IgE, perhaps sequentially. IL-13 also promotes isotype switching to IgE production. IL-5, IL-6, IL-9, and tumor necrosis factor-α (TNF-α) stimulate IL-4-mediated IgE synthesis, whereas interferon-α (IFN-α), IFN-γ, transforming growth factor-β (TGF-β), IL-2, IL-8, IL-10, and IL-12 inhibit IgE synthesis.

13. Characterize the receptors to which IgE binds.

IgE binds by its Fc portion to high-affinity IgE receptors (FcϵRI), present on the surface of mast cells, basophils, monocytes, eosinophils, non-B/non-T cells, and human skin Langerhans cells, and to low-affinity receptors (FcϵRII or CD23) present on B cells, some T cells, eosinophils, monocytes, macrophages, follicular dendritic cells, Langerhans cells, and platelets.

The high-affinity IgE receptor is formed by an α-chain, β-chain, and two γ-chains. The α-chain binds IgE, whereas the β- and γ-chains induce transmembrane

signals that mediate cellular activation following cross-linking of IgE by antigen. FcεRII is a single transmembrane chain that binds IgE about 1,000 times less firmly than FcεRI.

IL-4 up-regulates the expression of both high- and low-affinity IgE receptors. In dendritic cells, IL-4 induces the intracellular expression of the FcεRI α-chain.

14. How do serum IgE levels vary with age?

IgE-bearing B lymphocytes are detectable by the eleventh week of gestation, but IgE synthesis is negligible in utero. Serum IgE levels increase after birth, attain median adult levels at age 3 years, peak between ages 7 and 14 years, and decrease rapidly after age 15 years. IgE levels are less than 80 IU/mL in most nonallergic adults.

15. Which diseases are associated with elevated serum IgE?

Levels of IgE are elevated in patients with atopic diseases, including allergic rhinitis, allergic asthma, and atopic dermatitis. The quantity of IgE correlates with the severity of symptoms in patients with allergic rhinitis and atopic dermatitis. Total IgE levels are markedly elevated in allergic bronchopulmonary aspergillosis.

Increased levels of IgE are characteristic of Wiskott-Aldrich's syndrome, hyper-IgE syndrome, Hodgkin's disease, acute graft-versus-host disease, and IgE myeloma.

Infections with metazoan helminthic parasites (e.g., *Ascaris*, *Schistosoma*, and *Trichinella*) are frequently associated with elevated levels of serum IgE, whereas IgE levels are usually normal with protozoan infections (e.g., *Entamoeba*, *Giardia*, and *Toxoplasma*). An exception is malaria, caused by the protozoans plasmodia, in which serum IgE is typically increased. Most of the elevated IgE in parasitic infections is not specific for parasites.

16. What is the origin of mast cells?

Mast cells are derived from CD34+ hematopoietic progenitor cells. Mast cell-committed progenitors migrate from the bone marrow to mucosal or connective tissue sites, where they expand and differentiate into mature mast cells under the influence of stem cell factor (SCF) and perhaps other fibroblast-derived mediators.

17. List the mediators produced by mast cells.

PREFORMED MEDIATORS	NEWLY SYNTHESIZED MEDIATORS
Biogenic amines	Cyclooxygenase products
Histamine*	Prostaglandin D_2
Neutral proteases	Thromboxane A_2
Tryptase	Lipoxygenase products
Chymase	Leukotriene B_4
Carboxypeptidase A	Leukotrienes C_4, D_4, E_4
Cathepsin G	Platelet-activating factor
Hydrolases	Cytokines
Arylsulfatase	

(*Table continued on next page.*)

PREFORMED MEDIATORS	NEWLY SYNTHESIZED MEDIATORS
β-Galactosidase	
β-Glucuronidase	
β-Hexosaminidase	
Proteoglycans	
Heparan sulfate	
Chondroitin sulfate	
Chemotactic factors**	
Neutrophil chemotactic factors	
Eosinophilic chemotactic factor of anaphylaxis	
Cytokines	
IL-4	
TNF-α	

* Histamine is responsible for many of the phenomena associated with the early-phase reaction.
** Mast cell chemotactic factors initiate the late-phase reaction associated with allergic inflammation.

18. Define proteoglycans and identify the classes present in mast cells.

Proteoglycans are macromolecules composed of glycosaminoglycan (GAG) chains covalently linked to a protein core. The presence of acidic GAGs explains the affinity of mast cell and basophil granules for basic dyes such as toluidine blue, which leads to the metachromasia that characterizes these cells. Proteoglycans bind histamine, neutral proteases, and carboxypeptidases and may facilitate the packaging of these molecules within the secretory granules.

Mast cell granules contain two classes of proteoglycans: heparan and chondroitin sulfates. Within mature human pulmonary mast cells, the ratio of heparan to chondroitin is 2:1.

19. Identify the major enzyme present in mast cell cytoplasmic granules.

The major enzyme in the cytoplasmic granules is tryptase, a neutral protease stored in active form in association with heparan. Tryptase digests peptide and ester bonds on basic amino acids and accounts for the IgE-mediated kininogenase activity described in mast cells. Tryptase also functions as a growth factor for airway smooth muscle cells, epithelial cells, and fibroblasts. *Tryptase is present in all human mast cells, but is lacking in other cell types.*

20. Characterize serum tryptase isoenzyme levels in mastocytosis and allergic diseases.

Two forms of tryptase have been identified in humans: α-tryptase and β-tryptase. α-Tryptase is released constitutively from mast cells and represents a measure of mast cell mass or hyperplasia. In contrast, β-tryptase is stored in mast cell secretory granules and provides an indicator of mast cell activation. Accordingly, systemic mastocytosis and anaphylaxis may be associated with elevated levels of α-tryptase and β-tryptase, respectively. Peripheral blood tryptase levels are usually normal in patients with asthma and other allergic disorders.

21. **Explain the characteristics of MC_T and MC_{TC} mast cells.**

Mast cells have been subdivided into MC_T and MC_{TC} cells based on their neutral protease content. MC_T cells contain tryptase but not chymase, whereas MC_{TC} cells contain both tryptase and chymase. In addition, MC_{TC} cells contain carboxypeptidase and cathepsin G.

MC_T cells appear to play a major role in host defenses and constitute > 90% of the mast cells present in the alveoli, airway epithelium, and airway lumen. MC_{TC} mast cells are located in the submucosa of the respiratory tract and appear to be primarily involved with angiogenesis and tissue remodeling. MC_{TC} cells are also the predominant mast cells in skin, synovium, and gastrointestinal submucosa.

22. **Describe the stimuli that activate mast cells.**

Activation of mast cells is triggered by linking of adjacent FcεRI receptor-bound IgE molecules by bivalent or multivalent antigens, or by antibodies directed against either IgE or its receptor, resulting in the rapid release of preformed mediators and the synthesis of newly generated mediators.

Mast cells may also be activated by various biologic, chemical, and physical stimuli. For MC_{TC} cells, these stimuli include complement fragments C3a and C5a (anaphylatoxins), basic polypeptides (polyarginine and polylysine), peptide hormones, substance P, radiocontrast media, calcium ionophores, drugs (opiates and muscle relaxants), melittin in bee venom, and cold. Among these nonimmunologic stimuli, only calcium ionophores activate human lung mast cells.

23. **Compare mast cells to the least common granulocyte.**

Basophils represent the least common type of granulocyte in humans. Like mast cells, basophils are derived from CD34+ progenitor cells and constitutively express FcεRI surface receptors. However, basophils differentiate and mature in the bone marrow under the influence of interleukin-3, and circulate in the blood, rather than residing in the tissues.

Like mast cells, basophils store histamine, neutrophil chemotactic factor, and other preformed mediators in secretory granules. The predominant proteoglycan in human basophils is chondroitin sulfate A. Basophils also contain small amounts of Charcot-Leyden crystal protein and major basic protein. Following FcεRI-dependent activation, mature human basophils release IL-4 and IL-13. Activated basophils also generate LTC_4, LTD_4, LTE_4, and PAF. In contrast to mast cells, basophils contain negligible or undetectable amounts of tryptase, chymase, carboxypeptidase, and cathepsin G, and do not produce LTB_4 or PGD_2.

24. **What is the implication of an elevated histamine level without detectable PGD_2?**

The finding of an elevated histamine level in the absence of tryptase and PGD_2 suggests basophil activation, while elevated histamine in conjunction with either tryptase or PGD_2 implies mast cell activation.

25. **Identify the eosinophil progenitor cell.**

Eosinophils are produced in the bone marrow from a CD34+ progenitor cell capable of differentiating into basophils and eosinophils. Increased numbers of circulating

CD34+ eosinophil-basophil progenitor cells expressing the IL-5 receptor have been identified in atopic subjects.

26. How do cytokines regulate eosinophilopoiesis?
Eosinophils differentiate in the bone marrow under the influence of multiple cytokines, including IL-3, IL-5, and granulocyte-macrophage colony-stimulatory factor (GM-CSF), until they mature and are indistinguishable from eosinophils in the peripheral circulation. IL-5 is relatively specific for eosinophils and induces eosinophil-basophil progenitors to differentiate into eosinophils; IL-3 and GM-CSF stimulate basophils and neutrophils in addition to eosinophils. In contrast, TGF-β and IFN-α inhibit eosinophil proliferation and differentiation.

27. Discuss the kinetics of the eosinophil life cycle.
After circulating in the peripheral blood for a short time (average half-life 8–18 hours), eosinophils migrate by diapedesis at endothelial intercellular junctions into epithelial tissues such as the skin, lungs, and gastrointestinal tract, where they are exposed to the external environment. Following migration, most eosinophils remain in the tissues, where their life span typically ranges from 2 to 5 days. IL-3, IL-5, GM-CSF, and TNF-α may prolong eosinophil survival by inhibiting programmed cell death (apoptosis).

28. Describe cell adhesion molecules and their role in eosinophil migration.
Cell adhesion molecules (CAMs) are surface proteins essential for the recruitment of eosinophils and other leukocytes from the circulation to sites of inflammation. Subdivided into discrete groups, including selectins, integrins, and members of the immunoglobulin superfamily, CAMs regulate both cell-cell and cell-extracellular matrix protein interactions. This process occurs in sequential stages: leukocyte rolling and endothelial attachment, activation, firm adhesion, and migration.

29. What is the role of selectins?
Leukocyte rolling and the initial loose binding to vascular endothelium are mediated primarily by selectins. L selectin is expressed exclusively on the surface of leukocytes; E selectin is expressed on activated endothelial cells; and P selectin is present on platelets and endothelial cells. Eosinophils express P-selectin glycoprotein ligand I (PSGL-1), which binds to P selectin on endothelial cells. Through the combined effects of the cell adhesion molecules PSGL-1/P selectin and VLA-4/VCAM-1 (see below), eosinophils are tethered to endothelial cells, a requirement for migration into tissues.

30. Describe the structure and function of integrins.
Integrins and members of the immunoglobulin superfamily regulate firm adhesion and migration of eosinophils. Integrins, glycoproteins composed of noncovalently associated α and β subunits, are constitutively expressed on the surface of leukocytes, endothelial cells, and some other cells.

$β_1$-Integrins, the largest subfamily, represent a group of cellular receptors for extracellular matrix proteins such as collagen, fibronectin, and laminin. The $β_1$-integrin very-late-activation antigen-4 (VLA-4) is expressed on eosinophils, basophils,

lymphocytes, and monocytes, but lacking on neutrophils. Increased numbers of eosinophils bearing VLA-4 have been reported in sputum from asthmatic patients.

β_2-Integrins are composed of a β subunit called CD18 paired with one of four α subunits (CD11a–CD11d). Expression of β_2-integrins is limited to leukocytes. Activated eosinophils express the β_2-integrins leukocyte function-associated antigen-1 (LFA-1) and macrophage-1 antigen (Mac-1). Like VLA-4, these integrins are important for the firm adhesion of eosinophils to endothelial cells and their subsequent migration into the tissues.

31. What are the ligands for integrins?
The ligands for integrins include cell-surface molecules that are members of the immunoglobulin supergene family, such as intercellular adhesion molecules-1, -2, and -3 (ICAM-1, -2, and -3) and vascular cell adhesion molecule-1 (VCAM-1). These proteins are constitutively expressed on endothelial cells, neutrophils, and lymphocytes, among other cells. VCAM-1 binds to VLA-4, promoting adhesion of eosinophils, basophils, lymphocytes, and monocytes, whereas ICAM-1 binds to LFA-1 and Mac-1, enhancing adhesion of eosinophils and neutrophils.

32. How do cytokines modulate eosinophil recruitment?
Proinflammatory cytokines, such as IFN-γ, IL-1β, and TNF-α, augment the expression of ICAM-1 and VCAM-1, and the Th2 cytokines IL-4 and IL-13 up-regulate the expression of VCAM-1 on endothelial cells. This promotes VLA-4/VCAM-1–mediated adherence of eosinophils. Moreover, IL-5 selectively promotes adhesion of eosinophils—the only peripheral blood leukocytes with IL-5 receptors—to unstimulated endothelial cells.

33. Explain the classification and function of chemokines.
Chemokines are cytokines with chemotactic activity. These structurally related proteins are subdivided into four groups based on the number and appearance of conserved cysteine residues in the primary sequence. The two groups that include most identified chemokines are classified on the basis of the position of the first two of these cysteine residues into CC (containing adjacent cysteines) or CXC (containing another amino acid positioned between cysteine residues) subfamilies. The CC subset displays chemotactic activity for eosinophils, T lymphocytes, and monocytes, but not neutrophils. Members of this group include eotaxin, macrophage inflammatory protein-1α (MIP-1α), monocyte chemotactic protein-1 (MCP-1), and RANTES (regulated activation, normal T cell expressed and excreted). Eotaxin and RANTES are especially potent inducers of eosinophil migration. The CXC subfamily exerts chemotactic activity primarily toward neutrophils, although its member IL-8 also expresses chemotactic activity toward activated eosinophils.

34. List other mediators of eosinophil chemotaxis.
Histamine
LTD$_4$ (chemotactic for eosinophils, but not neutrophils)
Platelet-activating factor (PAF)
Platelet factor 4 (PF4)

Anaphylatoxins C3a and C5a
Cytokines GM-CSF, IL-2, IL-3, IL-4, and IL-5

35. Describe the surface receptors on eosinophils.

Human peripheral blood eosinophils express receptors for the Fc portion of IgG (FcγRII or CD32), IgA (FcαR), and IgE (FcεRI and FcεRII). Fcγ receptors mediate ADCC, degranulation, and phagocytosis. Increased numbers of Fcα receptors have been reported on eosinophils from patients with atopic diseases. Fcε receptors mediate killing of schistosomula. Surface receptors for C3a, C5a, C3b (CR1), CC chemokines, and CAMs (see above) have also been identified.

36. Characterize eosinophil secretory granules.

Eosinophils contain two principal types of secretory granules: specific granules and small granules. Specific secretory granules represent the primary source of major basic protein (MBP), localized to the crystalloid core of the granules, and eosinophil cationic protein (ECP), eosinophil-derived neurotoxin (EDN), eosinophil peroxidase (EPO), and β-glucuronidase, all identified within the matrix of the specific granules. Small secretory granules contain acid phosphatase and arylsulfatase B, among other enzymes. Eosinophils also contain lysophospholipase, neutrophil elastase, and collagenase.

37. Which protein causes the distinctive staining of eosinophils?

Major basic protein binds to acid dyes such as eosin, which stains the granules red.

38. Define Charcot-Leyden crystals.

Charcot-Leyden crystals are hexagonal bipyramidal crystals identified in the sputum of patients with asthma. (They have also been found in cervical smears and elsewhere.) Charcot-Leyden crystal protein possesses lysophospholipase activity and is present within eosinophils and basophils.

39. Discuss the biologic effects of the major eosinophil peptides.

MBP neutralizes heparin and induces the release of histamine from human basophils, lysozyme and superoxide from neutrophils, and serotonin (5-hydroxytryptamine) from platelets. MBP causes bronchoconstriction, impairs ciliary function, induces exfoliation of respiratory epithelial cells, and increases airway responsiveness. ECP neutralizes heparin and kills schistosomula and other parasites. Like MBP, this protein is toxic to airway epithelial cells. EDN damages myelinated neurons.

EPO and hydrogen peroxide (H_2O_2), in the presence of halide, kill a variety of microorganisms (including bacteria and protozoa) and tumor cells. In addition, EPO with H_2O_2 and halide trigger mast cell degranulation in an animal model. EPO also releases serotonin from platelets.

40. Describe the eicosanoids synthesized by eosinophils and their relevance to asthma.

LTC_4 is the most prevalent lipoxygenase metabolite produced by eosinophils, whereas only small amounts of LTB_4 are synthesized. Eosinophils also produce the

5-lipoxygenase metabolite 5-HETE. These mediators induce bronchoconstriction, mucus secretion, increased vascular permeability, and chemotaxis of eosinophils and neutrophils.

41. Which cytokines do eosinophils synthesize?

Eosinophils produce a variety of cytokines, including autocrine cytokines, such as IL-3, IL-5, and GM-CSF, which act upon eosinophils themselves. Eosinophils also have the capacity to synthesize IL-1, IL-4, IL-6, IL-8, IL-10, IL-16, MIP-1α, RANTES, TNF-α, TGF-α, and TGF-β1.

42. Summarize the stimuli that induce degranulation/activation of eosinophils.

Degranulation of eosinophils may be triggered by secretory IgA (sIgA), IgA, IgG, IgE, RANTES, MIP-1α, PAF, C3a, C5a, substance P, melittin, and β-integrin ligands. Among immunoglobulins, sIgA is the most potent mediator of degranulation. MBP and EPO also induce eosinophil degranulation, suggesting the presence of an autocrine degranulation pathway. Eosinophils may also be activated by cytokines, including IL-1, IL-3, IL-4, IL-5, GM-CSF, TNF-α, and IFN-γ.

43. What is the population of eosinophils of abnormal density identified in some diseases?

Analysis of circulating eosinophils in patients with eosinophilia has demonstrated a population of eosinophils of lower density than normal. Called hypodense eosinophils, these cells have been identified in subjects with parasitic infections, allergic diseases, and idiopathic hypereosinophilic syndrome. They are believed to represent primed or partially activated eosinophils.

44. Describe the kinetics and CAMs of neutrophil migration.

After release from the bone marrow, neutrophils circulate in the blood for 6 to 8 hours prior to being sequestered through margination, primarily in the lung capillaries. Migration of neutrophils from blood vessels into tissues requires the expression of cell adhesion molecules. Neutrophils express several adhesion proteins, including the integrins Mac-1 (important for binding to fibrinogen and degranulation) and LFA-1 (important for migration into tissues).

45. Which neutrophil products might contribute to allergic inflammation?

Neutrophils recruited to sites of allergic inflammation generate a number of molecules that may induce tissue damage, including collagenase, elastase, oxygen radicals, LTB$_4$, PAF, and thromboxane A$_2$ (TXA$_2$). In contrast to mast cells and eosinophils, neutrophils produce little LTC$_4$.

46. What evidence supports a pathogenic role for neutrophils in asthma?

Both PAF and LTB$_4$ have been identified in human airways following allergen challenge, consistent with neutrophil activation. Increased neutrophils have been reported in sputum during exacerbations of asthma. In patients who died from an acute asthma attack, neutrophils comprised the majority of cells infiltrating the airways, whereas in patients who died from hours to days after an asthma flare, most infiltrating cells were eosinophils.

47. Summarize the role of B and T cells in generating an immune response.

B lymphocytes play a crucial role in the immune response by virtue of their synthesis of specific IgE antibody after sensitization by antigen. T lymphocytes regulate B cells and contribute to the late-phase reaction and allergic inflammation through the release of cytokines and chemokines.

48. What is the function of membrane-bound immunoglobulin on B lymphocytes?

B cells utilize membrane-bound immunoglobulin molecules as receptors for soluble antigens. Immature B lymphocytes express IgM surface receptors, whereas most mature B cells display both IgM and IgD surface receptors.

49. Describe the events triggered by binding of antigen to B cell surface immunoglobulin.

Following antigenic stimulation, B cells proliferate and differentiate into immunoglobulin-secreting cells with the capacity to express various immunoglobulin isotypes, leading to the synthesis of different classes of antibody with the same antigenic specificity. The principal antibody produced in response to a primary antigenic challenge is IgM, followed by IgG, IgA, and IgE. During the secondary, or memory, response, IgG, IgA, and IgE account for most antibody synthesis.

50. What conditions are required for IgE synthesis?

In addition to IL-4 or IL-13, direct contact between B lymphocytes and activated T cells is required for switching to IgE production. B cells present processed antigen bound to major histocompatibility complex (MHC) class II molecules to T cell receptors. Other cell surface interactions are also necessary. These may occur between the B cell surface glycoprotein CD40 and its ligand CD40L on T cells and between CD23 on B cells and CD21 on T cells.

51. Characterize CD4+ a nd CD8+ T lymphocytes.

  CD4+ T cells, which comprise approximately 60% of circulating T cells, function as helper cells for B-cell differentiation and mediate delayed-type hypersensitivity (DTH) reactions. CD8+ T cells participate in the host response against intracellular microorganisms and mediate cytotoxic and suppressor activities. Although CD4+ T cells have been categorized as helper-inducer cells and CD8+ T cells as cytotoxic-suppressor cells, both CD4+ and CD8+ lymphocytes can act as helper-inducer and cytotoxic-suppressor cells and produce similar cytokines.

52. What is the primary difference between CD8+ and CD4+ T cells?

CD8+ T cells recognize antigens presented by class I MHC molecules (HLA-A, -B, and -C). CD4+ T cells recognize antigens presented by class II MHC molecules (HLA-DR, -DP, and -DQ in humans).

53. Describe the subsets of CD4+ T cells and their properties.

CHARACTERISTIC	T HELPER 1 (Th1) CELLS	T HELPER 2 (Th2) CELLS
Type of response	Cell-mediated	Humoral-mediated
Activators	Microbes	Allergens, parasites
Functions	Cytotoxicity, DTH, monocyte activation	B cell help, IgE synthesis, monocyte inhibition, eosinophil activation
Cytokines produced*	IFN-γ, IL-2	IL-4, IL-5, IL-6, IL-10, IL-13
Cytokine inducers	IFN-γ, IL-12	IL-4, IL-5
Cytokine inhibitors	IL-4, IL-10	IFN-γ, IL-12

* Both types of T helper cells secrete IL-3, TNF-α, and GM-CSF. CD4+ cells may also produce CC chemokines such as eotaxin, MCP-3, MIP-1α, and RANTES.

54. How do these subsets differ from the CD8+ T cell subsets?

CD8+ T cells are also divided into subsets based upon their cytokine profiles. CD8+ T cells that produce cytokines similar to CD4+ Th1 cells are designated T cytotoxic 1 (Tc1) cells, whereas those that produce cytokines similar to CD4+ Th2 cells are called T cytotoxic 2 (Tc2) cells.

55. What is the role of Th0 cells in the immune response?

Another type of T helper cell, Th0, secretes cytokines characteristic of both Th1 and Th2, and is considered a precursor to Th1 and Th2 cells. Infection of monocytes by bacteria or viruses induces the secretion of IFN-α and IL-12, which promote the formation of Th1 cells, and IFN-γ, which inhibits the development of Th2 cells. In contrast, IL-4 from mast cells or Th2 promotes the formation of Th2 cells and antagonizes the development of Th1 cells.

56. Describe the structure and function of the most characteristic type of T cell marker.

The most characteristic T cell surface markers are T cell receptors (TCRs), through which T cells recognize antigens. These receptors are composed of two polypeptide chains (α and β or γ and δ) that are associated with the CD3 complex. Each T cell expresses a single type of TCR, either αβ (> 90%) or γδ. In normal subjects, cells bearing γδ TCR rarely express either CD4 or CD8.

αβ T cell receptors are members of the immunoglobulin supergene family and recognize peptide fragments that have been processed by antigen-presenting cells (APCs). In contrast, γδ T cell receptors may recognize some antigens directly without processing and may comprise the first line of defense at mucosal surfaces.

57. How do antigens presented to TCRs on CD4+ cells differ from those presented to CD8+ cells?

Antigens presented to CD4+ T cells originate extracellularly and include allergens, such as pollens, molds, and house dust mites, in addition to extracellular bacteria, bacterial toxins, fungi, and vaccines. These exogenous proteins are internalized by antigen-presenting cells, degraded into peptides, bound to MHC class II molecules, and transported to the cell surface, where the peptide-MHC class

II molecule combination is recognized by specific αβ T-cell receptors on the surface of CD4+ T cells.

In contrast, antigens presented to CD8+ T cells originate in the cytoplasm. These endogenous antigens can include intracellular infectious agents, tumor-associated antigens, and transplantation antigens. Endogenous antigens are processed by APCs into peptides and bound to MHC class I molecules for transport to the cell surface, where the combination is recognized by specific αβ TCRs on CD8+ T cells.

58. What are the prerequisites for activation of T cells?

In addition to antigen recognition by TCRs, activation of αβ T cells requires stimulation by IL-1 (produced by macrophages and other APCs) and a second or costimulatory signal provided by binding of the T cell ligand CD28 to CD80 or CD86 on the surface of APCs. In the absence of costimulatory signals, the T cell-dependent immune response is considerably decreased or eliminated. (Another costimulatory molecule, CTLA-4, is expressed on the surface of T cells about 48 hours after activation. CTLA-4 also binds to CD80 or CD86 on APCs but, in contrast to CD28, inhibits the immune response.)

59. How does glucocorticoid treatment modify T cells in patients with allergic asthma?

Treatment of allergic asthma patients with corticosteroids markedly decreases pulmonary γδ T cells, probably due to steroid-induced apoptosis. Glucocorticoid therapy decreases the proportion of bronchoalveolar lavage fluid cells expressing IL-4 and IL-5, and increases the cells expressing IFN-γ, suggesting a shift toward a Th1 response.

60. Describe the kinetics of the monocyte life cycle.

Progenitors of monocytes/macrophages differentiate in the bone marrow over a period of about 6 days to form monocytes, which are released into the peripheral blood and circulate with a half-life of approximately 3 days. These cells then migrate into tissues such as the lungs and differentiate into macrophages, which have a life span that ranges from days to months. Monocytes may also differentiate under the influence of local tissue factors into dendritic cells, which display MHC class II antigens and are found in the lungs and other tissues.

61. Which mediators influence the production of monocytes?

Monocyte production is stimulated by GM-CSF, IL-3, and macrophage colony-stimulating factor (M-CSF) but inhibited by interferon-α/β and PGE_2.

62. What is the role of monocytes/macrophages in generating an immune response?

The monocyte-macrophage system—consisting of monocytes in the circulation and macrophages in tissues—plays a key role in generating the immune response by presenting antigen to lymphocytes, as described above. In addition, monocytes are the primary source of IL-12, which acts on T cells and natural killer (NK) cells to induce the production of IFN-γ, thereby promoting the Th1 pattern of differentiation. In contrast, IL-10 secreted by monocytes inhibits the synthesis of IFN-γ, which may counterbalance the effects of IL-12. Monocytes also produce the cytokines IL-1 and TNF-α;

chemokines MIP-1α, monocyte chemotactic proteins (MCPs), and RANTES; proinflammatory arachidonic acid metabolites PGD_2, LTB_4, and LTC_4; and PAF.

63. Identify the major antigen-presenting cells in the lungs.

Pulmonary dendritic cells are the primary antigen-presenting cells in the lungs. Although alveolar macrophages demonstrate potent phagocytic and antimicrobial properties, they are weak activators of T cells. In fact, alveolar macrophages may function as suppressors rather than inducers of the immune response.

64. Describe mechanisms by which macrophages may induce airway damage in asthma.

Macrophages represent potential inducers of airway damage through production of nitric oxide (NO), which may be triggered by either allergic or infectious processes. NO reacts with superoxide anions to form toxic hydroxyl radicals. Alveolar macrophages also synthesize fibroblast growth factors, platelet-derived growth factor, and transforming growth factor-β, which may contribute to irreversible airway remodeling in asthma.

65. Describe the structure of platelets.

Platelets contain three types of secretory granules: alpha granules, dense granules, and lysosomes. Alpha granules, the most numerous, contain fibronectin, fibrinogen, platelet factor 4, and β-thromboglobulin. Dense granules contain adenosine diphosphate (ADP), serotonin, calcium, and pyrophosphate. Lysosomes contain acid hydrolases. Resting platelets possess surface receptors for platelet agonists, collagen (gpIa/IIa), and fibrinogen/von Willebrand factor (gpIIb/IIIa).

66. Which stimuli induce platelet aggregation and activation?

Platelet aggregation occurs through platelet-platelet interaction and adhesion to fibrinogen, which induces the release of the contents of alpha granules and dense granules. Platelet activation may result from adhesion or soluble agonists such as ADP, epinephrine, serotonin, thrombin, substance P, C-reactive protein, complement components, eosinophil-derived MBP, interferon, and TNF. In addition, platelets possess FcϵRII receptors and are activated by aggregation of these receptors following binding of specific allergen or anti-IgE antibody.

67. List the mediators released by activated platelets.

Adenosine	Nitric oxide (NO)
β-thromboglobulin	PAF
Factor D	Platelet-derived growth factor (PDGF)
Free radicals	Platelet factor 4
12-HETE	RANTES
Histamine	Thromboxane A_2
Histamine-releasing factor (HRF)	Transforming growth factor-β

68. How is histamine synthesized and metabolized?

Histamine is synthesized in the Golgi apparatus of mast cells and basophils by decarboxylation of histidine. Histamine associates with the acidic residues of the

glycosaminoglycan (GAG) side chains of heparin and other proteoglycans. Human mast cells contain 3 to 6 pg of histamine per cell and secrete histamine spontaneously at low levels, producing a normal plasma level of 0.5 to 2 nM. Histamine is rapidly metabolized (usually within 1 or 2 minutes) following extracellular release by either of two mechanisms, methylation by histamine-n-methyltransferase or oxidation by diamine oxidase (histaminase).

69. Describe the biologic effects mediated by histamine.

The biologic effects of histamine are mediated by activation of specific cell surface receptors, of which three subtypes have been identified. Binding of histamine to H_1-receptors induces contraction of airway and gastrointestinal smooth muscle, mucus secretion, and increased vascular permeability. Stimulation of H2 receptors inhibits T cell cytotoxicty, IFN-γ production, and release of lysozymes, but increases suppressor T cell activity, expression of complement receptors for C3b (CR1) on human eosinophils, and eosinophil and neutrophil chemokinesis. H3 receptors are located presynaptically on histaminergic nerves and function as autoreceptors that regulate the synthesis and release of histamine from neurons.

70. How is arachidonic acid converted to prostaglandins and thromboxane?

Cyclooxygenase converts arachidonic acid to the intermediate compounds prostaglandin G_2 (PGG_2) and prostaglandin H_2 (PGH_2). PGH_2 is converted to the biologically active prostaglandins PGD_2, PGE_2, and $PGF_{2\alpha}$ by prostaglandin synthases and isomerases, to prostacyclin (PGI_2) by prostacyclin synthase, and to TXA_2 by thromboxane synthase.

71. Explain the differences between the isoenzymes cyclooxygenase-1 and cyclooxygenase-2.

Cyclooxygenase-1 (COX-1), which is present in most types of cells, is a constitutive isoenzyme that exerts cytoprotective effects on the gastric mucosa, regulates renal blood flow, and decreases platelet aggregation. In contrast, cyclooxygenase-2 (COX-2), which is present in mast cells, macrophages, and leukocytes, is an inducible enzyme activated by proinflammatory mediators.

72. What are the biologic effects of cyclooxygenase metabolites?

PGD_2, the major cyclooxygenase product generated by human pulmonary mast cells, is 30 times as potent a bronchoconstrictor as histamine in patients with mild allergic asthma. PGD_2 also induces pulmonary and coronary artery vasoconstriction and peripheral vasodilatation, mediates neutrophil chemotaxis, and decreases platelet aggregation. $PGF_{2\alpha}$, a metabolite of PGD_2, exerts similar effects on the airways and blood vessels. TXA_2 mediates vasoconstriction, increases platelet aggregation, and may represent a more potent bronchoconstrictor than PGD_2. In contrast, PGE_2 and prostacyclin induce bronchodilatation.

73. Describe the lipoxygenase pathway of arachidonic acid metabolism.

Metabolism of arachidonic acid by lipoxygenase yields unstable hydroperoxyeicosatetraenoic acids (HPETEs). 5-Lipoxygenase converts arachidonic acid to 5-HPETE and then to 5-HETE or leukotriene A_4 (LTA_4). In turn, LTA_4 is metabolized

to LTB_4 or LTC_4. Sequential amino acid cleavage from LTC_4 yields LTD_4 and LTE_4. Collectively known as cysteinyl-leukotrienes (cys-LTs), LTC_4, LTD_4, and LTE_4 comprise the major lipoxygenase products synthesized by mast cells. An alternative metabolic pathway catalyzed by 15-lipoxygenase produces 15-HETE from arachidonic acid but appears to be of lesser importance in mediating allergic reactions.

74. Explain the relevance of these mediators to allergic diseases.

Cysteinyl-leukotrienes exert potent bronchoconstrictor effects that are up to 1,000 times more potent than histamine and 100 times more potent than prostaglandins. In addition, cys-LTs increase postcapillary venule permeability, augment bronchial mucus secretion, and attract eosinophils.

LTB_4 possesses potent chemotactic activity for neutrophils, eosinophils, monocytes, lymphocytes, and fibroblasts—cells responsible for the late-phase response and tissue remodeling. LTB_4 also increases vascular permeability and may enhance production of IgE and cytokines.

75. Bronchoalveolar lavage fluid obtained during the late-phase allergic reaction has been reported to contain cys-LTs without PGD_2 or tryptase. What does this imply?

This finding suggests that the cys-LTs present at this stage are derived from eosinophils or basophils rather than from mast cells.

76. Describe the synthesis and actions of platelet-activating factor (PAF).

Platelet-activating factor is an ether-linked phospholipid (alkylacetyl-glycerylether-phosphorylcholine) produced in a two-stage reaction during which phospholipase A_2 hydrolyzes membrane phospholipid to form lyso-PAF. Acetylation of lyso-PAF yields PAF, which is inactivated by conversion back to lyso-PAF.

Platelet-activating factor is synthesized by activated human lung mast cells, eosinophils, neutrophils, mononuclear phagocytes, platelets, endothelial cells, and epithelial cells. Biologic effects of PAF include platelet aggregation, bronchoconstriction, increased vascular permeability, and chemotaxis for eosinophils and neutrophils.

77. How do kinins mediate allergic disorders?

Kinins are potent vasoactive peptides produced in tissues and airway secretions in patients with inflammatory airway diseases, including allergic rhinitis, viral rhinitis, and asthma. The nonapeptide bradykinin is generated from high-molecular-weight kininogens in plasma by kininogenases, including kallikrein and tryptase. In the upper airways, kinins stimulate submucosal glands, increase vascular permeability, and activate sensory nerves, producing symptoms of rhinitis such as rhinorrhea, nasal congestion, and pruritus. In the lower airways, kinins induce bronchoconstriction by stimulation of sensory nerve-parasympathetic bronchoconstrictor reflexes and release of neuropeptides, including tachykinins, from sensory nerves.

78. Describe tachykinins and their effects.

Tachykinins are peptides with rapid onset of action located in neuronal endings within the skin, mucosa, and viscera, where they may induce vasodilatation, increase vascular permeability, attract inflammatory cells, and produce pain. The tachykinins

identified within the mammalian nervous system are substance P, neurokinin A (NKA), neurokinin B (NKB), neuropeptide K (NPK), and neuropeptide (NP).

79. What are cytokines?

Cytokines are low-molecular-weight proteins that regulate immune and inflammatory responses. They are secreted by lymphocytes, mast cells, macrophages, and airway cells, among others. This diverse group of glycoproteins can modulate both nonspecific inflammatory and specific immune effects on target cells and may contribute to tissue remodeling in chronic asthma.

80. Describe the actions of cytokines relevant to allergic and immune responses.

CYTOKINE	EFFECTS
GM-CSF	Secreted by activated macrophages, T cells, mast cells, eosinophils, and other cells Promotes differentiation of neutrophils and macrophages Activates mature eosinophils Prolongs eosinophil survival
IFN-γ	Derived mainly from Th1 lymphocytes, but also from cytotoxic T cells and other cells Represents the most important cytokine activator of macrophages Increases expression of class I and II MHC antigens Stimulates B-cell proliferation and differentiation Inhibits IL-4-induced IgE synthesis Inhibits Th2 lymphocytes Induces ICAM-1 expression
IL-1	Produced mainly by monocytes and macrophages, but also by lymphocytes and other cells Induced by endotoxin, microorganisms, antigens, and cytokines Increases proliferation of B cells and antibody synthesis Promotes growth of Th cells in response to APCs Stimulates production of T cell cytokines and IL-2 receptors Without IL-1, tolerance develops or immune response is impaired Promotes formation of arachidonic acid metabolites, including PGE_2 and LTB_4 Induces proliferation of fibroblasts and synthesis of fibronectin and collagen Increases ICAM-1, VCAM-1, E-selectin, and P-selectin expression IL-1 receptor antagonist (IL-1ra) antagonizes proinflammatory effects of IL-1
IL-3	Derived primarily from Th cells, but also from mast cells and eosinophils Stimulates development of mast cells, lymphocytes, macrophages Activates eosinophils Prolongs eosinophil survival
IL-4	Preformed peptide in mast cells and eosinophils Also secreted by Th2 cells, cytotoxic T cells, and basophils Promotes growth of Th2 cells, cytotoxic T cells, mast cells, eosinophils, basophils Initiates IgE isotype switching Increases expression of class I and II MHC antigens and FcεR on macrophages Stimulates VCAM-1 expression
IL-5	Produced by Th2 cells and mast cells Attracts eosinophils Activates eosinophils Prolongs eosinophil survival

(Table continued on next page.)

CYTOKINE	EFFECTS
IL-6	Synthesized primarily by monocytes and macrophages, but also by T, B, and other cells Induces B cell differentiation into plasma cells Inhibits TNF and IL-1 synthesis
IL-8	Produced mainly by monocytes, phagocytes, and endothelial cells Exerts potent chemoattraction for neutrophils Attracts activated eosinophils Induces neutrophil degranulation and activation Inhibits IL-4-mediated IgE synthesis
IL-9	Produced by Th2 cells Promotes mast cell and T cell proliferation Stimulates IgE synthesis Produces eosinophilia Induces bronchial hyperreactivity
IL-10	Secreted primarily by monocytes and B cells Inhibits monocyte/macrophage function Stimulates growth of mast cells, B cells, and cytotoxic T cells Induces permanent tolerance in Th lymphocytes Decreases synthesis of IFN-γ and IL-2 by Th1 cells Inhibits IL-4-induced IgE synthesis Decreases eosinophil survival
IL-11	Produced in response to respiratory viral infections Promotes generation of mast cells and B cells Induces bronchial hyperreactivity
IL-12	Synthesized by monocytes/macrophages, dendritic cells, B cells, neutrophils, mast cells Induced by IFN-γ and microorganisms Promotes Th1 and inhibits Th2 cell development Inhibits IL-4 induced IgE synthesis Enhances activity of cytotoxic T cells and NK cells
IL-13	Produced by Th1 and Th2 cells, mast cells, and dendritic cells Exerts effects similar to IL-4 on B cells and macrophages but does not affect T cells Induces IgE isotype switching Increases VCAM-1 expression Suppresses production of proinflammatory cytokines and chemokines Decreases synthesis of nitric oxide
IL-16	Secreted by CD8+ T cells, eosinophils, mast cells, and epithelial cells Promotes growth of CD4+ T cells Provides major source of CD4+ T cell chemotactic activity after antigen challenge Induces IL-2 receptors and class II MHC expression on CD4+ T cells
IL-18	Produced by lung, liver, and other tissues, but not by lymphocytes Stimulates secretion of IFN-γ and GM-CSF Promotes Th1 responses and activates NK cells (similar to IL-12) Induces synthesis of TNF, IL-1, Fas ligand Decreases IL-10 synthesis
TGF-α	Synthesized by macrophages and keratinocytes Stimulates proliferation of fibroblasts Promotes angiogenesis

(Table continued on next page.)

CYTOKINE	EFFECTS
TGF-β	Secreted by platelets, monocytes, some T cells, and fibroblasts Stimulates monocytes and fibroblasts Attracts mast cells, macrophages, fibroblasts Inhibits B cells, T helper cells, cytotoxic T cells, mast cells Inhibits airway smooth muscle cell proliferation
TNF-α	Produced primarily by mononuclear phagocytes; stored preformed in mast cells Induced by endotoxin, GM-CSF, IFN-γ, IL-1, and IL-3. Enhances class I and II MHC expression Activates neutrophils Increases cytokine production by monocytes and airway epithelial cells Promotes ICAM-1 and VCAM-1 expression Stimulates COX-2 expression in airway smooth muscle Induces bronchial hyperreactivity

BIBLIOGRAPHY

1. Barnes PJ, Chung KF, Page CP: Inflammatory mediators of asthma: An update. Pharmacol Rev 50:515–596, 1998.
2. Busse WW: Respiratory infections: Their role in airway responsiveness and the pathogenesis of asthma. J Allergy Clin Immunol 85:671–683, 1990.
3. Church MK, Levi-Schaffer F: The human mast cell. J Allergy Clin Immunol 99:155–160, 1997.
4. Corrigan CJ: Biology of lymphocytes. In Middleton E Jr, Reed CE, Ellis EF, Adkinson NF Jr, Yunginger JW, Busse WW (eds): Allergy: Principles and Practice, 5th ed. St. Louis, Mosby, 1998, pp 228–236.
5. Costa JJ, Weller PF, Galli SJ: The cells of the allergic response. Mast cells, basophils, and eosinophils. JAMA 278:1815–1822, 1997.
6. Gleich GJ: Mechanisms of eosinophil-associated inflammation. J Allergy Clin Immunol 105:651–663, 2000.
7. Hamid QA, Minshall EM: Molecular pathology of allergic disease. I. Lower airway disease. J Allergy Clin Immunol 105:20–36, 2000.
8. Kalish RS, Askenase PW: Molecular mechanisms of CD8+ T cell-mediated delayed hypersensitivity: Implications for allergies, asthma, and autoimmunity. J Allergy Clin Immunol 103:192–199, 1999.
9. Nickel R, Beck LA, Stellato C, Schleimer RP: Chemokines and allergic diseases. J Allergy Clin Immunol 104:723–742, 1999.
10. Panettieri RA Jr: Cellular and molecular mechanisms regulating airway smooth muscle proliferation and cell-adhesion molecule expression. Am J Respir Crit Care Med 158:S133–S140, 1998.
11. Romagnani S: The role of lymphocytes in allergic disease. J Allergy Clin Immunol 105:399–408, 2000.
12. Schroeder JT, MacGlashan DW: New concepts: The basophil. J Allergy Clin Immunol 99:429–433, 1997.
13. Vignola AM, Gjomarkaj M, Arnoux B, Bousquet J: Monocytes. J Allergy Clin Immunol 101:149–152, 1998.
14. Wardlaw AJ: Molecular basis for selective eosinophil trafficking in asthma: A multistep paradigm. J Allergy Clin Immunol 104:917–926, 1999.
15. Weller PF: Human eosinophils. J Allergy Clin Immunol 100:283–287, 1997.

3. AEROALLERGENS AND OTHER ENVIRONMENTAL ALLERGENS

Sarah Kuhl, M.D., Ph.D.

1. What are allergens?

Allergens are antigens that elicit the production of IgE. The allergic person will have a positive immediate wheal-and-flare reaction when the allergen is introduced in skin testing, and will have allergen-specific IgE in serum, as measured by in vitro assays such as the RAST (radioallergosorbent test) or ELISA (enzyme-linked immunosorbent test). Skin tests or RAST tests must always be interpreted in the context of the patient's history and physical examination, so the allergist must have a working knowledge of the aeroallergens in the community.

2. How are allergens named or classified?

The International Union of Immunologic Societies has established a method for naming aeroallergens: the first three letters of the genus, followed by the first letter of the species and an Arabic numeral indicating the order of discovery. Thus, *Dermatophagoides pteronyssinis*, the first allergen discovered for the dust mite, is called Der p 1.

3. What are aeroallergens?

Aeroallergens are airborne antigens that can cause allergy. The aeroallergen must be present in significant quantities, and must be of relatively small size and buoyant. Inhalant allergens can be plant pollen; fungi or molds; animal products of mammalian or arthropod or acarid origin; organic or inorganic dusts; and, uncommonly, algae. Outdoor aeroallergens, such as pollen and fungal spores, tend to be released into the atmosphere during seasons specific to each aeroallergen. Most species occur abundantly; however, a single highly productive tree may cause a high local exposure. Sensitization to a specific pollen is unusual unless the pollen count exceeds $50/m^3$ for at least 2 weeks in the year. Temperature, humidity, and wind direction and speed influence the concentration of aeroallergens. Warmth increases pollination and sporulation, which typically occur during the middle of the day. Many fungal spores, and some pollens such as ragweed, increase with high levels of humidity. The concentration of aeroallergen typically increases with wind speed up to about 15 mph. Higher wind speeds tend to decrease the concentration of allergen. Smaller particles tend to be more buoyant than larger particles, although the shape of certain pollen grains is thought to influence their buoyancy.

4. Does allergen size have anything to do with the resulting disease?

The physical size of pollen and some fungal spores has been thought to restrict them to the eyes and upper airways, and to causing allergic rhinitis and conjuctivitis. However, both elevated pollen and fungal spore counts can exacerbate asthma. Whether this is due to a cytokine-mediated effect originating in the upper airway, or

is the result of the inhalation of pollen and fungal spores, is controversial. Pollen spores have been found in the lungs at autopsy of patients with asthma. Patients with allergy to molds such as *Aspergillus* typically experience asthma rather than allergic rhinitis. This is thought to be due to small fungal debris (particularly spores) that is able to penetrate all the way to the lungs.

5. Describe pollen.

Pollen is the male germinal cell necessary for the reproduction in most seed plants. Insect-pollinated (entomophilous) plants such as roses tend to be colorful in order to attract insects. Wind-pollinated (anemophilus) plants tend to more allergenic, as the pollen is in high concentrations in the outdoor air. Wind-pollinated plants tend to be plain trees, grasses, and weeds. Pollen is invisible to the naked eye, but can readily be seen under a microscope.

6. How is pollen counted?

Early pollen counts often used gravitational methods with a glass slide covered with glycerin. A covered slide support, or Durham "shelter," was adopted in the 1940s as the standard pollen sampler, and was used for many years because it was simple, economical, and durable. However, airspeed, wind direction, and turbulence on particle deposition have resulted in newer volumetric methods. Suction traps and rotating arm impactors recover comparable numbers of pollen and spores. Suction traps are used for monitoring viable and nonviable spores, and pollen in air, and are particularly useful indoors. Rotating arm impactors are not affected by wind direction, and are minimally affected by airspeed less than 15 mph. Smaller spores tend to be deflected by the airstream, and impact the rod with lower frequency. Both provide useful data.

7. Can different pollens be distinguished under a microscope?

Pollens have distinct shapes and structures that are recognizable under the microscope. The outer envelope may show apertures or pores, as well as elongate furrows that act like miniature wings, or otherwise help to distinguish different pollens under the microscope. For example, grass pollens all have a single germinal pore. Although there is variation in size of pollen, it is difficult to distinguish between grass species under the microscope.

8. How do allergists know what pollens are important in their community?

Clinicians should know the most prevalent pollens in their area, as well as the seasonal pattern. They need to know the most prevalent flora that is wind pollinated in the area where they practice. Pollen counts are useful in determining the local prevalence of common allergens, although a single tree in a pollen-allergic patient's yard may make that patient miserable for the few weeks of that pollen's season. Conversely, pollens such as ragweed have been detected many miles offshore (albeit in small quantities); thus, pollens can travel long distances. Ragweed and grass are particularly known to cause allergic symptoms dozens of miles away. Correlation of pollen counts with patient symptoms and skin or RAST tests is helpful. Pollen and spore counts for many localities can be obtained from the National Allergy Bureau at http://www.aaaai.org/nab or 1-800-9-POLLEN.

9. Name the most common cause of allergic disease and state why it is the most common cause allergic disease.

Grass pollen allergy is the most common cause of allergic disease because the grasses are wind-pollinated and distributed worldwide. Grass pollens show extensive cross reactivity between species. Allergic rhinitis was originally described in the nineteenth century in England as "hay fever" because of the association of nasal symptoms with the harvesting of hay from Timothy grass. The major grasses that produce abundant pollen in North America are Sweet, Vernal, Orchard, Timothy, Bluegrass, Fescue, Redtop, and Perennial Ryegrass. In the northern United States, Canada, and Europe, the grass pollen season typically lasts from approximately May to July. In warmer areas, the season can be considerably longer. However, in tropical or subtropical climates, grass and other pollens may be present perennially. The majority of grass pollens in the northern United States (Orchard, Bluegrass, Redtop, and Perennial Ryegrass) have antigens that cross-react. A person who is allergic to one of these grasses is typically allergic to all of them. Timothy also has cross-reactive antigens, as well as distinctive antigens. Bermuda, Johnson, and Bahia grasses are less cross-reactive with the above-mentioned grasses, and have more distinctive antigens. Bermuda grass is cosmopolitan, and present in warm areas of both hemispheres.

10. Is tree pollen season a problem?

Tree pollen season is shorter in most countries, so tends to be less of a problem. In North America and Europe, the tree pollen season is early spring, before grass and weed pollen season. There is some cross-reactivity between tree pollen allergens, but less than among the grass pollens. Most of the major tree pollens are from trees in the angiosperm family such as birch, elm, maple, ash, alder, hazel, and oak. The angiosperm family comprises two subclasses, the *Monocotyledonae* (which includes grasses) and *Dicotyledonae* (which includes flowering plants, deciduous trees, and weeds).

11. Are tree pollens cross-reactive?

Tree pollens are generally much less cross-reactive than grass pollens. Often there is cross-reactivity within the same genus, but not within the family. The exception appears to be the *Oleaceae* family, which includes olive, ash, and privet species. There is a high degree of cross-reactivity between these three pollen species, and the antigenic differences are said to be less than among grass species. This explains how a person who lives in Michigan, and who has never been exposed to olive pollen, can have olive-specific IgE.

The major (group I) tree pollen allergens are small, cytoplasmic, acidic proteins with immunologic cross-reactivity. Group II tree pollen allergens are less cross-reactive.

Birch pollen is another major allergen in North America. The major birch pollen allergen, Bet v 1, is highly allergenic, and cross-reacts with many of the group I tree pollens. Bet v 1 also cross-reacts with a low-molecular-weight allergen in apples, which explains why some people with birch allergy experience oral allergy syndrome.

12. What is oral allergy syndrome?

Oral allergy syndrome is caused by a cross-reaction of antigens between inhaled pollen and certain raw foods. Some people who experience allergic rhinitis to

inhaled pollens will experience itching and swelling of the mucous membranes at the point where a food touches the mouth: lips, tongue, throat, and roof of mouth. Patients with oral allergy syndrome can often eat the same foods cooked. Patients must avoid the raw food, particularly during pollen season. Foods that are known to cross-react are shown in the Table.

Oral Allergy Syndrome

POLLEN	FOODS THAT MAY CAUSE ORAL ALLERGY SYNDROME
Birch	Apple, pear, celery, carrot, parsnip, potato, hazelnut, kiwi
Ragweed	Gourd family: watermelon, cantaloupe, honeydew melon, zucchini, cucumber
Tree and grass	Apple, tree nuts, peach, orange, pear, cherry, fennel, tomato, carrot

13. Are nondeciduous trees allergenic?

The Gymnosperm family includes conifer and ginkgo orders of nondeciduous trees. Coniferales includes the orders *Pinaceae* (which includes pine, spruce, fir, and hemlock), *Cupressiaceae* (which includes juniper, cypress, cedar, and savin), and *Taxodiaceae* (which includes bald cypress). There are two major types of gymnosperm pollen. Pines, spruces, firs, true cedars, mountain or black hemlock, and golden larch (*Pseudolarix amabilis*) have large (50 to 90 µm) pollen grains with two air bladders. Members of the cypress-juniper, yew, and bald cypress-sequoia family have spherical pollen grains 20 to 35 µm in diameter with a thick exine or outermost layer, and a thick intine, or cellulose-rich middle layer. Larger pollens with similar shape include larch (*Larix* sp.), which is 40 to 70 µm, and Douglas fir (80 to 110 µm).

Conifers are wind-pollinated, and pollen can be present in significant quantities in certain regions. Pine pollen can form a yellow dust when in bloom, but is rarely allergenic. Most types of conifer pollen are not very allergenic, so most conifers do not cause problems in significant numbers of people. However, mountain cedar is an important cause of allergic rhinitis in areas where it has proliferated due to overgrazing (particularly from Texas to central Mexico), and sheds pollen from late fall to late winter. Other species of juniper and cypress may cause allergies further north. Bald cypress is known to cause allergic rhinitis in Florida, and a pine-allergic person living in the midst of a pine forest may experience rhinitis during pollen season. Japanese cedar ("sugi") is the major cause of tree pollen allergy in Japan, and other cedar species in the United States (such as Port Orford cedar in the Cascades) are known to cause rhinitis. Pine pollen has been documented as a cause of ocular and respiratory pollinosis.

14. Are people allergic to cottonwood seeds that are released with cotton-tufts?

People who believe they are allergic to cottonwood tufts and seeds are typically allergic to grass. Cottonwoods tend to shed their seeds at the height of grass pollen season in many areas. Cottonwood pollinates much earlier in the spring, and the pollen is invisible to the naked eye.

15. Do blooming roses cause allergies? Don't insects pollinate roses?

Roses are insect-pollinated, and do not tend to cause high rates of allergy in the general population. An allergy attributed to blooming roses is often due to grass

pollen. The grass pollen season coincides with the rose season in many areas. Persons with high levels of exposure due to their occupation or hobbies can rarely become allergic to flowering plants.

16. Are people allergic to goldenrod in the fall?

Allergy attributed to goldenrod is more likely due to ragweed. Again, the season that goldenrod blooms coincides with ragweed pollen season, and goldenrod is a more colorful insect-pollinated plant.

17. Can mowing the lawn exacerbate allergies?

People who believe that mowing the lawn exacerbates their allergies are often allergic to mold.

18. Are people who are allergic to the pollens of food-producing trees (such as olives and tree nuts) allergic to the foods produced by these trees?

Not usually.

19. Name other plants that cause allergic symptoms.

Weeds such as ragweed, sagebrush, lamb's quarter, and English plantain cause allergic symptoms in many people. Ragweed is the most notorious pollen in North America, but it is not a problem in the Pacific Northwest, northern California, and other parts of the world. Sagebrush is another member of the composite family that can cross-react with ragweed; it is typically found in desert areas of the western United States and Mexico. Russian thistle and burning bush are found in the same areas, and may cross-react. The pollens of lamb's quarter and pigweed are microscopically similar, as well as members of the Chenopod-Amaranth family, and are widespread in agricultural areas and vacant lots. English Plantain is a common lawn weed in North America that pollinates from May to July. Members of the dock-knotweed and nettle families also can be allergenic. *Parietaria* species, members of the nettle family, are the main allergen in the Mediterranean basin.

20. What are the recommendations for pollen avoidance?

Wear a mask or respirator when exposed to outdoor triggers, such as mowing lawn, gardening, or if you must be outdoors. Remain indoors on warm, windy days when pollen counts are high, and during the middle of the day when pollen counts are highest. Grasses typically release their pollen late in the day, so grass-allergic persons may want to stay indoors late in the day. Air conditioners typically exclude outside air, and decrease pollen counts indoors, so allergists recommend closing windows and using air conditioners.

21. Are molds or fungi major outdoor or indoor allergens?

They can be both. Allergenic molds or fungi can be divided into storage (indoor, perennial) versus field (seasonal) molds, although a few species are major allergens both indoors and outdoors. Airborne mold spores can be collected like pollen, and show seasonal variation in many temperate areas. Warm weather increases the numbers of airborne mold spores, while frozen or snow covered ground prevents growth. *Alternaria* and *Cladosporium* (or *Hormodendrum*) are the most prominent outdoor

molds, and increase in number in late summer and early fall, and during the daytime. They are typically found on decaying plants and leaves. Other common outdoor molds include *Aspergillus*, *Penicillium*, and *Botrytis*. Fungal spores can be detected year-round except in polar regions. High levels are found in areas of crop production.

Alternaria spores are particularly prominent in grain growing areas. *Cladosporium* often outnumbers other outdoor fungi in North America. They are common saprophytes and parasites of spinach, bananas, and tomatoes. *Helminthosporium* form species includes plant parasites, particularly in the southern United States. Species such as *Curvularia* may cause allergic fungal sinusitis as well as allergic rhinitis and asthma. *Epicoccum* is widespread in grassland and agricultural areas, and reach high levels during dry fall periods in midwestern United States. *Fusarium* is a cosmopolitan genus of mold, which includes spoilage organisms and plant pathogens. *Aspergillus* is another spoilage organism that is widely present in rotting vegetation and compost piles. *Aspergillus* may be present in higher numbers indoors than outdoors.

The perennial molds *Aspergillus* and *Penicillium* are the major indoor or storage molds, which can grow in lower humidity, and in barns, sheds, and indoors, especially in basements. *Aspergillus* is also commonly found in rotted grains or vegetables, and in rotting leaves and compost piles. *Penicillium* can occur in abundance indoors, and is typically a green mildew found on items stored in damp basements, and on decaying food. *Rhizopus* and *Cladosporium* are also often found indoors, particularly if there is any rotting wood. Molds can often be found in damp bathrooms and on windowsills. Vaporizers and humidifiers contaminated with mold become a source of mold spores.

22. Is mold allergy implicated in asthma exacerbations?

Yes, it can be. *Alternaria* has been recognized as a risk factor for death due to asthma. About 25% of asthmatics have positive skin tests to *Aspergillus*. Patients with mold allergy (often children) usually experience asthma because the small fungal debris (particularly spores) can penetrate all the way to the lungs.

23. Can a patient be allergic to *Aspergillus* and not have allergic bronchopulmonary aspergillosis (ABPA)?

Yes. People can have specific IgE with allergic rhinitis and asthma symptoms due to *Aspergillus*. Patients with ABPA will also have specific IgE to *Aspergillus*.

24. Can *Aspergillus* cause invasive fungal infection?

Yes. *Aspergillus* causes a spectrum of disease from allergic rhinitis and asthma to ABPA and allergic fungal sinusitis to invasive aspergillosis. Other molds can cause parenchymal lung disease. Thermophilic *Actinomyces* can cause hypersensitivity pneumonitis.

25. Are people who are allergic to the mold *Penicillium* also allergic to the antibiotic penicillin?

No. Penicillin is a product of the mold *Penicillium*, but there is no cross-reactivity between the mold *Penicillium* and the drug penicillin. Although a person could be allergic to both, there is no increased risk of penicillin allergy in people who are allergic to the mold *Penicillium*.

26. Does *Penicillium* cause food allergies?

Penicillium is also found in blue-veined cheeses such as Roquefort and on the surface of cheeses such as Camembert. Eating these cheeses can occasionally cause symptoms in *Penicillium*-allergic people.

27. What can be done to avoid mold and fungi?

• Avoid raking leaves, mowing lawns, farming activities, and hiking in forested areas, and avoid compost piles.

• Wear a mask or respirator if you must be exposed to molds, or if mold spore counts are high.

• Decrease indoor humidity. Cleaning damp areas indoors regularly with bleach effectively kills and controls mold growth. Typically a solution of one part bleach with three parts water is effective, but should be tested on a small part of the area to be cleaned. Other household fungicides are also effective.

28. Name the major indoor allergens.

Dust mites and insect emanations, fungal or mold spores, and animal danders.

29. Describe the history of dust allergies.

House dust has been recognized as an allergen for centuries. Dust mites were recognized as the cause of most dust allergy in the 1960s, and the potency of house dust allergen was eventually recognized to correlate with the number of house dust or mattress mites in the dust. Pure cultures of the mites were used to make mite extracts, which were 10 to 100 times more potent than house dust.

30. Are dust mites insects?

Dust mites are technically a subclass of the Acarid class, which includes spiders and scabies, so they are not insects. They can be seen only with the aid of low-power magnification. The family Pyroglyphidae includes the house dust mite species *Dermatophagoides pteronyssinus*, *D. farinae*, and *Euroglyphus maynei*. The tropical dust mite *Blomia tropicalis* is found in areas such as Florida and Brazil. The family Pyroglyphidae contains the storage mites, another subclass of acarids that can cause allergy.

31. Where are dust mites found?

House dust mites are found worldwide. The house dust mite species *Dermatophagoides pteronyssinus* is more numerous in European homes, while North American homes contain mainly *D. farinae*, although both species may be found in the same home. There are numerous cross-reactive antigens and allergens.

Storage mites are mainly found in stored grain, but can cause allergy in farm or grain workers, and are occasionally associated with dust allergy in homes.

House dust mites feed mainly on human or animal dander, fungi, and other debris found in human environments. High concentrations of dust mites are found in mattresses, pillows, carpeting, and upholstered furniture.

32. If someone is allergic to dust, can they vacation in or move to an area of the world without mites? Are there specific environments that dust mites like?

A relative humidity of greater than 50% and a temperature of 65 to 80°F are optimal for mite propagation. Mite levels appear to rise with the peak humidity in July

in Virginia, and stay high until after January. Dust mites are rarely found in arid climates or at high altitude. So, a person who is allergic only to dust mites will often find relief in northern Sweden, central Canada, and the mountain states of the United States.

33. Does the concentration of an allergen predispose to sensitization? Is there a relationship between dust mite exposure and the development of asthma?

Levels of about 2 µg of group 1 mite antigen or about 100 mites per gram of dust increases the risk of sensitization in genetically at-risk individuals. In areas in which all houses contain mites, sensitivity to mites is a major risk factor for hospital admission for asthma.

Exposure to the house dust mite allergen Der p I is an important factor in the development of pediatric asthma. In the United States and England, 80 to 90% of allergic asthmatics and 10% of the population have immediate skin test reactivity to house dust mites.

34. Which part of the mite is most allergenic?

The major mite allergen is found in mite fecal particles. These are spherical particles of approximately 10 to 35 microns, so they are approximately the size of many pollen granules. A chitinous peritrophic membrane surrounds mite fecal proteins. Mite allergen is also found in the cuticle of the mite. However, host dust mite fecal particles are the most important reservoir of allergens, and the major form in which Der p 1 becomes airborne.

35. Describe avoidance measures for mite allergen.

Cover mattresses and pillows with impermeable covers. Wash bedding (including blankets, comforters, and bedspreads) in hot water (130°F); dry in dryer or sunlight. Reduce relative humidity to 45% or less. Remove carpets, stuffed animals, and clutter, especially from bedrooms.

Vacuum at least weekly, using a HEPA bag. Minimize carpets and upholstered furniture (vinyl or leather preferred). Treating carpets with tannic acid to denature mite allergen, or benzyl benzoate to kill mites may decrease allergen concentrations for weeks to months. Freezing stuffed toys in a freezer bag at –20°C for 24 hours kills mites. HEPA air filters are not as useful for dust mites as they are for pollen and other aeroallergens, as airborne Der p 1 is detected only after disturbance of a house.

36. Are feather pillows more mite-ridden than foam pillows?

Allergic patients have often been told to avoid feather pillows, as they may become sensitized to the feathers. Furthermore, feather pillows were long thought to harbor higher concentrations of dust mites, but this has not proved true. The tightly woven covers needed to contain the down may be a barrier to other allergens, such as dust mites. Most allergists recommend encasing pillows and mattresses in dust mite pillow covers.

37. Which insects are sources of indoor allergens?

Cockroaches are a major cause of inner-city asthma in the United States. The German cockroach (*Blattella germanica*) is common in inner cities with hot climates

or with central heating. The highest level of cockroach antigens Bla g 1, Bla g 2, and Bla g 4 are found on kitchen floors, and in bathrooms. As with dust mites, the major allergens are related to the GI tract or feces, and little or no allergen is present in undisturbed air.

The American cockroach (*Periplaneta americana*) and the Oriental cockroach (*Blattella orientalis*) are hardier, and are found indoors and outdoors, particularly in the southern United States. Allergen Per a 1 cross-reacts with Bla g 1.

The prevalence of cockroach allergy is inversely proportional to socioeconomic level in inner cities. Cockroaches are difficult to eradicate, but frequent cleaning and eliminating shelter, food, and water availability help to control them. Killing cockroaches has not been proven to reduce cockroach antigen levels. However, extermination followed by aggressive cleaning does appear to be effective in decreasing antigen levels. Spraying kills few roaches, and traps catch few roaches. Boric acid is relatively nontoxic to humans, but effectively kills roaches, and other baits more toxic to humans and roaches are available.

One of the most effective methods for cockroach control is a cat. However, this is not a method recommended by allergists due to the potential for developing cat allergy.

38. Can other insects be allergens?

Mayfly and caddis fly scales and body parts can cause respiratory allergy in the eastern Great Lakes (particularly Lake Erie) in late summer. Respiratory allergy has been reported to the green nimmiti midge in the Sudan, and to the moth *Pseudoaletia unipuncta* in Minnesota. The major allergen is thought to be in the insect body. In Japan, many asthmatics are allergic to silkworm moth wings. Bed quilts are often filled with crude silk. Occupational exposure may result in allergy to crickets used for frog food.

39. Is patient history a reliable indicator of allergy to mammalian dander?

A positive patient history is often a reliable indicator of cat allergy, as patients will report erythema or urticaria where licked by a cat, or eye irritation if they rub their eyes after petting a cat. These reactions may also be seen in patients who are dog allergic, although cats cause more allergic symptoms than dogs or other indoor animals. While this was initially attributed to animal hair or fur, the desquamated epithelium has been found to be the culprit in certain cases. The most important cat allergen, Fel d 1, is found in saliva and in sebaceous glands of the skin. All breeds of cat produce Fel d1, although nonneutered male cats are reported to produce more than females. Other cat proteins such as albumin can be allergenic to patients. Cat dander particles tend to be smaller than 25 microns, and some particles are smaller than 0.25 microns, so can be inhaled into the lungs. Cat allergen is airborne: cat-allergic patients often report rapid onset of eye and respiratory tract symptoms when entering a home where a cat lives.

40. How can cat dander be avoided?

Cat dander can best be avoided by removing the cat from the home, a difficult, if not impossible, achievement in some homes. After a cat is removed from the home, it typically takes 12 to 16 weeks for allergen levels to fall below the typical

allergic threshold. If the cat cannot or will not be removed from the home, it should be kept outdoors. If it cannot be kept outdoors, the cat must be kept out of the bedroom, and a HEPA filter and pillow and mattress covers can be used to decrease Fel d 1 concentrations in the bedroom, although this may not be to sufficiently low levels. Weekly cat washing has also been recommended as a method for decreasing exposure in patients who cannot or will not remove the cat from the home. However, there are conflicting reports as to the success of cat washing in decreasing allergen exposure.

41. What is the major dog allergen?

Dog allergy is less common than cat allergy. The major allergen, Can f 1, is a protein found in dog saliva and hair in all breeds. The levels of this allergen vary between different breeds of dogs, and some breed-specific allergens exist, although their significance is unknown. Dog allergy causes asthma exacerbation less often than cat allergen. HEPA filters and dog washing can decrease levels of Can f 1.

42. Name the major rodent allergens.

The urinary proteins of laboratory rodents such as mice and rats can cause allergic reactions, in addition to mouse dander. Rodent aeroallergens can also be found at high levels in rodent-infested apartment buildings. The major mouse (*Mus musculus*) allergen is Mus m 1, a prealbumin found in mouse urine and dander. The major allergens in the rat (*Rattus norvegicus*) are Rat n 1A and Ratn1B, both variants of alpha-globulin, and found in rat dander, urine, and saliva. Serum and urine levels of major allergens in both rats and mice are higher in males. These allergens may be airborne, so respirators, good ventilation, frequent washing of cages, and laminar flow caging may be helpful.

Allergens from pets such as gerbils, guinea pigs, rabbits, ferrets, and the like, are less well characterized, but may cause symptomatic allergy. Farm animals such as horses, cattle, and pigs may also cause allergy, and a horse-allergic individual can react to the horsehair stuffing in antique furniture.

Feathers can be allergenic, either from pet birds or in feathers used to make down pillows, comforters and other bedding, and clothing.

43. Is it worthwhile for an individual who is allergic to Orchard grass pollen to move to an area of the country where another grass species such as Kentucky Blue grass is predominant?

Because there is a high level of allergenic cross-reactivity between grass pollens, the person would most likely be allergic to all of the common grasses discussed earlier. They could consider moving to a desert area where grass does not grow. Many people who moved to a desert area such as Arizona found relief earlier in this century. However, as many of these areas have been irrigated and planted with anemophilous plants, they are no longer havens for allergic persons. Allergic individuals may have few symptoms the first season they are in an area with new trees and weeds, but then find themselves allergic during the second pollen season in an area with vastly different fauna.

The Arctic and Antarctic are too cold for both fungi and plants to proliferate. Also people who spend many months on the high seas may find a reprieve from seasonal

allergens. However, the increased humidity may foster dust mites in the ship's bedding. At high altitudes in arid areas, there are also fewer dust mites. Colder climates also have a shorter growing season.

44. Can latex be a cause of indoor inhalant allergy?

Yes. Latex allergen can be present in high levels in operating rooms and clinics. Latex gloves are the major source of allergen. In traffic-congested urban areas, tire fragments may account for high levels of latex aeroallergen in outdoor air. There are currently no standardized extracts available in the United States for latex skin testing. A latex-free hospital and clinic environment is recommended for latex-allergic individuals.

45. Are foods causes of indoor inhalant allergy?

Inhalation of the aeroallergens from cooking shrimp has been known to cause anaphylaxis. The inhalation of flour can cause rhinitis or "baker's asthma."

46. Are there inhalant airborne allergens associated with certain occupations?

Yes. There are more than 250 agents in the workplace associated with occupational asthma.

47. Do perfumes and other strong odors cause allergic reactions?

Perfume and cologne typically have an irritant effect, and affect patients with nonallergic rhinitis, as well as exacerbates allergic rhinitis. Strong odors and fumes, such as fumes from petroleum products and organic solvents, as well as diesel exhaust, can also exacerbate rhinitis and asthma. Fumes from cooking oils can also exacerbate asthma.

48. Does air pollution cause asthma and allergy?

Cigarette smoking (passive or active) is implicated in the causation of asthma and allergies. Other air pollutants are implicated in acute exacerbations of asthma and other respiratory symptoms, but it appears that pollutants and irritants are not implicated in causation.

49. Name the major indoor pollutants and describe their source.

Unfortunately, tobacco smoke remains one of the most serious air pollutants in some households and in some areas of the world. Passive smoking may have an adjuvant effect on allergic response.

Formaldehyde is an indoor pollutant that is released from new particleboard, furnishings, tobacco smoke, gas stoves, foam insulation, and carbonless carbon paper. Levels may be particularly high in manufactured or mobile homes. Formaldehyde causes mucous membrane irritation in some people at levels of 1 to 3 parts per million (ppm), and lower in atopic individuals.

"Sick building syndrome" occurs in energy-efficient buildings with poor ventilation and little outdoor air exchange. Irritated conjunctiva and respiratory tract are the most common complaints. Irritants include hydrocarbons, ammonia, and acetic acid from office machines; insecticides; rug shampoo; tobacco smoke; and combustion gases. Sometimes the pollutants originate outdoors. For example, the location

of air intake for a building is next to a loading dock where trucks are kept running, thus accounting for high ozone and nitrogen dioxide levels inside the building.

50. Name the major outdoor pollutants and their sources.

Sulfur dioxide and particulate black smoke result from burning fossil fuels, as well as from natural phenomenon such as volcanoes. These cause respiratory and conjunctival symptoms, although levels have improved since the 1960s in the United States, and are reportedly improving in Eastern Europe.

The increased use of motor vehicles has resulted in increased ozone, oxides of nitrogen, and fine-particulate matter less than 10 μm in diameter. Increased levels of ozone can exacerbate asthma. Pollutants such as nitrogen dioxide and ozone can increase the response of persons with asthma or allergic rhinitis to inhaled allergens. Human and animal studies have shown that diesel exhaust particles enhance IgE production by a number of mechanisms.

51. Can a newborn be allergic?

The general teaching is that it takes one season of exposure to become allergic to a seasonal allergen. So, infants are typically not allergic in their first year of life to seasonal allergens.

BIBLIOGRAPHY

1. Bousquet J, Guérin B, Hewitt B, Lim S, Michel FB: Allergy in the Mediterranean area. III: Cross-reactivity among Oleaceae pollens. Clin Allergy 15(5):439–448, 1985.
2. Gossage DL: Airborne allergens. In Altman LC, Becker JW, and Williams PV (eds): Allergy in Primary Care. Philadelphia, W.B. Saunders, 2000, pp 65–75.
3. Horwitz RJ, Bush RK: Allergens and other factors important in atopic disease. In Patterson R, Grammer LC, Greenberger PA (eds): Allergic Diseases, Diagnosis and Management, 5th ed. Philadelphia, Lippincott Williams & Wilkins, 1997, pp 75–130.
4. Kernerman SM, McCullough J, Green J, Ownby DR: Evidence of cross-reactivity between olive, ash, privet, and Russian olive tree pollen allergens. Ann Allergy 69(6):493–496, 1992.
5. Solomon WR, Platts-Mills TAE: Aerobiology and inhalent allergens. In Middleton E Jr, et al (eds): Allergy Principles and Practice, 5th ed. Philadelpha, W.B. Saunders, 1998, pp 367–403.

4. EVALUATION OF ALLERGIC DISEASE

Kristina Hoffman Philpott, M.D., and Joshua Jacobs, M.D.

CLINICAL EVALUATION

1. What clues in the patient's clinical history are pertinent to asthma and/or allergic rhinitis?

- Age of onset of symptoms (typically asthma and allergic rhinitis begin in childhood or early adulthood, whereas chronic obstructive pulmonary disease becomes symptomatic after age 40).
- Family history of atopic conditions in close relatives.
- History of comorbid conditions (e.g., gastroesophageal reflux, bronchopulmonary dysplasia, tobacco exposure) that may contribute to the severity of atopic respiratory conditions.
- Onset, duration, severity, and frequency of symptoms (although asthma and/or allergic rhinitis may be episodic, many individuals have perennial symptoms that may wax or wane, depending on other factors).
- Diurnal or seasonal variation in cough or rhinitis symptoms or correlation with pollen counts in the geographic area.
- Symptoms related to specific location, whether indoor or outdoor.
- Coughing or wheezing triggered by physical activity or strong emotion (laughing or crying very hard).
- Chronic and/or recurrent sinus complaints, snoring, or mouth breathing.
- Past clinical improvement with proper use of medications for treatment of asthma or allergic rhinitis (e.g., inhaled corticosteroids, bronchodilators, leukotriene modifiers, antihistamines).
- History of hospitalizations, emergency department visits, and/or urgent care visits due to symptoms.
- In women, variation in symptoms with menstrual cycle or during pregnancy.
- Symptoms with concurrent viral infections.
- Exposure to indoor pets, dust mites, or molds.
- Occupational or social exposures to chemicals, irritants, or latex glove powder.
- Symptoms occurring after medication usage (e.g., aspirin, beta-blockers).
- Symptoms occurring after ingestion of food additives or preservatives (e.g., sulfites).

2. What aspects of general appearance require specific attention in the physical examination of a potentially atopic and/or asthmatic patient?

- Level of distress, need for immediate attention
- Nasal voice quality or vocal hoarseness
- Work of breathing
- General state of nutrition
- In children, appropriate growth and development for age

3. What dermatologic findings are relevant?
- Distribution and severity of eczema (extensor and facial involvement is more common in children; flexural involvement is typically seen in adults).
- Pruritus may be only historical if patient is taking medications, but it is critical in the diagnosis of atopic dermatitis.
- "Soft signs" or minor skin findings in atopic patients include: keratosis pilaris, mild xerosis, palmar hyperlinearity, dermatographism, and pityriasis alba.

4. What aspects of the eye and ear examinations are important?
Eyes
- Allergic "shiners" or creases.
- Conjunctival inflammation.
- Baseline ophthalmoscopic exam (anterior subcapsular cataracts may be present in 8–12% of patients with atopic keratoconjunctivitis and severe atopic dermatitis).
- Trantas' dots or Horner's points may be seen in vernal conjunctivitis.
- White ropy discharge is characteristic of an allergic etiology, whereas mucopurulence may indicate infection.

Ears
- Tympanic membrane appearance.
- Pneumatic otoscopy to check for potential eustachian tube dysfunction or middle ear effusion.
- Look for cholesteatoma.

5. What clues may be found in the examination of the nose and pharynx?
Nose
- Transnasal crease (especially in atopic children).
- Color and quality of secretions.
- Nasal mucosal color and presence of edema.
- Visible nasal polyps. (The true incidence of nasal polyps in allergic disorders is unknown. If they are seen in children under age 10, the diagnosis of cystic fibrosis should be considered. Nasal polyps also occur in association with immotile cilia syndrome.)
- Transillumination of the sinuses is considered to be of limited usefulness in the diagnosis of sinusitis.

Pharynx
- High-arched palate may be associated with atopic disorders.
- Size, symmetry, and appearance of tonsils.
- Uvula (bifid uvula may be associated with a soft-palate cleft).
- "Cobblestoning" on the pharyngeal mucosa may be seen in atopic patients.
- Any visible postnasal drainage.

6. What findings are important in the chest and lung examination?
- Chest deformity, thoracic hyperexpansion, hunched shoulders.
- In children, respiratory rate appropriate for age

Age	Normal rate (awake)
< 2 months	< 60/minute
2–12 months	< 50/minute
1–5 years	< 40/minute
6–8 years	< 30/minute

- Use of accessory muscles during respiratory cycle may indicate respiratory distress (e.g., intercostal retractions).
- Audible inspiratory stridor may indicate an upper airway obstruction (e.g., croup, epiglottitis, laryngeal angioedema, or foreign body).
- Bibasilar wheezing on auscultation and/or prolonged expiratory phase are usually indicative of asthma, in conjunction with other diagnostic criteria. The absence of wheezing does not exclude the diagnosis of asthma; audible wheezing may not be present in mild intermittent asthma or cough-variant asthma.

7. **What are the differential diagnoses for patients with asthma-type symptoms?**
Infants and children
  Upper airway diseases
  Allergic rhinitis and sinusitis
  Obstruction involving large airways
  Foreign body in trachea or bronchus
  Vocal cord dysfunction
  Vascular rings or laryngeal webs
  Laryngotracheomalacia, tracheal stenosis, or bronchostenosis
  Enlarged lymph nodes or tumor
  Obstructions involving small airways
  Viral bronchiolitis or obliterative bronchiolitis
  Cystic fibrosis
  Bronchopulmonary dysplasia
  Heart disease
  Other causes
  Recurrent cough not due to asthma
  Aspiration from swallowing mechanism dysfunction or gastroesophageal reflux
Adults
  Chronic obstructive pulmonary disease (chronic bronchitis or emphysema)
  Congestive heart failure
  Pulmonary embolism
  Laryngeal dysfunction
  Mechanical obstruction of the airways (benign and malignant tumors)
  Pulmonary infiltration with eosinophilia
  Cough secondary to drugs (e.g., angiotensin-converting enzyme [ACE] inhibitors)
  Vocal cord dysfunction

From National Asthma Education and Prevention Program Panel Report II: Guidelines for the Diagnosis and Management of Asthma. Rockville, MD, National Institutes of Health, NIH Publication 97-4051, 1997.

8. According to the 1997 National Asthma Education and Prevention Program Panel Report, what are the criteria for the diagnosis of asthma?
- Episodic symptoms of airflow obstruction are present.
- Airflow obstruction is at least partially reversible.
- Alternative diagnoses are excluded.

9. When is a total serum IgE a useful diagnostic test?

Although it is commonly used as a screening test for allergic disease, total serum IgE is best reserved for specific indications (e.g., as part of the diagnostic criteria for allergic bronchopulmonary aspergillosis). When total serum IgE is used as a screening test for allergic disease, be aware of the potential pitfalls:
- Levels vary with age.
- There is a significant overlap in levels between nonatopic and atopic patients.
- The reported sensitivity and specificity of total IgE in serum cord blood to predict atopy in infants varies widely compared with a strong family history of atopy and eventual development of atopy in children.
- Total serum IgE is often extremely high in parasitic disease, specific immunodeficiencies, allergic bronchopulmonary aspergillosis, and in children with severe atopic dermatitis and food allergies.

10. What are the general indications for in vivo percutaneous and intradermal testing with allergenic extracts?
- Clinical history consistent with possible IgE-mediated hypersensitivity.
- Need to exclude IgE-mediated hypersensitivity as the cause of clinical manifestations in a particular patient.

11. What are the medical contraindications to in vivo skin tests?
- Inability to discontinue medications that interfere with skin test interpretation (e.g., antihistamines).
- Severe uncontrolled atopic dermatitis or other generalized skin disease.
- Severe dermatographism.
- History of life-threatening anaphylaxis to particular antigens (usually venom or food antigens), when alternative in vitro tests may be safer.
- Medical conditions and/or medications that may decrease a patient's ability to survive an anaphylactic reaction (e.g., patient with unstable asthma or a patient taking a beta-blocker medication).

12. Is it diagnostically feasible to perform skin prick tests on infants?

Yes. When clinically indicated, skin prick tests may be useful in infancy, but the size of the wheal is often reduced. Therefore, the criteria for interpretation for each allergen should be based on comparison with the size of the wheal of the positive control.

13. Is there an upper age limit for performing skin tests?

No. However, over the age of 50, skin test wheal size may decline, and positivity always should be interpreted relative to control values.

14. Are there gender differences in skin test responses?
No. Although wheal size in response to histamine may vary in women during the menstrual cycle, the variation is not considered clinically significant.

15. Describe the seasonal variation in skin tests to specific pollen allergens.
Skin test responses peak after a specific pollen season and gradually decline until the subsequent season.

16. Do skin test reactions vary with which part of the body is tested?
Yes. The back is more reactive than the forearm. The upper back is more reactive than the lower back. Forearm reactivity increases from lateral wrist to medial antecubital fossa.

17. What are appropriate controls for percutaneous skin testing?
Positive control: histamine phosphate at the equivalent of 1 mg/ml histamine.
Negative control: the diluent used to prepare antigens used in testing.

18. Which common medications interfere with in vivo skin tests? What is the duration of suppression of full wheal formation after discontinuing the medication?

DRUG	DEGREE	DURATION (DAYS)
H₁ antagonists		
1st generation		
Chlorpheniramine	++	1–3
Clemastine	+++	1–10
Azelastine	++++	3–10
Cyproheptadine	0–+	1–8
Diphenhydramine	0–+	1–3
Hydroxyzine	+++	1–10
Promethazine	++	1–3
Tripelennamine	0–+	1–3
Doxepin	++	3–11
2nd generation		
Astemizole	++++	30–60
Cetirizine	++++	3–10
Loratadine	++++	3–10
Terfenadine	++++	3–10
H₂ antagonists		
Cimetidine	0–+	Unlikely to be clinically significant
Ranitidine	+	Unlikely to be clinically significant
Others		
Imipramines	++++	> 10
Phenothiazines	++	
Corticosteroids (oral)		
Long term	possible	
Corticosterioids (topical)	0–++	
Theophylline	0–+	
Cromolyn	0	
Clonidine	++	

Modified from Middleton E, Reed C, Ellis E, et al (eds): Allergy Principles and Practice, 5th ed. St. Louis, Mosby, 1998.

19. What concentrations of allergen extracts are used in prick and intradermal testing?

In general, **percutaneous tests** are performed with a glycerinated extract of 1:10 or 1:20 w/v. Standardized extracts should be tested at 10,000 to 100,000 BAU/ml.

Intracutaneous tests can be performed with a dilution of 1:100 or 1:1,000 of the strength used in percutaneous tests, if the percutaneous tests are negative. In cases of an historically severe reaction, particularly to venom or a drug, even higher dilutions may be indicated for the initial intracutaneous test. Potent grass extracts may produce a large number of false-positive results in intracutaneous tests. Intracutaneous testing with food antigens is not indicated because of the high false-positive rate and the risk of causing a systemic reaction.

20. What effect does previous immunotherapy have on skin tests?

The effect of specific allergen immunotherapy on the immediate skin test response is variable, with some studies suggesting a decrease in wheal and erythema. Decreases in wheal and erythema have been demonstrated most consistently with venom immunotherapy, not with aeroallergen immunotherapy. Specific venom skin tests, which become negative after a course of venom immunotherapy, often are used as criteria to discontinue venom immunotherapy in individual patients. However, the same criteria have not been found to be reliable with respect to aeroallergen immunotherapy.

21. How safe is skin testing to allergens?

The risk of adverse reaction to **percutaneous testing** is low; no systemic allergic reactions to percutaneous tests were observed in 16,000 persons undergoing testing for aeroallergens. Anaphylaxis during percutaneous skin testing has been reported as a rare occurrence; the risks are higher in percutaneous food, venom, or drug skin testing.

The risk of adverse reactions for patients undergoing **intracutaneous testing** with anaphylactic sensitivities (penicillin and venom) is 1–2%. Fatalities have been reported with intracutaneous testing, but, in many instances, patients had not undergone previous percutaneous tests.

22. What is the correlation between in vivo tests and in vitro tests?

In general, percutaneous skin tests are the most specific, convenient, and least expensive method of testing for the presence of allergen-specific IgE. Intracutaneous tests are more sensitive but less specific than percutaneous tests. In vitro methods of detection of allergen-specific-IgE correlate with percutaneous testing in 85–95% of cases, depending on the allergen being tested, although values can be as low as 50%.

23. How is an in vitro assay for allergen-specific-IgE performed?

Two commonly used assay methods, radio-allergo sorbent test (RAST) and enzyme-linked immunosorbent assay (ELISA) are based on nearly identical principles. In the figure below, an allergenic protein with multiple epitopes (triangles) is bound to a solid phase, often in a multi-well plate (A). The bound allergen is then incubated with serum from the allergic patient, and specific IgE, if present, binds to

the allergen (*B*). After washing away nonbound proteins, an anti-IgE antibody is used to detect the presence of bound allergen specific antibody (*C*). The anti-IgE may be linked to a radioactive isotope (radioactivity measured) or an enzyme that catalyzes a colorimetric reaction, measured photometrically (*D*). The concentration of specific-IgE present is calculated from the comparison of the measurement found in the serum sample with known concentrations in the control samples.

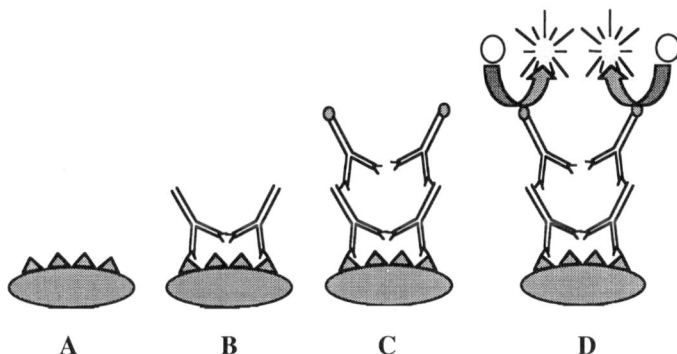

A   B   C   D

24. What are the advantages and disadvantages of in vivo vs. in vitro testing?

IN VIVO SKIN TEST	IN VITRO SERUM RAST, FAST, ELISA
Less expensive	No patient risk
Greater sensitivity	Specific and quantitative
Greater antigen availability	Not affected by drugs
Prompt results	Antigen stability
Technically easier	Patient convenience
Visible result useful for teaching	Useful in patients with skin conditions (e.g., dermatographism)
Good correlation with history and RAST tests	Good correlation with history and skin tests

Adapted from Bierman CW, Pearlman DS, Shapiro GG, Busse W (eds): Allergy, Asthma, and Immunology from Infancy to Adulthood, 3rd ed. Philadelphia, W.B. Saunders, 1996.

25. What is considered the gold standard in the diagnosis of food allergies?
- The double-blind, placebo-controlled food challenge (DBPCFC) is considered the gold standard in the diagnosis of food allergies.
- Percutaneous tests can be useful in screening out IgE-mediated food allergies (very low false-negative rate), but positive results must be correlated with clinical history to determine if a DBPCFC is indicated.
- The CAP-FEIA test (Pharmacia) for measurement of specific IgE (kUa/L) for milk, egg, and peanut has an excellent positive predictive value for clinical reactivity, above specific measured values.

26. Why is spirometry recommended in the diagnosis of asthma?
Because clinical history and physical examination by themselves are not reliable in excluding other diagnoses, objectively measuring degree of airflow obstruction,

or assessing reversibility, spirometry is recommended as part of the diagnostic evaluation of asthma in children and adults capable of performing the test. Obviously this requirement excludes infants, toddlers, and people with specific handicaps.

27. Why is spirometry recommended over peak flow measurement in the diagnosis of asthma?
There is less variability in published spirometry reference values than in peak expiratory flow reference values. In addition, peak flow meters are designed as monitoring, not as diagnostic, tools for patient self-management and periodic assessment.

28. How are the "spaces" of the lung divided with respect to volume for the purposes of pulmonary function testing?
• IRV = inspiratory reserve volume
• TV = tidal volume
• ERV = expiratory reserve volume
• RV = residual volume

29. What are the relationships of these volumes to total lung capacity (TLC)?
$$TLC = VC + RV$$
$$VC = IRV + TV + ERV$$
where VC = vital capacity, IRV = inspiratory reserve volume, TV = tidal volume, and ERV = expiratory volume.

30. Which lung volume cannot be measured by spirometry alone?
RV and TLC cannot be measured spirometrically. Because only VC can be determined spirometrically, restrictive ventilatory defects should be interpreted with caution. The diagnosis of restrictive lung disease cannot be made in the setting of moderate-to-severe obstruction based on spirometry alone.

31. What spirometric measurements are used most commonly in evaluating asthma?
• FEV_1 (forced expiratory volume at 1 second) is the most reproducible and sensitive value that can be measured with a simple office spirometer.
• PEFR (peak expiratory flow rate) can be measured with a handheld device, correlates with FEV_1, and is useful for monitoring asthma status.
• A ratio of the FEV_1 to FVC (forced vital capacity) of > 0.80 generally indicates normal airflow without significant obstruction.
• When flow rates (L/sec) are plotted on the y axis against volumes (L) on the x axis, specific appearances of flow-volume curves become evident both in the expiratory and inspiratory phases. In asthma, the descending expiratory curve, instead of being straight, becomes concave or "scooped out."

32. What measurement constitutes significant reversibility of small airway obstruction after bronchodilator administration, according to the American Thoracic Society?
In adults, improvement in $FEV_1 \geq 12\%$ and an absolute change ≥ 200 ml.

33. Describe the characteristic spirometric findings in vocal cord dysfunction.

Flow limitation (flattened areas or variable spikes) on the *inspiratory* flow-volume curve, when symptomatic. Inspiratory flow-volume loops are usually (but not always) normal when the patient is asymptomatic. If the diagnosis of vocal cord dysfunction is suspected by clinical history and spirometry, direct visual laryngoscopy is usually recommended to rule out anatomic pathology and also to visualize (while symptomatic) the abnormal adduction of the cord during the inspiratory cycle.

34. How can asthma be differentiated from chronic obstructive pulmonary disease (COPD) by pulmonary function testing?

TEST	ASTHMA	COPD
FEV_1	↓	↓
FVC	↓	↓
FEV_1/FVC	↓	↓
Postbronchodilator increase in FEV_1 > 12%	++	±
Total lung capacity (TLC)	Normal (or ↑ during acute episode)	Normal or ↑
Residual volume (RV)	↑	↑
RV/TLC	↑	↑
Diffusing capacity of lung for carbon monoxide	Usually normal	Usually ↓

Adapted from NAEPP Working Group Report: Considerations for Diagnosing and Managing Asthma in the Elderly, Rockville, MD, National Institutes of Health, NIH Publication No. 96-3662, 1996.

35. What are the pathologic findings demonstrated by the spirometric curves below?

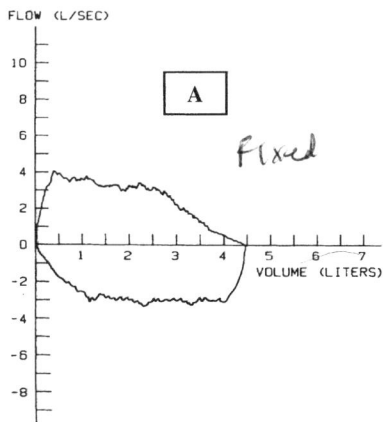

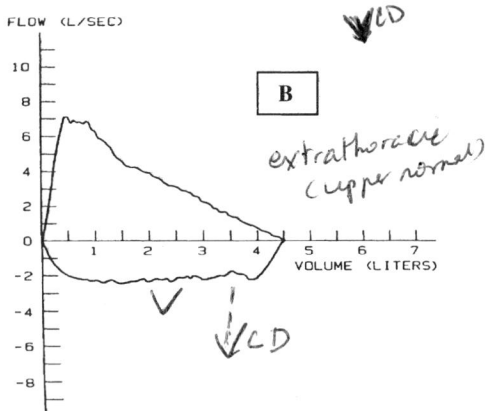

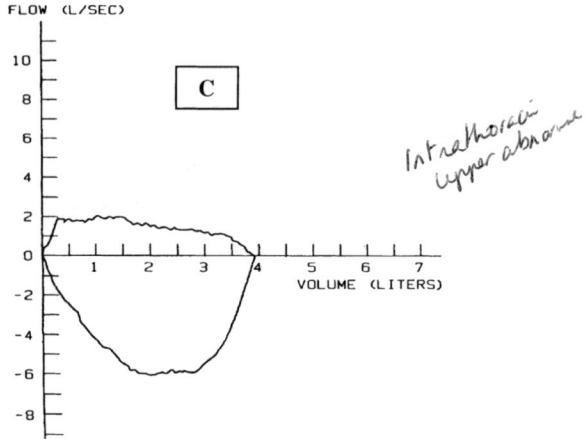

FLOW (L/SEC)

C

Intrathoracic
upper abnormal

VOLUME (LITERS)

A, Fixed intra- or extrathoracic obstruction, such as may be caused by tracheal stenosis. *B*, Variable extrathoracic obstruction, as may be caused by vocal cord paralysis. *C*, Variable intrathoracic obstruction, as may be caused by a tumor in trachea. (From Enright PL, Hyatt RE: Office Spirometry: A Practical Guide to the Selection and Use of Spirometers, Philadelphia, Lea & Febiger, 1987, with permission.)

36. How is airway hyperresponsiveness measured in a chemical bronchoprovocation challenge test? How are the results interpreted?

Methacholine or histamine is the most frequently used agent in bronchoprovocation challenges, and the techniques for administration and measuring response are well standardized. The patient inhales increasing amounts of the agent, and spirometry is performed between inhalations until a drop in the $FEV_1 > 20\%$ relative to the initial saline nebulization occurs (referred to as the PC_{20} or PD_{20}). If this drop does not occur after the inhalation of the highest concentration in the protocol, the challenge is completed.

The PC_{20} refers to the noncumulative concentration of the agent inhaled (mg/ml) at which the FEV_1 dropped by more than 20% relative to the initial saline nebulization. The PD_{20} refers to the cumulative dose of the agent inhaled (in micromoles or breath units) at which the drop occurred. Standard tables correlate the degree of airway hyperresponsiveness with PC_{20} or PD_{20}. Measurement of airway hyperresponsiveness to pharmacologic agents is *not* the gold standard in diagnosing asthma; it is only an additional test that may be useful in specific clinical situations.

37. In what clinical situations is bronchoprovocation challenge testing useful?

The most common clinical situation in which bronchoprovocation (usually with methacholine) is useful is to evaluate a patient in whom asthma is suspected by the clinical history, but whose *baseline spirometry is normal*. ($FEV_1 > 65\%$ of predicted normal at baseline is the usual safety limit before undergoing bronchoprovocation testing). Exercise challenge is less sensitive than methacholine or histamine challenges in screening for airway hyperresponsiveness. Bronchoprovocation usually is not used to distinguish between asthma and COPD because bronchial hyperresponsiveness can be found in many patients with COPD.

Antigen bronchoprovocation challenges are performed less often than chemical bronchoprovocation challenges and may be helpful in specific cases of suspected asthma due to occupational exposure. Antigen challenges are potentially more dangerous than chemical bronchoprovocation studies because of the risk of inducing anaphylaxis and/or a severe late-phase response. Bronchoprovocation challenges are used more often in research settings for comparing efficacy, duration, and dose responses of asthma medications, determining severity of asthma, studying mechanisms, and evaluating the epidemiology of airway reactivity.

38. Name four "diagnostic" tests of no proven value or efficacy that often are used by practitioners of controversial methods.
   1. Provocation–neutralization (not to be confused with bronchoprovocation): a substance is given subcutaneously or sublingually until the patient reports cessation of the "sensations."
   2. Cytotoxic tests: whole blood is mixed with food antigens, and the examiner looks for leukocyte changes.
   3. Electrodermal diagnosis: machine measures changes in skin electrical conductance caused by "allergies."
   4. Applied kinesiology: subjectively measures muscle strength while allergen contacts patient.

LABORATORY EVALUATION

39. What is tryptase? When is its measurement useful in the diagnosis of allergic disease?
   Tryptase is a protease found in human mast cells and to a lesser extent (< 500-fold) in basophils. It is stored in the secretory granules of these cells and released after cell activation. Because it is relatively stable compared with histamine, increased serum typtase levels persist 2–4 hours after mast cell release. Therefore, if blood is drawn at the appropriate time interval, tryptase levels are useful in the diagnosis of anaphylaxis, in active cases of mastocytosis, and in monitoring allergen challenge testing.

40. What is the fluorescence-activated cell sorter (FACS)?
   FACS uses a flow cytometer (see figure, next page) to identify a particular cell type based on its physical characteristics and specific surface markers. Two nonfluorescent parameters (blue light) are monitored. Forward scatter is related to cell size, whereas side (90°) scatter is related to the internal complexity of the cell. Three fluorescent parameters (green, orange and red) also can be monitored. Fluorochromes can be coupled to monoclonal antibodies specific for cell surface markers. Therefore, cells can be defined by as many as five separate parameters. A cell meeting specific criteria can be sorted by deflection in an electric field and separated from dissimilar cells in the sample.

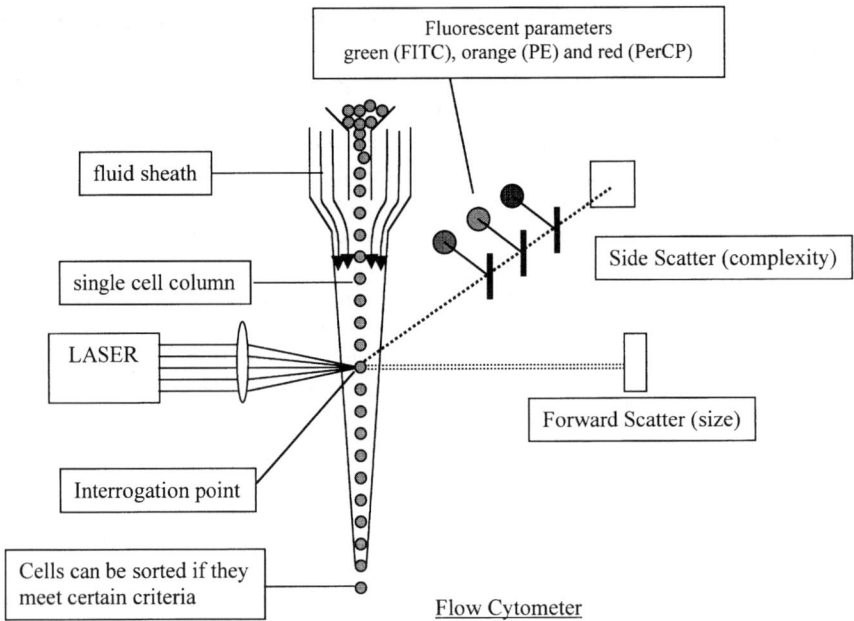

Flow Cytometer

41. What is a Western blot test?

Western blots (also known as immunoblots) are used to characterize a particular protein antigen when it is in a mixture with other protein antigens. First the proteins are separated by sodium-dodecyl sulfate (SDS)-polyacrilamide gel (PAGE) electorphoresis so that their positions in the gel are determined by molecular size. The proteins then are transferred from the gel to a support membrane by capillary action ("blotting"). The location of the antigen on the membrane can be determined by binding labeled antibody (either enzyme-linked or radiolabeled).

42. What is meant by cluster of differentiation (CD)?

The CD nomenclature is a uniform system that assigns to a cell surface marker a number that identifies a particular lineage or differentiation stage, which has a defined structure and is recognized by a group or "cluster" of monoclonal antibodies.

For example, CD3 is a surface structure on T cells and is associated with the T-cell antigen receptor. Monoclonal antibodies that recognize the T-cell antigen receptor CD3 on a cell surface define the cluster of differentiation. Cells that possess the CD3 molecule can then be defined as T cells. Combinations of surface markers can define specific functional groups of cells. For example, CD3+, CD4+, and CD8− cells are considered helper T cells. Some surface markers are expressed on many cell types; CD45 (leukocyte common antigen), for example, is found on all leukocytes and therefore is less specific in defining a unique cell type.

43. Define polymerase chain reaction (PCR).

This laboratory technique was developed to amplify or create multiple copies of a particular sequence of DNA that is defined by two oligonucleotide primers. The

two primer sites need to be approximately within 1 kb of each other for the reaction to be successful.

In a PCR many copies (molar excess) of the sense and antisense primer are combined with double-stranded DNA containing the sequence of interest, thermostable DNA polymerase (Taq), and deoxynucleotide (A, T, G, and C) triphosphates. The mixture is heated, causing denaturation of the double-stranded DNA. Upon cooling, the primers that are present in great excess can aneal to the native sense and antisense strands. The primers then can be elongated by DNA polymerase, producing a copy of the sense and antisense strand. The reaction mixture can be reheated and the newly synthesized strands used as templates for the next cycle of synthesis, hence doubling the number of templates with each cycle. A single copy of a DNA sequence can be greatly amplified, allowing its detection. For example, the DNA from a single cell is sufficient to allow detection of a particular sequence in that cell.

44. How is PCR used?

PCR usually is automated using commercially available thermal cyclers. The reaction is repeated from 25–35 times, resulting in exponential amplification of the target sequence. A modified form of PCR, known as reverse transcription PCR, can be used to amplify specific RNA sequences. This technique uses the enzyme reverse transcriptase to synthesize DNA from RNA, then uses PCR to amplify the DNA sequence, hence allowing the detection of specific gene expression and RNA-based pathogens.

PCR has many applications, such as detection of specific HLA types, prenatal screening for many genetically based diseases, and detection of many pathogens, including Chlamydia spp., human immunodeficiency virus 1 (HIV_1), and *Mycobacterium tuberculosis.*

45. How is complement measured?

An intact complement cascade can be measured qualitatively by a CH50 test, also known as a total hemolytic assay. The solid-phase method involves use of agarose gels embedded with antibody-coated erythrocytes. The serum sample is placed in a small well and diffuses into the gel. The serum complement hemolyzes the erythrocytes, creating a clear area around the well. The measured diameter of the clear zone is proportional to the logarithm of the number of CH50 units of complement.

Quantitative measurements of individual complement components are usually made by nephelometry or immunodiffusion.

46. What is HLA typing?

HLA molecules are expressed on the surface of all nucleated cells. The designation HLA (human leukocyte antigen) was used because this system of heterogeneous gene products was first recognized in recipients of blood transfusions who experienced reactions (became sensitized) to the white blood cells contained in the transfusions.

Subsequently, using alloantisera from various sources, six polymorphic gene loci were identified on the short arm of chromosome 6. This region is known as the major histocompatibility complex (MHC). The MHC contains the genes for class I

(HLA-A, B, and C) and class II (HLA-DP, DQ, and DR) molecules. The set of HLA genes present on each chromosome is known as an MHC haplotype. Each person inherits one haplotype from each parent.

HLA typing refers to the identification of the specific set of HLA gene products expressed in an individual. In the past it was accomplished primarily by assessment of specific serologic complement-dependent cytotoxicity. Isoelectric focusing (IEF) has been used to define the variation in more detail by detecting amino acid substitutions that affect overall charge but not serologic binding sites. Most HLA typing is done with DNA-based techniques (PCR). Using sequence-specific oligonucleotide primers, the presence or absence of a specific allele can be confirmed and the HLA type rapidly determined.

47. What tests are used in assessment of immune complex disease?

The tests used most commonly in assessing immune complex disease include the C1q binding assay and the Raji cell assay. Neither of these assays differentiates between aggregated immunoglobulin and actual immune complexes (antibody bound to antigen). See the chapter "Serum Sickness" for additional reading.

48. How is the C1q binding assay performed?

The C1q binding assay is performed in the solid or fluid phase. In the fluid-phase assay, radiolabeled C1q added to the serum binds to the complexes. It is separated from the unbound fraction by polyethylene glycol. In the solid-phase assay, complexes bind to C1q bound to plastic surfaces and subsequently are measured by a radiolabeled or enzyme-labeled anti-Ig antiserum. Rheumatoid factor can interfere with the results of the solid-phase assay. The presence of heparin may cause a false-positive result in the fluid-phase assay.

49. How is the Raji cell assay performed?

The Raji cell assay uses a cell line derived originally from a patient with Burkitt's lymphoma. The cells have no surface immunoglobulin, but they have receptors for the Fc fragment and complement receptors. Complexes containing complement bind to the surface of the Raji cells. Radiolabeled anti-Ig is added, and the amount of bound radioactivity is measured.

50. What in vitro test is most commonly used to assess T-lymphocyte function?

The test most commonly used to assess T-lymphocyte function is the mitogenic stimulation assay. Normally functioning T lymphocytes proliferate (undergoing mitogenesis) in vitro when exposed to certain plant lectins. Phytohemagglutinin (PHA), concanavalin A (con A), and pokeweed mitogen (PWM) are the most commonly used in laboratory assays. The degree of proliferation and differentiation caused by exposure to the lectins on lymphocytes can be quantified by measuring the amount of 3H-thymidine uptake by the stimulated cells in vitro. The mitogen is added to lymphocytes purified from a freshly drawn peripheral blood sample. Incubation takes place for 48–72 hours at 37°C in 5% carbon dioxide. A small amount of 3H-thymidine is added for a few hours, and the cells are washed. The amount of radiolabeled thymidine, which was incorporated by the proliferating cells, is determined by scintillation counting. The results are expressed as counts per

minute (cpm) and/or as a ratio of stimulated to control cultures, known as the stimulation index.

51. How are eosinophils stained for microscopic evaluation?

Eosinophils are important effector cells in allergic disease. Ehrlich first coined the term eosinophil in 1879. He noted that a certain leukocyte type avidly bound acidic dyes. The granules of eosinophils have a marked affinity for eosin, a reddish-orange acidic dye.

Eosinophils can be identified by their characteristic orange granules and bilobed nuclei. Electron micrographs demonstrate unique secondary granules, which contain a dense core surrounded by a less dense matrix. Small granules are uniform in appearance and contain acid phosphatase and arylsulfatase. Primary granules are found in eosinophilic promyelocytes. Hansel's stain or Wright's stain typically is used to look microscopically for eosinophils in dried nasal smears. A finding of >10% eosinophils is considered to be indicative of allergic disease.

52. How are mast cells characterized?

Mast cells are tissue resident cells with eccentric, nonsegmented nuclei that contain numerous cytoplasmic granules that stain in a metachromatic fashion. The granules of certain mast cells vary at the ultrastructural level as viewed by electron microscopy. In humans, two subpopulations possess different granule morphology, which correlates with protease content. Mast cell granules contain tryptase or tryptase and chymase and are designated MC_T and MC_{TC}, respectively. Granules that contain chymase demonstrate a lattice pattern, whereas granules that contain tryptase alone demonstrate a scroll pattern.

53. What assays are available to test for phagocytic function?

The most common test is the **nitroblue tetrazolium (NBT) test** for chronic granulomatous disease (CGD), which is designed to evaluate the ability of granulocytes to generate superoxide and hydrogen peroxide. The NBT test requires less specialized laboratory facilities than bactericidal assays but should be performed in laboratories with expertise. The test is performed on leukocytes from freshly drawn specimens (including a freshly drawn normal control). Oxidized NBT is colorless. When NBT is reduced by superoxide, it precipitates in the cytosol as blue formazan, which can be identified by direct microscopic visualization or spectrophotometrically. Because neutrophils from patients with CGD have an impaired respiratory burst and inability to produce superoxide, no colorimetric change is seen. Patients with CGD have less than 1% NBT-positive granulocytes. Normal subjects have > 90% NBT-positive granulocytes. Heterozygous carriers of X-linked recessive CGD have 50% NBT-positive granulocytes. Because of the molecular genetic heterogeneity in CGD, confirmatory molecular genetics tests for these defects should be done in laboratories specializing in such disorders.

Chemiluminescence assays may be used adjunctively in measuring oxidative metabolism during phagocytosis. Neutrophils during phagocytosis chemically produce light, which can be measured with a beta-scintillation spectrophotometer. This test may be abnormal in CGD or in cases of severe glucose-6-phosphate dehydrogenase deficiency.

BIBLIOGRAPHY

1. Abbas AK, Lichtman AH, Pober JS: Cellular and Molecular Immunology, 4th ed. Philadelphia, W.B. Saunders, 2000.
2. Bernstein IL, Storms WW, et al: Practice parameters for allergy diagnostic testing. Ann Allergy Asthma Immunol 75:553–625, 1995.
3. Bierman CW, Pearlman DS, Shapiro GG, Busse W (eds): Allergy, Asthma, and Immunology from Infancy to Adulthood, 3rd ed. Philadelphia, W.B. Saunders, 1996.
4. Crapo RO: Pulmonary function testing. N Engl J Med 331:25–30, 1994.
5. Creticos PS, Lockey RF (eds): Immunotherapy: A Practical Guide to Current Procedures. Milwaukee, American Academy of Allergy, Asthma and Immunology, 1994.
6. Enright PL, Hyatt RE: Office Spirometry: A Practical Guide to the Selection and Use of Spirometers, Philadelphia, Lea & Febiger, 1987.
7. Lee GR, Foerster J, Lukens J, et al (eds): Wintrobe's Clinical Hematology. Baltimore, Williams & Wilkins, 1999.
8. McMillan, JA, DeAngelis CD, Feigin RD, Warshaw JB (eds): Oski's Pediatrics: Principles and Practice. Philadelphia, Lippincott Williams & Wilkins, 1999.
9. Middleton E, Reed C, Ellis E, et al (eds): Allergy Principles and Practice, 5th ed. St. Louis, Mosby, 1998.
10. National Asthma Education and Prevention Program Panel Report II: Guidelines for the Diagnosis and Management of Asthma. Rockville, MD, National Institutes of Health, NIH Publication 97-4051, 1997.
11. National Asthma Education and Prevention Program Panel Working Group Report: Considerations for Diagnosing and Managing Asthma in The Elderly. Rockville, MD, National Institutes of Health, NIH Publication 96-3662, 1996.
12. Noe DA, Rock RC (eds): Laboratory Medicine: The Selection and Interpretation of Clinical Laboratory Studies. Baltimore, Williams & Wilkins, 1994.
13. Official Statement of the American Thoracic Society: Lung function testing: Selection of reference values and interpretive strategies. Am Rev Respir Dis 144:1202–1218, 1991.
14. Sampson HA, Ho DG: Relationship between food-specific IgE concentrations and the risk of positive food challenges in children and adolescents. J Allergy Clin Immunol 100:444–451, 1997.
15. Stiehm ER: Immunologic Disorders in Infants & Children, 4th ed. Philadelphia, W.B. Saunders, 1996.

5. ALLERGIC RHINITIS

Gordon Garcia, M.D.

1. Define rhinitis.

Generally, rhinitis is defined as inflammation of the mucus membranes of the nose. Within this term resides a heterogeneous group of disorders characterized by one or more of these symptoms: sneezing, rhinorrhea, congestion, or nasal itch.

2. What is the differential diagnosis of rhinitis?

Allergic rhinitis accounts for approximately 50% of the cases of chronic rhinitis. Causes of nonallergic rhinitis are diverse and can be categorized as:

- Idiopathic nonallergic syndromes
  - a) Nonallergic rhinitis with eosinophlia syndrome (NARES)
  - b) Perennial nonallergic rhinitis (Vasomotor)
  - c) Cholinergic syndromes; for example, gustatory rhinitis, cold air rhinitis
- Infectious
- Endocrinologic
  - a) Pregnancy
  - b) Hypothyroidism
- Drug-induced
  - a) Topical decongestants (rhinitis medicamentosa)
  - b) Antihypertensives
  - c) Oral contraceptives
  - d) Aspirin or NSAIDs in aspirin-sensitive rhinosinusitis
  - e) Cocaine abuse
- Granulomatous diseases
  - a) Sarcoidosis
  - b) Wegener's granulomatosis
  - c) Midline granuloma
  - d) Rhinoscleromatosis
  - e) Relapsing polychondritis
- Anatomic or mechanical obstruction
  - a) Septal deviation
  - b) Nasal polyps
  - c) Hypertrophic turbinates
  - d) Tumors
  - e) Adenoidal hypertrophy
  - f) Choanal atresia
- Miscellaneous
  - a) Ciliary dyskinesis
  - b) Atrophic rhinitis
  - c) Nasal CSF leak

3. What is the prevalence and natural history of allergic rhinitis?

Most studies estimate the cumulative prevalence of allergic rhinitis in the United States to be between 10% and 20%; however, one study documented that 42% of 6-year-old children had doctor-diagnosed allergic rhinitis. The mean age at onset is 10 years old, with 80% of cases starting before age 20 years. In childhood, males are more frequently effected than females, however the gender-specific prevalence equalizes in adulthood. Once established, the disease generally persists for many years.

4. List some risk factors for developing allergic rhinitis.
- Family history of allergy
- Serum IgE > 100 IU/ml before age 6 years
- Higher socioeconomic status
- Exposure to indoor allergens, such as animals and dust mites
- Presence of a positive allergy skin test

5. List the physiologic functions of the nose.
- Provides a conduit for airflow
- Warms, humidifies, and filters air. By the time it reaches the larynx, nasally inspired air is warmed to 35 to 37°C and humidified to 75 to 95% saturation. Airborne particles 10 microns or greater are completely filtered.
- Antimicrobial defense. Innate or natural immunity includes the presence of the antibacterial proteins lysozyme and lactoferrin. Phagocytic cells enter the mucosa in response to invasion by foreign organism. Acquired immunity is provided by secretory IgA and to a lesser extent, IgG.
- Olfaction

6. Describe the nasal cycle.
Approximately 80% of humans have a cyclic, reciprocal alteration in blood content of the turbinate vasculature. This cycle averages 1 to 4 hours and results in reciprocal increasing and decreasing nasal airway caliber. The sympathetic, alpha-adrenergic nervous system is believed to be an integral part of this process because it reduces blood pooling in the venous sinusoids of the submucosa.

7. Name some factors that affect turbinate size.
- Increases turbinate size: lying supine, chilling skin, cold air, sexual stimulation
- Decreases turbinate size: exercise, warming skin, fear

8. What is the primary physiologic method of controlling nasal secretions?
Cholinergic nerves innervate the submucosal glands, arterial vessels, and sinusoids. The primary effect of cholinergic stimulation is to increase glandular secretion.

9. Explain the role of the mast cell in the pathophysiology of allergic rhinitis.
Mast cells in the nasal epithelium of the atopic individual are coated with allergen-specific IgE. Within minutes of allergen contact, the cross-linked IgE causes mast cell degranulation of preformed mediators such as histamine, tryptase, kininogenase, and heparin. Leukotrienes C_4, D_4, and E_4, and prostaglandin D_2 are also

newly produced and secreted. These, along with several other mediators lead to the **early phase** symptoms of sneezing, itching, rhinorrhea, and congestion.

Additionally, some of these mediators, including chemokines and cytokines up-regulate adhesion molecules on vascular endothelium and attract inflammatory cells such as eosinophils, basophils, neutrophils, and T-lymphocytes to migrate into the mucosa, leading to the **late phase** response, 4 to 8 hours after the initial reaction.

10. What are the physiologic effects of histamine release in the nose?

SYMPTOM	MECHANISM
Sneeze, itch	Direct sensory nerve stimulation
Rhinorrhea	Direct and reflex stimulation of glandular mucus secretion
Congestion	Vascular engorgement and increased plasma transudation

11. Explain the priming effect.

With repeated nasal allergen challenges, the dose of allergen needed to induce symptoms decreases. The etiology of this effect is thought to be due to the influx of inflammatory cells into the nasal mucosa resulting in repeated and prolonged late phase responses.

12. Discuss the utility of measuring total IgE level in the evaluation of chronic rhinitis, and differentiate this from assessing allergen-specific IgE.

While a clear association exists between elevated serum IgE level and allergic rhinitis (versus nonallergic rhinitis), no dividing line can be created to adequately differentiate the allergic from the nonallergic individual. Therefore, measurement of total IgE is of limited value.

Assessment of allergen-specific IgE by skin testing or by in vitro technique, by contrast, is the defining test for the confirmation of allergy in a patient suffering from chronic rhinitis. Importantly, the results of the test must be correlated with the history, as positive skin tests alone do not prove a cause-and-effect relationship. In studies of teenage and college students, 15 to 25% of the group who had no symptoms had at least one positive skin test. In vitro testing has a greater incidence of false negative results when compared to skin testing, but reduced false positive results.

13. List some common triggers for seasonal and perennial allergic rhinitis.
- Seasonal
  - a) Pollen—Trees will pollinate earliest in the season in most areas of the country, with the specific start month determined by climate and tree type. Grass usually pollinates later in spring and early summer, and weeds may pollinate from spring through fall.
  - b) Certain outdoor molds are released into the air in a seasonal fashion, common examples being Alternaria and Cladosporium.
- Perennial
  - a) Dust mites are prevalent throughout much of the country and live in bedding, carpeting, and upholstered furniture.
  - b) Indoor pets.

    c) Perennial molds.

    d) Pollens may also be present perennially in certain areas of the country.

14. What is vasomotor rhinitis? How is it differentiated from NARES and allergic rhinitis?

Vasomotor rhinitis, also known as nonallergic or idiopathic rhinitis describes a perennial condition with nasal congestion and/or rhinorrhea as the predominant symptoms. Typical symptom triggers include fumes/odors, temperature or humidity changes, alcohol ingestion, emotion, and bright light.

Patients with NARES and allergic rhinitis have elevated eosinophils in their nasal mucosa, which is not true for vasomotor rhinitis. In contrast to allergic patients, both vasomotor and NARES patients have negative allergen skin tests.

15. Can nasal cytology be evaluated? What purpose does it serve?

Material for cytologic staining may be obtained by blowing the nose into plastic wrap, a cotton swab of the mucosa, or by using a flexible plastic curette (Rhino-Probe®). The presence of eosinophils suggests allergic rhinitis or NARES, both of which respond well to treatment with topical intranasal steroids.

16. List some occupations and their allergens that are associated with IgE-mediated occupational rhinitis.

OCCUPATION	ALLERGEN
Baker	Flour
Lab worker	Animals
Spray painter	Isocyanates
Plastics/resin worker	Anhydrides
Woodworker	Western red cedar
Healthcare provider	Latex

17. List some of the key points to be reviewed when obtaining a rhinitis history.

- Symptoms
    a) What? (sneeze; itch, drip—clear vs. purulent; congestion—bilateral vs. unilateral; associated ocular symptoms)
    b) When? (seasonality; age at onset)
    c) Where? (indoors vs. outdoors; effect of travel out of the home area)
- Triggering or exacerbating factors, including:
    a) Allergens (animals; pollen; house dust)
    b) Irritants (smoke; odors; fumes)
    c) Miscellaneous (weather; emotion; food/alcohol)
- Home environmental and occupational exposures
- Other medical history including medications
- Response to current and prior medications
- Personal or family history of other atopic conditions (asthma; eczema; conjunctivitis)

18. What value does the nasal exam provide in differentiating allergic rhinitis from other causes of rhinitis?

No features of the nasal exam are found exclusively in allergic patients. Exam findings in allergic rhinitis are quite variable; while the mucosa is classically pale and edematous in the allergic patient, this may also be found in the nonallergic patient as well. Conversely, the mucosa may appear hyperemic in both types of rhinitis.

Mucus, when apparent, is typically clear and thin; mucopurulent discharge suggests infection.

The exterior of the nose may show a transverse nasal crease or wrinkle at the point at which the nasal septal cartilage attaches to the bone. This occurs after chronically rubbing the nose upward (termed the "allergic salute") in childhood.

Perhaps the most important role of the exam is to look for structural causes of obstruction, such as septal deviation, polyps, tumors, or hypertrophied turbinates.

19. What are nasal polyps?

Nasal polyps are smooth, pale, semitranslucent structures composed of edematous stroma infiltrated with inflammatory cells including activated eosinophils, lymphocytes, plasma cells, mast cells, and, in some cases, neutrophils. Few mucous glands are present. They most commonly arise from the ethmoid sinuses and are seen in the area of the middle meatus.

Edematous turbinates are sometimes confused with polyps on exam; however, if a topical decongestant such as phenylephrine is applied to the mucosa, the turbinate, unlike the polyp, will shrink. Additionally, polyps are mobile and insensitive to touch.

20. What is the association of allergic rhinitis and nasal polyps?

While nasal polyps do occur in patients with allergic rhinitis, allergy does not appear to predispose to polyp formation. In fact, nasal polyps are considerably more common in nonallergic patients.

21. When nasal polyps are seen in a child, what disease should be suspected?

Polyps rarely occur in children under age 10 years. Cystic fibrosis (CF) should be considered in these patients, as the prevalence of polyps in CF is at least 20%.

22. Discuss the treatment of nasal polyps.

Medically, systemic and topical corticosteroids are used to shrink polyps. Large polyps respond more consistently to a 10- to 14-day burst of prednisone, followed by long-term corticosteroid nasal spray. If the polyps are severe or do not respond well to corticosteroid treatment, endoscopic polypectomy should be considered. Despite therapy, recurrence of polyps is common.

23. How might a patient present with a nasal CSF leak? What screening test should be performed?

Typically, such a patient would present with copious unilateral or bilateral watery nasal discharge. Often there is increased flow with leaning forward or straining. A history of head trauma or surgery is suggestive, but spontaneous leaks may occur. The presence of glucose in the fluid (> 30 mg/dl) suggests a CSF leak. A more sensitive and specific test is to measure beta$_2$ transferrin.

24. What is rhinitis medicamentosa and how is it treated?

Rhinitis medicamentosa occurs with prolonged use of nasal decongestant sprays. Tachyphylaxis occurs rapidly with this class of medication; thus, patients commonly use increasing doses to maintain nasal patency. The nasal exam classically shows erythematous swollen turbinates. Intranasal steroids are recommended as the patient weans off the decongestant spray. In more severe cases, a 5- to 10-day course of prednisone may be required.

25. Review the role of environmental control measures in treating patients with allergic rhinitis.

All patients with allergic rhinitis should undertake measures to reduce their exposure to allergen and irritant triggers. These environmental measures are usually combined with appropriate pharmacologic treatment, as many allergens are difficult to completely avoid.

ALLERGEN	CONTROL MEASURES
Pollen	Close home and car windows in season and use air conditioning Shower after outdoor activities Wear dust mask if yard work is performed
Mold (outdoor)	Similar to pollen; avoid leaf raking and working with compost
Mold (indoor)	Keep indoor humidity below 50% Avoid indoor plants Clean mold with commercial fungicide or 10% bleach in water
Animals	Remove allergenic pet from home, then thoroughly clean (even with extensive cleaning, allergen may remain for months)
Dust mite	Cover mattress, box spring, and pillows in mite-proof encasings Wash all bedding in hot (130°F) water at least biweekly Remove items that collect dust from the bedroom Use a high quality vacuum (e.g., HEPA) to decrease dust dispersal during vacuuming Consider removal of carpeting, especially in the bedroom Keep indoor humidity below 50%

26. Explain the pharmacologic and clinical actions of antihistamines.

All antihistamines competitively bind to the H_1 histamine receptor blocking histaminic effects. In addition, many antihistamines inhibit the release of mast cell mediators in response to a variety of triggers. The clinical relevance of this mast cell effect is uncertain. Clinically, antihistamines reduce sneeze, itch, and rhinorrhea, but have little effect on nasal congestion. Taking an antihistamine prior to contact with an allergen enhances the effectiveness of the drug.

27. List the six chemical classes for the first-generation antihistamines and provide specific examples of each class.

- Ethylenediamine: generally lower incidence of sedative and anticholinergic effects
  1. Pyrilamine
  2. Tripelennamine

- Ethanolamine: generally higher incidence of sedation, especially diphenhydramine
  1. Diphenhydramine
  2. Clemastine
  3. Carbinoxamine
- Alkylamine: most common class used in OTC products
  1. Chlorpheniramine
  2. Brompheniramine
  3. Triprolidine
- Piperazine
  1. Hydroxyzine
  2. Meclizine: used primarily for motion sickness and vertigo
- Piperidine
  1. Cyproheptadine: considered the drug of choice for cold-induced urticaria
  2. Azatadine
- Phenothiazine: marked sedative effects
  1. Promethazine

28. What are the advantages and disadvantages of second-generation antihistamines as compared to their predecessors?

The primary advantage of most second-generation antihistamines is that they do not cross the blood-brain barrier, and hence do not cause sedation, nor reduce psychomotor performance. Loratadine (Claritin) and fexofenadine (Allegra) have side-effect profiles indistinguishable from placebo, while cetirizine (Zyrtec) has mild potential for sedation. The Joint Task Force on Practice Parameters in Allergy, Asthma, and Immunology specifically recommends that second-generation antihistamines be considered before sedating antihistamines in the treatment of allergic rhinitis.

The primary disadvantage of these products is their high cost when compared to available generic formulations of the classical antihistamines.

Terfenadine (Seldane) and astemizole (Hismanal) were the first nonsedating antihistamines introduced, but were both removed from the US market due to the potential for causing a prolongation of the Q-T interval, and hence ventricular arrhythmias (particularly torsades de pointes). Cetirizine, fexofenadine, and loratadine do not prolong the Q-T interval.

29. Discuss the safety and performance issues associated with use of first-generation antihistamines.

In general, approximately one-third of patients using a first-generation antihistamine will complain of drowsiness. The magnitude of this side effect is highly variable from one patient to another. Several studies demonstrate that many patients have psychomotor impairment even when no sedation is perceived. Specific techniques used to document this impairment include measuring sleep latency period, reaction time, driving performance (both simulated and actual road tests), memory, learning, and visual-motor coordination. Epidemiologic studies have linked first-generation antihistamines to fatal automobile accidents, as well as to occupational injuries. In a majority of US states, people taking sedating antihistamines are legally considered to be "under the influence of a drug" while driving. Although it is commonly

reported that tolerance to the soporific side effect will develop with continued antihistamine use, objective studies of this belief have had inconsistent results.

30. Discuss the pharmacokinetics of antihistamines.

Antihistamines are rapidly absorbed from the gastrointestinal tract, and most reach their peak plasma concentration within 1 to 3 hours. All antihistamines, except cetirizine and fexofenadine, are metabolized predominantly by the cytochrome P450 system in the liver. Cetirizine is excreted predominantly in the urine, while 80% of fexofenadine is found unmetabolized in the feces. Terminal half-lives are quite variable, ranging from 2 to > 24 hours for currently available products, with children having more rapid rates of clearance. Tissue half-life is greater than serum half-life as demonstrated by suppression of histamine-induced wheal-and-flare reactions on skin testing. Astemizole (Hismanal), when available, was well known for suppressing skin-test reactivity for up to 6 weeks.

31. What is unique about the antihistamine azelastine?

Azelastine (Astelin) was the first antihistamine nasal spray in the US. It is dosed twice daily and has an onset of action in approximately 3 hours when compared to placebo. Despite its topical formulation 11% of patients report somnolence and 20% report a bitter taste.

32. Discuss the types, actions, and side effects of oral and topical decongestants.

Decongestants are alpha-adrenergic agonists that cause nasal vasoconstriction, thus reducing blood volume in the venous sinusoids. Specific oral decongestants include pseudoephedrine, phenylpropanolamine, and phenylephrine. Topical products include oxymetazoline, xylometazoline, naphazoline, phenylephrine, and tetrahydrozoline. The most common side effects of oral decongestants include nervousness, palpitations, loss of appetite, insomnia, and urinary hesitancy. Caution should be used in patients with hypertension, glaucoma, hyperthyroidism, and coronary artery disease. Topical products should be limited to 3 to 5 days of continuous use because tachyphylaxis develops rapidly and may lead to rebound nasal congestion with resultant rhinitis medicamentosa.

Because decongestants treat only nasal congestion, these medications are frequently combined with antihistamines. Decongestants, particularly the nasal sprays, are also useful in treating sinusitis and viral URIs.

33. What is the mechanism of action and role of cromolyn sodium nasal spray in the treatment of allergic rhinitis?

Cromolyn sodium (Nasalcrom) inhibits mediator release from mast cells. It thus prevents the allergic reaction rather than alleviating symptoms after they have begun. The protective effect of a single dose of cromolyn lasts for 4 to 8 hours. It is best to start cromolyn before the onset of the allergy season because the onset of sustained benefit takes several days to 2 weeks. Suggested dosing is 1 spray in each nostril every 4 hours during the day. Cromolyn may also be used as an intermittent medication to pretreat occasional exposures to known allergic triggers, such as a visit to a home containing a cat. Similar to antihistamines, cromolyn is more effective for reducing sneeze, itch, and rhinorrhea than it is for nasal congestion.

Potential side effects are few and mild, and include sneezing and stinging/burning. There is no evidence that cromolyn benefits patients with nonallergic rhinitis, including NARES.

34. What is the most effective class of medication used to treat allergic rhinitis?

A recent meta-analysis of 16 studies comparing intranasal steroid sprays to antihistamines showed a highly significant superiority of nasal steroids in controlling sneeze, itch, congestion, nasal discharge, and total nasal symptom score. In addition, compared to antihistamines, nasal steroids were equally effective at controlling ocular symptoms. The authors' conclusion based on efficacy, safety, and cost was that intranasal steroids are preferred as the first-line therapy for allergic rhinitis. Nasal steroids are more efficacious than cromolyn spray.

35. What are the currently available intranasal steroid sprays? How are they dosed in an average adult patient?

GENERIC NAME	TRADE NAME	DOSE RANGE (PER NOSTRIL)
Beclomethasone	Beconase, Vancenase (aerosol or AQ)	1–2 sprays b.i.d.
	Vancenase AQ, double strength	1–2 sprays q.d.
Budesonide	Rhinocort (aerosol or aqua)	2–4 sprays q.d.
Flunisolide	Nasalide, Nasarel (aqueous)	1–2 sprays b.i.d.
Fluticasone	Flonase, Flixonase (Europe) (aqueous)	1–2 sprays q.d.
Mometasone	Nasonex (aqueous)	2 sprays q.d.
Triamcinolone	Nasacort (aerosol or AQ)	1–2 sprays q.d.

With all products, once control of nasal symptoms has been attained, the dose is weaned to the lowest effective dosage.

36. How do intranasal steroid sprays work?

Topical intranasal steroids have multiple physiologic effects including:
• Reduced of the inflammation of the cellular infiltrate in the nasal mucosa
• Reduced vascular permeability and mucus secretion
• Reduced early and late phase allergen responses with chronic use

Some nasal steroids show statistically significant symptom reduction within 12 hours, although peak effects generally take up to 2 weeks to occur.

37. Discuss the potential side effects of intranasal steroid sprays.

The most common adverse effects of the steroid sprays are due to local irritation and include stinging or burning, sneeze, mild epistaxis, and, rarely, nasal septal perforation. To reduce the chance of septal perforation, the patient should be instructed to direct the spray slightly away from the septum. Additionally, patients who develop nosebleeds should discontinue the spray until a nasal exam can be performed. Mucosal thinning has not been reported, even in biopsy specimens from patients using beclomethasone spray for 5 years.

The potential for systemic effects is controversial. One recent study of beclomethasone spray in children showed a 0.9-cm decrement in growth rate over a 1-year period for the beclomethasone group as compared to the placebo control group.

There are no long-term studies of the effect of nasal steroids on growth, but in asthma, long-term inhaled budesonide has not been shown to effect final height. Some concern has been raised about the association of intranasal steroids with glaucoma and posterior subcapsular cataracts, but adequate studies have not been performed to document a clear association. Suppression of the hypothalamic-pituitary-adrenal axis has not been shown to occur.

38. What would be the preferred therapy for a patient complaining of isolated watery rhinorrhea?

Ipratropium bromide (Atrovent) nasal spray is an anticholinergic agent that is indicated to treat rhinorrhea only. With its quaternary amine structure, it is poorly absorbed and has few potential side effects other than excessive nasal drying. It is available in a 0.03% concentration for allergic and nonallergic rhinitis and a 0.06% concentration that can be used to reduce rhinorrhea associated with the common cold. Dosing is usually 2 to 3 sprays in each nostril b.i.d. to t.i.d. Atrovent is particularly useful for patients with gustatory or cold air-induced rhinorrhea, where the spray can be administered prophylactically.

39. Design a stepwise therapeutic approach for the managing rhinitis.

For all levels of severity, allergen avoidance should be instituted to the degree possible.

SEVERITY	TREATMENT OPTIONS
Mild and intermittent	Oral antihistamines and/or decongestants as needed Topical decongestants and saline sprays may also help
Mild persistent	Daily use of antihistamines with/without decongestant Cromolyn nasal spray Low-dose intranasal steroid spray
Moderate persistent	Intranasal steroid spray as first-line therapy Add antihistamine with/without decongestant if needed Immunotherapy may be considered
Severe persistent	Intranasal steroid spray plus antihistamine-decongestant Possibly burst of oral or intramuscular steroid Immunotherapy

40. List some complications of allergic rhinitis.

- Abnormal facial development in childhood leading to elongated midface ("adenoid facies") and high-arched palate with dental malocclusion. Chronic mouth breathing, which results in the lack of normal tongue contact with the palate, is the presumed mechanism of these abnormalities.
- Otitis media and sinusitis due to eustachian tube and sinus ostia obstruction, respectively.
- Decreased sense of smell.
- Sleep disturbance.

41. What are the preferred medications to treat allergic rhinitis in pregnancy?

Antihistamine: chlorpheniramine (FDA class B).

Decongestant: pseudoephedrine (class C) (avoid all decongestants in first trimester).

Nasal spray: saline and cromolyn (class B) are preferred, while beclomethasone (class C) is preferred when an intranasal steroid is required.

42. What role do rhinoscopy and CT scanning have in the evaluation of rhinitis?

Upper airway endoscopy (rhinoscopy) is used to examine the middle and superior meatal areas for polyps or mucopurulent sinus discharge, structures in the posterior portion of the nasal airway, as well as the nasopharynx. Anatomic problems that would be invisible with routine anterior nasal examination may be diagnosed with this technique. It is particularly valuable in evaluating nasal obstruction. CT scanning also provides detailed information on the nasal and sinus anatomy, and can detect pneumatization of the turbinates (concha bullosa).

BIBLIOGRAPHY

1. Bomer KV, Naclerio RM: Embryology, anatomy, and physiology of the upper airways. In Middleton E Jr. et al (eds): Allergy: Principles and Practice, 5th ed. St. Louis, Mosby, 1998, pp 544–558.
2. Druce HM: Allergic and nonallergic rhinitis. In Middleton E Jr. et al (eds): Allergy: Principles and Practice, 5th ed., St. Louis, Mosby, 1998, pp 1005–1016.
3. Dykewicz MS, Fineman S (eds): Diagnosis and management of rhinitis: Complete guidelines of the Joint Task Force on Practice Parameters in Allergy, Asthma, and Immunology. Ann Allergy Asthma Immunol 81:478–518, 1998.
4. Lieberman P: Rhinitis. In Slavin RG, Reisman RE (eds): Expert Guide to Allergy and Immunology. Philadelphia, American College of Physicians, 1999, pp 23–40.
5. Simons FER: Antihistamines. In Middleton E Jr. et al (eds): Allergy: Principles and Practice, 5th ed. St. Louis, Mosby, 1998, pp 612–637.
6. Skoner DP, Rachelefsky GS, Meltzer EO, et al: Detection of growth suppression in children during treatment with intranasal beclomethasone dipropionate. Pediatrics 105:e23, 2000.
7. Slavin RG: Nasal polyps and sinusitis. In Middleton E Jr. et al (eds): Allergy: Principles and Practice, 5th ed. St. Louis, Mosby, 1998, pp 1024–1027.
8. Weiner JM, Abraham MJ, Puy RM: Intranasal corticosteroids versus oral H_1 receptor antagonists in allergic rhinitis: Systematic review of randomised controlled trials. BMJ 317:1624–1629, 1998.

6. ASTHMA

Nicholas J. Kenyon, M.D., and Samuel Louie, M.D.

1. When should antibiotics be prescribed in acute exacerbations of asthma?

Evidence suggests that viral upper respiratory tract infections, namely rhinovirus, cause > 80% of asthma exacerbations in adults. Need for diagnostic chest radiographs or antibiotics in the treatment of such exacerbations is very uncommon. Indications for antibiotic use include concomitant acute pyogenic sinusitis or acute bacterial bronchitis in patients with underlying COPD (chronic obstructive pulmonary disease).

2. Is challenge testing useful in diagnosing asthma?

Pulmonary function testing (PFT) is an insensitive screen for obstructive airway disease in helping diagnose asthma. Although routine spirometry might suggest impairment to expiration (i.e., decreased FEV_1 and FEV_1/FVC) and a decreased flow volume can be indicative of obstruction, these parameters commonly will be normal in mild or intermittent asthmatics. In new patients with symptoms worrisome for asthma, but in whom the diagnosis remains unclear, bronchoprovocation testing should be performed. Airway hyperresponsiveness is shown by a 20% reduction in FEV_1 with serial increasing doses of methacholine or histamine. Exercise provocation testing via treadmill or ergometer for patients with symptoms of exercise-induced bronchospasm may also be beneficial. The absence of hyperresponsiveness with challenge testing is highly specific for ruling out asthma. Monitoring airway hyperresponsiveness may offer an additional guide for long-term control of asthma in addition to FEV_1 measurements and symptoms.

3. Are short-acting β_2-agonists associated with asthma deaths?

High doses of short-acting β_2-agonists have been associated with increased morbidity and mortality due to asthma. Tolerance to frequent β_2-agonist administration may occur due to down-regulation of airway receptors; overreliance on these agents for symptom management at the expense of controller medications place the patient at increased risk for fatal asthma. Despite several studies that correlate β_2-agonist usage with increased risk of asthma death, many clinicians do not believe this is a causal relationship. Short-acting β_2-agonists remain the drugs of first choice for rapid symptom relief in asthma, but disease control with prevention of acute exacerbations must be gained with appropriate anti-inflammatory and long-acting bronchodilator medications.

4. Can inhaled corticosteroid drugs cause systemic effects?

Concern has been raised by patients and physicians alike about the potential prolonged effects of chronic inhaled steroid usage in younger asthmatic patients. A host of pharmacologic studies show that high-dose inhaled corticosteroids may have systemic effects such as pituitary-adrenal axis suppression and growth inhibition. For example, children 6 to 16 years of age who receive doses of 400 to 800 μg per day of beclomethasone experience significantly slower annual growth (0.3 to 1.8 cm/yr). Inhaled budesonide (400 μg/day) causes a reduction in growth velocity of

~20% during the first year of treatment. However, growth subsequently recovers, and children treated with budesonide are expected to attain a normal adult height. Adult asthmatics are affected little by doses of inhaled steroids of 1500 µg or less per day. In general, the risk of these deleterious side effects with inhaled agents is significantly less than with long-term oral steroids. Once disease control is achieved, inhaled steroids should be reduced to lowest effective dose (see Table).

Estimated Comparative Daily Dosages for Inhaled Corticosteroids

DRUG	LOW DOSE	MEDIUM DOSE	HIGH DOSE
Adults			
Beclomethasone dipropionate	168–504 µg	504–840 µg	> 840 µg
42 µg/puff	(4–12 puffs–42 µg)	(12–20 puffs–42 µg)	(> 20 puffs–42 µg)
84 µg/puff	(2–6 puffs–84 µg)	(6–10 puffs–84 µg)	(> 10 puffs–84 µg)
Budesonide Turbuhaler	200–400 µg	400–600 µg	> 600 µg
200 µg/dose	(1–2 inhalations)	(2–3 inhalations)	(> 3 inhalations)
Flunisolide	500–1,000 µg	1,000–2,000 µg	> 2,000 µg
250 µg/puff	(2–4 puffs)	(4–8 puffs)	(> 8 puffs)
Fluticasone	88–264 µg	264–660 µg	> 660 µg
MDI: 44, 110,	(2–6 puffs–44 µg) or	(2–6 puffs–110 µg)	(> 6 puffs–110 µg) or
220 µg/puff	(2 puffs–110 µg)		(> 3 puffs–220 µg)
DPI: 50, 100,	(2–6 inhalations–	(3–6 inhalations–	(> 2 inhalations– 250 µg)
250 µg/dose	50 µg)	100 µg)	
Triamcinolone acetonide (Azmacort)	400–1,000 µg	1,000–2,000 µg	> 2,000 µg
100 µg/puff	(4–10 puffs)	(10–20 puffs)	(> 20 puffs)
Children			
Beclomethasone dipropionate	84–336 µg	336–672 µg	> 672 µg
42 µg/puff	(2–8 puffs–42 µg)	(8–16 puffs–42 µg)	(> 16 puffs–42 µg)
84 µg/puff	(1–4 puffs–84 µg)	(4–8 puffs–84 µg)	(> 8 puffs–84 µg)
Budesonide Turbuhaler	100–200 µg	200–400 µg	> 400 µg
200 µg/dose		(1–2 inhalations– 200 µg)	(> 2 inhalations– 200 µg)
Flunisolide	500–750 µg	1,000–1,250 µg	> 1,250 µg
250 µg/dose	(2–3 puffs)	(4–5 puffs)	(> 5 puffs)
Fluticasone	88–176 µg	176–440 µg	> 440 µg
MDI: 44, 110,	(2–4 puffs–44 µg)	(4–10 puffs–44 µg) or	(> 4 puffs–110 µg) or
220 µg/puff		(2–4 puffs–110 µg)	(> 2 puffs–220 µg)
DPI: 50, 100	(2–4 inhalations–	(2–4 inhalations–	(> 4 inhalations–100 µg)
250 µg/dose	50 µg	110 µg)	(> 2 inhalations–250 µg)
Triamcinolone acetonide	400–800 µg	800–1,200 µg	> 1,200 µg
100 µg/puff	(4–8 puffs)	(8–12 puffs)	(> 12 puffs)

5. How is severity of illness determined in asthma?

In 1997, the National Asthma Education and Prevention Program (NAEPP) sponsored by the National Institutes of Health (NIH) published comprehensive guidelines to assist physicians in classifying the severity of their patients' asthma

and to focus treatment. Their recommendations are readily available on the Internet at: http://www.nhlbi.nih.gov/nhlbi/lung/asthma/prof/asthgdln.htm. Mild intermittent asthmatics experience symptoms once or twice per week, and have near normal spirometry and peak expiratory flow rates (PEFR). Their infrequent symptoms can often be treated with as-needed bronchodilators. Patients with regular daytime and nocturnal symptoms are classified as having mild, moderate, or severe persistent asthma, depending on the degree of PEFR or FEV_1 variability and frequency of exacerbations. All patients with persistent asthma deserve controller therapy, such as inhaled corticosteroids, antileukotriene drugs, and other anti-inflammatory agents, or in combination with long-acting bronchodilator agents.

6. What is status asthmaticus and who is susceptible?

Status asthmaticus is defined as a severe asthma exacerbation that does not respond readily to aggressive, bronchodilator therapy. Descriptive terms for status asthmaticus include "life-threatening asthma" or "near-fatal" asthma, but a more specific definition with physiologic and gas exchange parameters is lacking. Patients in status asthmaticus are on the verge of acute respiratory failure and are at risk for mechanical ventilatory support and respiratory arrest. Most asthma deaths and episodes of status asthmaticus occur in patients with prolonged, poorly treated exacerbations. All asthmatics are potentially at risk for developing status asthmaticus and signs of deterioration in lung function must be treated promptly by patients and physicians.

7. What is airway remodeling in asthma and how is it associated with progressive lung function decline?

Many chronic asthmatics experience a decline in lung function faster (i.e., decline in FEV_1) than the general population and a subset of this group develop "irreversible" airways disease that is refractory to treatment with bronchodilator and anti-inflammatory therapy. This acknowledgment is a departure from previous beliefs that asthma remained a fully reversible bronchospastic disease throughout life. Remodeling of the airways is seen in biopsies of long-term asthmatics and is characterized by airway wall thickening, subepithelial fibrosis, myofibroblast proliferation, and mucous metaplasia. Markers of this response have not been clearly defined, and the true relationship between these physical changes and the irreversible nature of long-standing asthma is unclear. There is strong interest in altering the remodeling response through inhibition of various growth factors and other mediators, yet this research is in its infancy. This area may represent a focus of future therapy.

8. What should be considered in the differential diagnosis of new-onset asthma and what concomitant illnesses should be considered in acute exacerbations of preexisting asthma?

Several diagnoses must be entertained when confronted by a patient with apparent new-onset asthma. The adage that "all that wheezes is not asthma" continues to be true. Mimics of asthma include COPD, chronic bronchiectasis, bronchiolitis, congestive heart failure, pulmonary embolism, vocal cord dysfunction, upper-airway tumors, and foreign-body aspiration. In those patients with firmly established diagnoses of asthma, several concomitant conditions must be considered when symptoms prove refractory to standard care. Chronic postnasal drip, gastroesophageal reflux

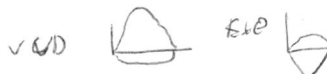

disease (GERD), congestive heart failure, or even rarer diseases, such as allergic bronchopulmonary aspergillosis and Churg-Strauss syndrome, should be considered potential confounding diseases in difficult to control asthmatics. Subxiphisternal tenderness elicited on firm palpation using the thumb or index finger is a helpful physical finding that can heighten the diagnostic possibility of GERD (Trudeau sign). Appropriate treatment of these diseases will enable better asthma control.

9. Describe the indications for leukotriene inhibitors.

The antileukotriene-receptor antagonists, montelukast (Singulair) and zafirlukast, and the 5-lipoxygenase inhibitor zileuton represent the most significant advancements in asthma therapy in recent years. These anti-inflammatory agents block the deleterious effects of specific leukotrienes. The strongest indications for these drugs are aspirin-sensitive asthma and exercise-induced asthma. In addition, difficult-to-control asthmatics who need to decrease their steroid dose, or who require increased β_2-agonist therapy while on appropriate steroids, may benefit from the addition of a leukotriene inhibitor. Lastly, the few patients who are unable to cooperate with metered-dose inhaler therapy would benefit from these oral drugs. In general, leukotriene-blocking drugs alone are not as efficacious as inhaled corticosteroids in the treatment of moderate persistent asthma. These newer medications should be considered in mild persistent asthma and as adjuncts to inhaled steroids for moderate and severe persistent asthma.

10. What future therapies may be useful in targeting mediators of inflammation?

Future therapy in asthma will target specific mediators that govern the chronic bronchial inflammation or suppress the allergic response to given allergens. Recent reports have shown that intravenous monoclonal anti-IgE therapy may benefit a subset of steroid-resistant atopic asthmatics with high serum IgE levels. In addition, inhibitors directed at eosinophil stimulants, such as humanized anti-IL-5 antibodies, their adhesion molecules and other immune mediators are being manufactured. The proper role of these medications is unclear, but they will likely serve as adjuncts to corticosteroids in select patients.

IL-4 plays a strong role in defining the asthma phenotype by promoting the differentiation of T-helper (Th0) cells to the Th2 phenotype, increasing IgE receptors on mast cells and signaling eosinophil infiltration into the lung. A link has been found between specific alterations in the IL-4 promoter gene and the severity of asthma, based on FEV_1, in several ethnic groups. A trial of nebulized recombinant IL-4 receptor to block the biologic effects of IL-4 in 25 moderately persistent atopic asthmatics who abruptly discontinued inhaled corticosteroids was very encouraging. Study subjects were randomized to receive either a single inhaled dose of IL-4 receptor (500 µg or 1500 µg) or placebo. High-dose IL-4 receptor prevented any deterioration in asthma symptom scores or decline in FEV_1 compared to placebo. These results are prelminary, but this therapy holds some promise for atopic asthmatics with inadequate clinical response to inhaled corticosteroid therapy.

11. In an outpatient clinic visit, which patient education objectives should be stressed in asthmatics?

Patient education is key to successful management of chronic asthma. First, patients must be instructed on the proper method of metered-dose inhaler (MDI) use

with a spacer device. Studies repeatedly show that as little as 10% of administered dose via MDI may reach the constricted bronchioles that may be further compromised by mucus plugging. Without proper technique, any prescribed MDI therapy will be ineffective. The more user-friendly dry powder inhaler (DPI) delivery device should help to improve compliance and efficacy. Second, patients must have a clear written "action plan" to follow when signs of deterioration become evident. Inherent in this is patient of PEF monitors and their rescue medications. Third, patient avoidance and control of triggers, especially in strongly atopic patients, is very important. For example, asthmatics allergic to common dust mite antigens must learn to clean their household regularly and, at times, cover their pillowcases in readily washable fabrics. Patient education remains an integral part of asthma clinics and should be stressed in follow-up visits in all settings.

12. How is occupationally associated asthma diagnosed?

Asthma is the most common occupational lung disease. The diagnosis requires the temporal association of symptoms and evidence of airway obstruction with exposure to the workplace environment. A host of agents have been shown to trigger asthma including isocyanates, latex, and baker's yeast. The low-molecular-weight-compound toluene diisocyanate, which is commonly found in paints and adhesives, may promote asthma in 5 to 30% of chronically exposed workers.

Patients with apparent occupational asthma should be asked to keep a symptom diary. Episodes of dyspnea, cough, and wheezing that arise at or soon after work and that improve while removed from this environment, are suggestive of occupational asthma. In addition, serial PEFRs and FEV_1 measurements that consistently worsen during and soon after work, but that improve at other times, provide strong evidence for this condition. Treatment obviously consists of removal from the offending work environment.

13. Define RADS.

Reactive airway dysfunction syndrome (RADS) is a separate entity from asthma. This condition is defined by persistent airway hyperreactivity after massive exposure to offending irritants such as acid, ammonia, and other fumes. Despite removal from the irritant symptoms may persist for years and methacholine challenge testing may remain abnormal. Treatment with inhaled steroids and bronchodilators is routinely recommended, but efficacy evidence is slim.

14. Are certain demographic populations at increased risk of asthma death?

While all asthmatics are at risk of dying of their disease, certain disturbing demographic trends in asthma deaths have been noted. A correlation between age and death from asthma appears clear. Likelihood of dying from asthma is 25 times higher for those greater than 75 years of age when compared to younger adults. Likewise, mortality rates from asthma in African Americans are approximately twice that of Caucasians. Death from asthma also loosely correlates with socioeconomic status; clusters of asthma deaths are noted in poor, inner-city populations particularly. Lastly, women have a higher relative risk of severe exacerbations and death when compared to men. Insight into these demographic trends is lacking, but many contend that some of these populations have poor access to medical care.

Misinformed patients frequently underestimate the severity of their asthma and physicians are often guilty of similar misjudgments. Together, misunderstanding and misdiagnosis may contribute to undue morbidity and mortality from asthma.

15. Do dry-powder inhalers have any benefits for patients?

Dry-powder, breath-activated delivery devices are available for both inhaled steroid and bronchodilator medications; combination formulations will soon be manufactured. They have gained favor among patients and physicians because of their ease of use. Dry-powder inhalers may benefit patients unable to master the hand-breath coordination of a MDI. Airway deposition of drug may be improved in many patients with poor MDI technique by employing a Diskus device. In addition, the automatic doses counter and simple packaging of dry-powder inhalers make them appealing to patients and physicians.

16. How can nocturnal awakenings be better controlled?

Nocturnal symptoms of sleep wakefulness, coughing, and wheezing are signs of poorly controlled asthma. The chronobiology of asthma in adults and children is well documented. Typically, PEFRs decrease significantly between 2 A.M. and 6 A.M. because of a natural diminution in circulating catecholamines and a rise in vagal tone. Because many medications lose their effect at these hours, nocturnal symptoms are often challenging to control. Moving the dose of inhaled corticosteroids to the afternoon hours, adding an inhaled long-acting β_2-agonist or anticholinergic bronchodilator, or offering a trial of a leukotriene inhibitor or theophylline before the patient retires to sleep are all appropriate measures. A stepwise approach is often needed for these persistent asthmatics and if one intervention does not ameliorate the symptoms, then another agent should be added to the regimen.

17. What are the effects of pregnancy? Should any particular medications be avoided during pregnancy?

Asthma is the most commonly encountered lung disease during pregnancy. Although only 1% of pregnancies are complicated by asthma, 1 of every 500 of asthma-complicated pregnancies experience life-threatening consequences. In general, approximately one-third of pregnant women experience worsening of their asthma during gestation, one-third remain the same, and one-third improve. Drugs commonly used to treat asthma are generally classified as Category B (no evidence of risk in humans) or Category C (risk cannot be ruled out). Three exceptions are triamcinolone and subcutaneous epinephrine, which are both Category D (evidence of risk), and methotrexate, which is category X (absolutely contraindicated in pregnancy) (see the Table). It is important to remember that despite a known association between chronic moderate-dose systemic steroid use and premature delivery and low birth-weight, pregnant asthmatics suffering an exacerbation should be treated with systemic corticosteroids. Morbidity and mortality from asthma is a much greater risk to the mother and fetus than is a short treatment course of oral steroids.

FDA Intrauterine Pregnancy Category Ratings for Asthma Drugs

Bronchodilator	Category	Inhaled Corticosteroid	Category
Albuterol	C	Beclomethasone	C
Metaproterenol	C	Budesonide	C
Salmeterol	C	Flunisolide	C
Terbutaline	B	Fluticasone	C
Theophylline	C	Triamcinolone	D
Epinephrine	D	Prednisone	C
Nonsteroidal	**Category**	**Antileukotriene**	**Category**
Cromolyn	B	Montelukast	B
Nedocromil	B	Zafirlukast	B
		Zileuton	C
Cytotoxic drugs	**Category**	**Anticholinergics**	**Category**
Methotrexate	X	Atropine	C
Cyclosporine	C	Ipratropium	B

A: controlled studies show no risk to fetus; B: no evidence of risk in humans; C: risk cannot be ruled out; D: positive evidence of risk to fetus; X: absolute contraindication during pregnancy

18. Is asthma associated with vocal cord dysfunction?

Vocal cord dysfunction (VCD) is a condition of unclear etiology in which patients manifest an abnormal abduction of the true vocal cords with inspiration. Failure to fully open the cords causes inspiratory stridor and a sensation of an obstructed upper airway. Approximately 50% of VCD patients have asthma, but the two diseases are not causally related. It is frequently difficult to differentiate VCD from asthma when faced with a distressed patient with apparent compromised airflow in the emergency department. Despite their distress, VCD patients should have normal gas exchange and airway resistance. A flow-volume loop showing truncation of the inspiratory limb of a flow-volume loop suggests VCD, but definitive diagnosis requires direct visualization of the abnormal vocal cord movement via rhinoscopy or bronchoscopy. Treatment consists of speech therapy, but this variably successful. VCD patients with asthma require standard treatment for asthma as well.

19. When should patients be referred to an asthma consultant?

Referral to an asthma consultant is a treatment option in all patients with moderate and severe persistent asthma. Recurrent emergency department visits, or failure to control symptoms despite moderate dose combination therapy, are indications for referral to an allergist, pulmonologist, or any physician with expertise in treating asthma. Prescribing of cytotoxic drugs, such as methotrexate or cyclosporine, allergen immunotherapy, or anti-IgE therapy should be done by asthma consultants only. In addition, a consultant should see any patient in whom the diagnosis of asthma is in doubt.

20. Is immunotherapy efficacious in asthma?

Many atopic asthmatics have exacerbations triggered by common environmental allergens. Studies of immunotherapy in these patients have produced conflicting results, and this treatment strategy cannot be routinely recommended. Select asthmatics with concomitant allergic rhinitis may note improvement in their asthma symptoms by treatment of their rhinitis with immunotherapy. In addition, patients

who cannot control their living environment by rigorous cleaning may benefit from immunotherapy. In general, though, this treatment plan should be pursued by a consulting allergist only and should not be considered until standard therapy has failed.

21. Name and describe the key effector cell in asthma.

Eosinophils, T lymphocytes, mast cells, and antigen-presenting cells such as alveolar macrophages, among others, play key roles in the pathogenesis of asthma. A single key effector cell that drives the inflammatory response in the airway cannot be identified because a host of native airway and recruited inflammatory cells secrete mediators that trigger a detrimental edematous response. For example, Th-2–differentiated lymphocytes release specific cytokines, such as IL-4 and IL-5, that promote the recruitment and activation of eosinophils and differentiation of helper lymphocytes. Activated eosinophils characteristically infiltrate bronchioles and release granule enzymes that promote airway edema and stimulate repair mechanisms. Mast cells, through the release of histamine and leukotrienes, further trigger airway inflammation and microvascular leak. All identified cells in the airways of asthmatic patients appear to have the capability to compound the detrimental inflammatory response through mediator release. The complexity of this cascade clearly hampers efforts to target a single cell or mediator for therapeutic means.

22. What is meant by the phrase "asthma is a Th-2 lymphocyte-mediated disease"?

Atopic asthmatics produce an overabundance of CD4+ T-helper lymphocytes in response to repeated allergen stimulation. These terminal lymphocytes are termed Th-2 cells because they resemble a previously defined subpopulation of mouse lymphocytes that secrete specific cytokines, including IL-4, IL-5, IL-9, IL-10, and IL-13. Bronchial biopsies of atopic asthmatics have shown a marked influx of such CD4+ cells and lymphocytes isolated from bronchoalveolar lavage fluid of asthmatics generate increased levels of Th-2 cytokines compared to normal controls. Th-2 cytokines play key roles in the airway inflammation of asthma (see Figure, next page). IL-5, for example, stimulates proliferation and differentiation of eosinophils from bone marrow progenitor cells and promotes eosinophil degranulation in the lungs. IL-4, in turn, triggers B-cell differentiation and IgE production, thereby reinforcing the atopic phenotype. Recent evidence suggests that IL-13 helps to sustain airway inflammation without eosinophil recruitment and encourages subepithelial matrix deposition. While it is clear that Th-2 cytokines are fundamentally important to the allergic asthma phenotype, their role in nonatopic asthmatics and elderly asthmatics, among others, is less well understood. Results from preliminary human studies using anti-IL-4 and anti-IL-5 antibodies therapeutically have been only modestly optimistic.

23. How is asthma differentiated from allergic rhinitis?

Researchers have tried to elucidate the differences between asthma and other atopic diseases, such as allergic rhinitis. Allergic rhinitis is fourfold more prevalent in the United States than asthma, yet much of the pathogenesis is common. What prompts differentiation to either the allergic rhinitis or asthma phenotype is unclear. Similarities between the two diseases include the effector cells (eosinophils, T lymphocytes, and mast cells), inflammatory mediators (histamine, prostaglandins, leukotrienes), and cytokine profiles. Relative differences in the up-regulation of

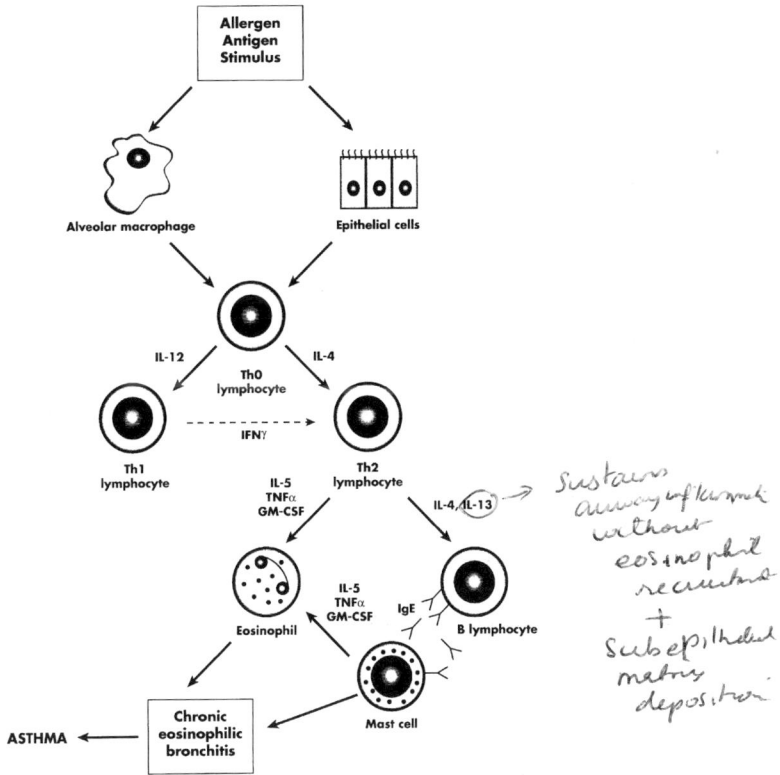

Handwritten annotation (right side): Sustains airway inflammation without eosinophil recruitment + subepithelial matrix deposition

certain cytokines, the role of bronchial airway smooth-muscle tone, and epithelial shedding and remodeling in asthmatic airways, may help to distinguish these diseases. Further understanding of the programmed cellular events in the airway may reveal a key mediator that serves as a marker for asthma. This biochemical marker would be useful clinically and remains an important focus of research.

24. Is there an association between asthma and chronic obstructive pulmonary disease?

Lung disease specialists have long noted similarities between asthma and COPD as defined by both chronic bronchitis and emphysema. Indeed, the outdated term *asthmatic bronchitis* reflects this belief. Pathologically, COPD derives from neutrophil infiltration with resultant airway epithelial metaplasia and alveolar destruction from the neutrophil's proteolytic enzymes. Like asthma, however, one histologic description does not uniformly characterize the spectrum of COPD. Overlapping phenotypic and pathologic features in a subset of asthma and COPD patients is well recognized. One example of this is recent evidence suggests that chronic asthma patients lose lung function, as measured by reduction in FEV_1 (mL/yr), at a rate more comparable to COPD patients than normal controls. Future understanding of the cellular mechanisms involved in asthma and COPD may uncover further similarities between these common lung diseases.

25. Why is the prevalence and mortality from bronchial asthma increasing?

Approximately 17 million people in the United States (7% of the population) have asthma. In 1996, the National Center for Health Statistics reported an increase in self-reported asthma of nearly 80% since 1980. The prevalence of asthma increased from 30.7 per 1,000 persons in the United States to 55.2 per 1,000 persons, and an increase in hospitalization rates of 120% between 1978 and 1994. Although deaths from asthma average 5,000 to 6,000 people annually, mortality is three to four times higher in African-Americans than among Caucasians, particularly among individuals 5 through 34 years of age. While boys have more asthma difficulties than do girls, women have more frequent and severe exacerbations when compared to men.

All of these alarming statistics have taken place despite unprecedented public health initiatives to better manage asthma. Factors that may account for the increase in asthma prevalence and incidence include more accurate diagnosis, air pollution, obesity, dietary habits, and more concentrated exposure to indoor allergens such as dust mites and cockroaches.

26. What type of collagen is deposited in airway remodeling in asthma?

Collagen types I, III, and V have been identified in the lamina reticularis and subepithelial matrix. Fibroblasts in connective tissues are responsible for the production of collagen reticular and elastic fibers. In asthma, fibroblasts may differentiate into myofibroblasts through a host of mediators, including IL-4 and IL-13, and myofibroblasts may contribute to the up-regulation of bronchial inflammation through the release of cytokines and matrix components such as elastin, fibronectin, tenascin, laminin. Myofibroblasts are found in increased numbers beneath the reticular basement membrane in asthma. The clinical significance of increased airway collagen is unclear, but it may relate to the development of fixed airway obstruction leading to a decrement in lung function. Whether current therapy can alter the course of airway remodeling is not known.

27. What is the current treatment of status asthmaticus?

Acute severe asthma refractory to medical treatments and accompanied by evidence of acute respiratory failure defines status asthmaticus. The treatment is both supportive and therapeutic with critical care respiratory monitoring, supplemental oxygen, early institution of systemic corticosteroids, nebulized or MDI-delivered albuterol and ipratropium bromide, and in certain young and refractory adult patients, parenteral β agonists such as subcutaneous epinephrine.

Aerosolized albuterol or albuterol with ipratropium bromide is first-line therapy. Nebulized therapy is preferred over MDI in status asthmaticus patients because of ease of administration. Doses of 2.5 mg of nebulized albuterol repeated two to three times per hour, or 0.4 mg/kg/hour continuously, are routinely prescribed in this situation. The difference between continuous and intermittent aerosol treatments is controversial. Any individual older than 40 years of age should have close cardiac monitoring for tachyarrhythmias (HR > 120/minute) and chest pain with high doses of albuterol are given (2.5 mg and higher). Levalbuterol may prove to provide better bronchodilator effect than racemic albuterol. An early improvement in PEFR or FEV_1 after 30 minutes of treatment is the most important predictor of a good outcome. If patients do not respond to inhaled $β_2$ agonist, subcutaneous epinephrine 0.3

ml of 1:1,000 solution subcutaneously every 20 minutes for three doses, or terbu-taline 0.25 to 0.5 mg subcutaneously every 4 hours may be given. Airway obstruction from bronchial inflammation and mucus plugging may prevent adequate delivery of aerosolized β_2-agonists and ipratropium bromide in acute severe asthma. Intravenous montelukast has been reported to be of benefit in clinical trials but its use requires further testing.

Endotracheal intubation with mechanical ventilation is indicated when acute respiratory failure ensues with acute respiratory acidosis (pH < 7.35), hypercarbia ($PaCO_2$ > 45 mm Hg) and hypoxemia (PaO_2 < 60 mm Hg) that does not readily improve with bronchodilator therapy. The place for noninvasive positive pressure ventilation in acute severe asthma is unclear but might, in selected cases, obviate the need for invasive ventilatory support. Clearly, prevention of attacks is the best remedy of all.

28. Name the five key components for long-term asthma control.

Easy access to professional help; frequent self-assessment and PEFR monitoring; simplified and effective pharmacologic therapy patients can adhere to; control of factors that contribute to worsening asthma severity; and patient education for a partnership are key components to long-term asthma control and an excellent quality of life.

29. Does physical examination aid in the evaluation of asthma patients?

Physical examination findings in patients with exacerbations of their asthma do not correlate well with the degree of airflow obstruction. Diffuse expiratory wheezing is a nearly ubiquitous finding, but the most severely impaired patients may have dramatically decreased breath sounds that limit auscultatory wheezing—often termed the "quiet chest." Simple observation of the respiratory pattern and recording of the vital signs provide much of the relevant physical exam in status asthmaticus patients. Distressed patients will be tachypneic, sitting upright and using their accessory muscles of respiration. Heart rates typically exceed 110 beats per minute, but blood pressure can fluctuate significantly depending on the degree of hemodynamic embarrassment secondary to high intrathoracic pressures. The pulsus paradoxus, a reflection of these high intrathoracic pressures, may prove the most helpful examination finding in status asthmaticus patients. An exaggerated pulsus paradoxus, defined as the difference in systolic blood pressure between expiration and inspiration, of > 15 mm Hg that does not improve after initial therapeutic efforts has been suggested as a parameter for intensive care monitoring.

30. Describe the natural history of wheezing in infancy and the development of asthma.

Although this issue has not been fully resolved, longitudinal data from several large population studies provide important evidence on this topic. Children less than 3 years of age who develop viral respiratory illnesses with wheezing have poorer lung function than children who do not have a wheezing episode. It is unclear, however, whether this a causal relationship or whether infants with wheezing illnesses were predisposed to such episodes because of diminished airway function at birth. An Arizona population study has shown that most infants with wheezing viral

respiratory infections before the age of 3 years do not develop subsequent asthma by the age of 6 years. A significant minority of infants (25 to 40%) with wheezing is diagnosed ultimately with asthma, and identification of this subset is difficult. Factors associated with an increased risk of a wheezing infant developing persistent asthma include maternal smoking and a history of maternal asthma or atopy.

BIBLIOGRAPHY

1. Agertoft L, Pedersen S: Effect of long-term treatment with inhaled budesonide on adult height in children with asthma. N Engl J Med 343:1064–1069, 2000.
2. American Thoracic Society. Guidelines for methacholine challenge and exercise challenge testing. Am J Respir Crit Care Med 161:309–329, 2000.
3. Barnes PJ: Mechanisms of glucocorticoids in asthma. Am J Respir Crit Care Med 154:S21–S26, 1996.
4. Barnes PJ, Chung F, and Page CP: Inflammatory mediators of asthma. An update. Pharmacol Rev 50:515–596, 1998.
5. Borish LC, Nelson HS, Lanz MJ, et al: Interleukin-4 receptor in moderate atopic asthma. Am J Respir Crit Care Med 160:1816–1823, 1999.
6. Busse WW, Elias J, Sheppard D, et al: Airway remodeling and repair. Am J Respir Crit Care Med 160:1035–1042, 1999.
7. Childhood Asthma Management Program Research Group: Long-term effects of budesonide or nedocromil in children with asthma. N Engl J Med 343:1054–1063, 2000.
8. Corbridge TC, Hall JB: The assessment and management of adults with status asthmaticus. Am J Respir Crit Care Med 151:1296–1316, 1995.
9. Creticos PS, Reed CE, Norman PS, et al: Ragweed immunotherapy in adult asthma. N Engl J Med 334:1380–1388, 1996.
10. Dempsey OJ, Wilson AM, Sims EJ, et al: Additive bronchoprotective and bronchodilator effect with single doses of salmeterol and montelukast in asthmatic patients receiving inhaled corticosteroids. Chest 117:950–953, 2000.
11. Doerschug KC, Peterson MW, Dayton CS, et al: Asthma guidelines. An assessment of physician understanding and practice. Am J Respir Crit Care Med 159:1735–1741, 1999.
12. Drazen JM, Israel E, O'Byrne PM: Treatment of asthma with drugs modifying the leukotriene pathway. N Engl J Med 340:197–206, 1999.
13. Laviolette M, Malmstrom K, Lu S, et al: Montelukast added to inhaled beclomethasone in treatment of asthma. Am J Respir Crit Care Med 160:1862–1868, 1999.
14. Milgrom H, Fick RB, Su JQ, et al: Treatment of allergic asthma with monoclonal anti-IgE antibody. N Engl J Med 341:1966–1973, 1999.
15. Rosenwasser LJ: New immunopharmacologic approaches to asthma: Role of cytokine antagonism. J Allerg Clin Immunol 105:S586–S592, 2000.
16. Shapiro G, Lumry W, Wolf J, et al: Combined salmeterol 50 µg and fluticasone propionate 250 µg in the Diskus device for the treatment of asthma. Am J Respir Crit Care Med 161:527–534, 2000.
17. U.S. Department of Health and Human Services. National Asthma Education and Prevention Program. Management of asthma during pregnancy. Bethesda, MD, NHLBI/NIH Publication No. 93-3279A, 1993.
18. Verberne APH, Frost C, Dulverman EJ, et al: Addition of salmeterol versus doubling the dose of beclomethasone in children with asthma. Am J Respir Crit Care Med 158:213–219, 1998.
19. Wenzel SE, Schwartz LB, Langmack EL, et al: Evidence that severe asthma can be divided pathologically into two inflammatory subtypes with distinct physiologic and clinical characteristics. Am J Respir Crit Care Med 160:1001–1008, 1999.

7. SINUSITIS

E. Bradley Strong, M.D.

DEFINITION

1. How are the terms "acute," subacute," and "chronic sinusitis," defined?

Acute sinusitis is defined as a sinus infection lasting less than 4 weeks. **Subacute sinusitis** is defined as a sinus infection lasting 4 weeks to 3 months. **Chronic sinusitis** is defined as a sinus infection lasting greater than 3 months.

Two other less-commonly used terms are **recurrent acute sinusitis** (greater than four episodes of acute sinusitis per year, each lasting 7 to 10 days, with an absence of intervening symptoms) and **acute exacerbations of chronic sinusitis** (a sudden worsening of chronic sinusitis symptoms with return to baseline symptoms after treatment).

CLINICAL PRESENTATION

2. What are the most common disease processes that predispose patients to sinusitis?
- **Viral upper respiratory tract infections** are probably the most common cause of acute bacterial sinusitis. Viral infections result in diffuse nasal mucosal edema, obstruction of sinus ostia, poor mucociliary clearance, and bacterial overgrowth.
- **Allergic rhinitis** also results in mucosal edema, obstruction of ostia, and a predisposition for bacterial sinusitis.
- **Rhinitis medicamentosa** secondary to overuse of topical vasoconstrictors.
- **Anatomic abnormalities** including septal deviation or concha bullosa (aerated middle turbinate).
- **Neoplastic diseases** such as benign polyps or inverted papilloma.
- **Genetic disorders** such as cystic fibrosis and immotile cilia syndrome.
- **Immunologic diseases** such as IgA deficiency.

3. Discuss the pathophysiology of bacterial sinusitis.

Normal sinuses are air-filled cavities with small ostia (1–2 mm) for drainage. The nasal lining secretes mucous and IgA. The mucus absorbs any particulate matter or bacteria and the IgA offers an initial barrier to bacterial infection. The cilia beat toward the natural ostia and move any foreign material into the nasal cavity.

When ostial obstruction occurs, an infectious cycle begins. The mucus stagnates and becomes thick, the pH drops, ciliary function decreases, mucosal edema occurs, and bacterial overgrowth results. The local immune response may exacerbate the ostial obstruction by further increasing mucosal edema.

4. What are the two most common causes of acute bacterial sinusitis in children?

Viral upper respiratory tract infection and nasal foreign body.

5. What symptoms are strongly indicative of sinusitis?

A thorough and accurate history is extremely important in the diagnosis of sinusitis because the physical examination can be unremarkable, even in the face of active infection.

Major symptoms of sinusitis:

- **Facial pressure/pain:** While the symptoms of facial pressure/pain are *consistent* with sinusitis, the differential diagnosis of facial pressure/pain is very broad. It also includes intracranial lesions (such as tumors, hematoma, and infection); peripheral cranial nerve neuralgia; migraine; hypertension; muscle tension headache; orbital abnormalities (eye strain, glaucoma); ear lesions (otitis media, mastoiditis); temporomandibular joint (TMJ) dysfunction, and myofacial syndrome. However, when facial pressure/pain is present in combination with the other major symptoms listed below, it becomes a strong historical finding.
- **Nasal obstruction** is a common complaint in sinusitis patients. However, the nature and timing of nasal obstruction must be clarified. Nasal obstruction secondary to infection is most often bilateral and relatively symmetric. It occurs during an active infection and resolves when the infection clears. Other types of obstruction are more constant. Septal deviation usually results in a unilateral, fixed obstruction. Nasal polyps are generally bilateral and slowly progressive. Dynamic nasal valve collapse can be unilateral or bilateral, but is relieved by lateralization of the nasal ala with a Q-tip or by lateralizing the ala with digital pressure on the cheek.
- **Purulent nasal discharge** from the middle meatus is highly suggestive of sinusitis. Foreign bodies can result in purulent nasal discharge in children, but this is usually localized to one nostril. Purulent secretions should be cultured whenever possible. Unfortunately, "blind" nasal cultures with a headlight are notoriously unreliable. Endoscopic guidance is required to obtain reliable cultures from the middle meatus.
- **Hyposmia/anosmia:** Mucosal edema may result in diminished airflow and obstruction of the odorant molecules from reaching the olfactory bulb located above the nasal roof (cribriform plate). This is most commonly seen with nasal polyposis.
- **Fever** is more common in patients with acute sinusitis than in patients with chronic sinusitis.
- **Dental pain** is a strong indicator of *acute* maxillary sinusitis; however it is less common in chronic sinusitis.

6. Which symptoms are moderately suggestive of sinusitis?

The symptoms listed below support the diagnosis of sinusitis only when they are present in association with other major symptoms.

Minor symptoms of sinusitis:

- **Generalized headache** can be a sign of sinusitis, but it is uncommon when other symptoms of sinusitis are lacking (see facial pressure/pain above).

    Halitosis: Purulent nasal secretions can result in halitosis. Patients will more commonly complain of a foul nasal smell.
- **Fatigue**

• **Cough:** Purulent nasal discharge and postnasal drainage can result in cough. Patients with underlying asthma or bronchitis are at risk for exacerbations of their pulmonary disease.

7. Name the most common symptoms of pediatric sinusitis.

Pediatric sinusitis patients are more difficult to evaluate. They often give a less-detailed history with more atypical or "minor" symptoms. The most common complaints are chronic cough, rhinorrhea, and nasal congestion.

ANATOMY

8. Where are the nasal turbinates located and what is their function?

There are three nasal turbinates: inferior, middle, and superior. A fourth turbinate is commonly found posterosuperior to the superior turbinate. When present, this is called the "supreme turbinate." The turbinates are bony projections from the lateral nasal sidewall that are covered with pseudostratified, ciliated, columnar epithelium. The turbinates act to warm, humidify, and clean the inspired air. Each turbinate contains a venous plexus that periodically engorges, resulting in an increase in nasal resistance. This occurs on alternating sides of the nose at varying frequencies (hours to days). This "nasal cycle" is thought to allow one side of the nose to "rest" while the contralateral side "works." Patients can often sense these changes and may perceive them as abnormal. A brief explanation generally alleviates any anxiety.

9. Define the superior, middle, and inferior meatuses.

The superior, middle, and inferior meatus are air passageways located beneath the turbinate of the same name.

10. Which sinuses drain into the superior, middle, and inferior meatus?

The superior meatus drains the posterior ethmoid air cells.

The middle meatus contains the ostia of multiple sinuses. The maxillary sinus ostia is located on the lateral nasal side wall and is generally less than 2 mm in diameter. The normal maxillary ostium is not visible with nasal endoscopy because the uncinate process obscures it. There may be accessory maxillary sinus ostia located posterior to the true ostia that can be visualized. The frontal sinus also drains into the middle meatus via the nasofrontal recess or duct. Finally, the anterior ethmoid air cells are honeycomb-shaped sinuses that drain into the middle meatus. The openings are too numerous and variable to anatomically detail.

The inferior meatus drains the nasolacrimal apparatus. The nasolacrimal duct runs from the lacrimal fossa, through the maxillary bone, and exits into the anterior third of the middle meatus. Nasal polyps obstructing the inferior meatus can result in epiphora (watery eyes).

11. What is the osteomeatal complex (or osteomeatal unit)?

The osteomeatal complex (OMC) is located in the anterior third of the middle meatus. It is the final common drainage pathway from the frontal, anterior ethmoid,

and maxillary sinuses. Therefore, it is important to examine this area when performing nasal endoscopy. Mucosal edema, nasal polyps, and postoperative scarring can all obstruct the OMC and result in sinusitis.

12. Where does the sphenoid sinus ostia drain?
The sphenoid sinus drains into the sphenoethmoidal recess located on the sphenoid rostrum, lateral to the septum and medial to the superior turbinate.

13. Where is the olfactory bulb located?
The olfactory bulb is located in the anterior cranial fossa, just above bony nasal roof (cribriform plate). The sensory fibers of the olfactory bulb traverse the cribriform plate to enter the nasal cavity. Odorant molecules enter the nostrils and stimulate the olfactory bulb. Nasal polyps can obstruct normal nasal airflow and result in a decreased or absent sense of smell (hyposmia/anosmia). Because the sense of smell is integral to taste, patients with hyposmia/anosmia often have complaints of poor taste.

PATHOGENESIS/MICROBIOLOGY

14. Name the most common organisms that cause acute bacterial sinusitis.
- *Streptococcus pneumoniae* 20–35%
- *Haemophilus influenzae* 6–26%
- *Moraxella catarrhalis* 2–10%
- Anaerobes 0–8%
- *Staphylococcus aureus* 0–8%

Streptococcus pneumoniae, *Haemophilus influenzae*, and *Moraxella catarrhalis* are traditionally taught as the most common organisms causing acute bacterial sinusitis. Viral cultures are difficult to obtain, and the exact incidence of viral sinusitis is not clearly defined.

15. Name the most common organisms that cause chronic bacterial sinusitis.
- Coagulase-negative staphylococcus 24–80%
- *Staphylococcus aureus* 9–33%
- Anaerobes 0–8 %
- *Streptococcus pneumoniae* 0–7%
- Gram-positive and anaerobic organisms are more common in chronic sinusitis. However, anaerobes are difficult to culture, and the exact incidence is difficult to quantify.

16. Which sinuses are most commonly involved in acute bacterial sinusitis?
The maxillary sinuses are most commonly involved, followed by the frontal and ethmoid sinuses. Isolated sphenoid sinusitis is uncommon.

17. What is the most common fungal pathogen resulting in sinusitis?
Aspergillus fumigatus

18. How is fungal sinusitis classified?

Acute fulminant fungal sinusitis is a rapidly invasive, life-threatening fungal infection that is seen in immunocompromised hosts. Mucoraceae is the most common fungal species causing this disease. Acute fulminant fungal sinusitis requires aggressive surgical debridement with a margin of normal tissue and systemic antifungal therapy (amphotericin B). Mortality rates have dropped from greater than 90% before 1970 to less than 20% today.

Chronic indolent fungal sinusitis occurs in an immunocompetent, nonatopic host. Aspergillus is the most common fungal etiology. Tissue invasion can occur. The most appropriate treatment is conservative surgical debridement and systemic antifungal therapy (e.g., fluconazole).

A **fungus ball** results from a long-standing fungal infection in an immunocompetent, nonatopic host. The most common fungal pathogen is Aspergillus. The fungus ball is usually unilateral and located in the maxillary sinus. Tissue invasion does not occur. The most appropriate therapy is surgical debridement and aeration of the sinus cavity.

Allergic fungal sinusitis results from an inflammatory response of the nasal mucosa to a fungal allergen (most commonly Aspergillus and Bipolaris species). The host is immunocompetent and atopic. There is generally no fungal overgrowth or invasion seen. The most appropriate treatment is not clearly defined but likely includes surgical debridement and systemic antifungals, as well as topical and systemic steroids. The role of immunotherapy is unclear.

DIFFERENTIAL DIAGNOSIS

19. What is in the differential diagnosis of patients presenting with sinus complaints?
- Viral upper respiratory tract infection
- Allergic rhinitis
- Nonspecific rhinitis
- Rhinitis medicamentosa
- Nasal septal deviation
- Bacterial sinusitis

20. Why should unilateral maxillary sinusitis be of particular concern?

Sinusitis is generally a mucosal disease that effects all of the sinuses. While some isolated sinus cavities may be spared, it is uncommon to have unilateral maxillary sinusitis. When this occurs, a neoplastic process must be considered. The differential diagnosis includes both benign and malignant lesions. Therefore, isolated maxillary sinusitis should be considered the result of an obstructing malignant lesion until proven otherwise.

21. What are three common etiologies of nonrhinogenic headache?

Temporomandibular joint (TMJ) dysfunction is a very common cause of facial pain that can be mistaken for sinus pain. TMJ pain is usually localized to the joint or ear, but it can be referred to the maxilla, orbit, temple, vertex, mastoid, or

neck. These patients may present with isolated maxillary sinus discomfort masquerading as sinusitis. Therefore, facial pain without other major symptoms of sinusitis must raise suspicion for TMJ dysfunction.

Migraine headaches are also associated with facial pain. Classic migraine symptoms include a brief prodromal period with irritability, visual changes, or paraesthesias. Severe headache, nausea, and photophobia follow. Cluster headaches are a migraine variant. They include severe, sharp periorbital pain associated with ipsilateral pupillary constriction, local vasodilatation, rhinorrhea, and lacrimation.

Muscle tension/stress headaches are very common. They often begin at the occiput or shoulders and radiate to the fronto-orbital area.

While TMJ pain and headache pain can be mistaken for sinusitis, there will be no associated sinus symptoms (i.e., purulent rhinorrhea, nasal obstruction) and the timing will not be consistent with an infectious etiology.

22. Describe four common causes of nasal obstruction besides sinusitis.

Rhinitis medicamentosa occurs with long-term use of topical vasoconstrictor sprays (oxymetazoline, phenylephrine). These sympathomimetic agents result in marked vasoconstriction of the venous plexuses in the nasal turbinates. While this provides a short-term increase in nasal airflow, the ultimate result is rebound vasodilatation and nasal obstruction. Continuous use for greater than 7 to 10 days can result in chronic inflammation and addiction. The mainstay of therapy is nasal steroid spray. The nasal steroid spray should be applied daily for 1 week and then the topical decongestant should be stopped. Discontinuing the use of the topical decongestant in one nostril at a time may be easier for some patients. Systemic steroids may be indicated in the most severe cases.

Allergic rhinitis is a common cause of nasal obstruction. Inhaled allergens result in chronic turbinate hypertrophy and reduced nasal airflow. Common treatments include topical nasal steroids, topical and systemic antihistamines, cromolyn sodium, as well as immunotherapy. Surgical reduction of the inferior turbinates can increase nasal airflow in refractory cases. Unfortunately, the turbinate hypertrophy may slowly recur in a minority of patients (months to years).

Nonallergic vasomotor rhinitis is a poorly defined term referring to chronic nasal obstruction and rhinorrhea. Common etiologies include pregnancy, temperature-induced rhinitis, and idiopathic rhinitis. A detailed discussion of this topic is beyond the scope of this chapter. Treatment is generally symptomatic and includes nasal steroid sprays or ipratropium nasal spray.

Nasal septal deviation generally results in a unilateral, fixed nasal obstruction. However, an "S"-shaped septal deviation that results in fixed, bilateral nasal obstruction is often seen. Initial treatment includes a trial of nasal steroid spray. Significant obstruction that is refractory to nasal steroids may require surgery.

23. What is the most common etiology of anosmia/hyposmia?

The most common definable cause of anosmia/hyposmia is paranasal sinus disease (i.e., nasal polyps, sinusitis). An equal number of patients will have an idiopathic etiology. Head trauma is also a common cause.

EVALUATION

24. What are the key components to an anterior rhinoscopic examination?
While the history is extremely important in the diagnosis of sinusitis, anterior rhinoscopy is probably the most important part of the physical examination. Anterior rhinoscopy can be performed with either an otoscope or a nasal speculum and head mirror. The otoscope offers a narrower field of view but provides magnification of the posterior nasal vault. The nasal speculum offers a more thorough examination of the anterior nasal cavity. The structures that should be examined include (a) the inferior, middle, and superior turbinates, (b) the inferior and middle meatus (superior meatus if possible), (c) the nasal septum, and (d) the choana. Any evidence of nasal polyposis, turbinate hypertrophy, nasal bleeding, mucosal lesions, or mucopurulent discharge should be documented.

25. How does transillumination work and is it efficacious?
Transillumination works on the assumption that fluid-filled sinuses transmit less light than air-filled sinuses. The maxillary sinuses can be transilluminated by instructing the patient to purse their lips around a light source placed in the mouth. The left and right side of the frontal sinus can be evaluated by placing the light source on the inferomedial aspect of each supraorbital rim. Unfortunately, not all sinuses are symmetric and it has been shown that transillumination does not correlate well with other diagnostic studies.

FIBEROPTIC RHINOSCOPY

26. Is fiberoptic rhinoscopy superior to standard anterior rhinoscopy?
Yes. Fiberoptic nasal endoscopy enables the physician to closely examine the entire nasal vault. Rigid or flexible fiberoptic endoscopes can be passed from the nasal vestibule to the choana. While the examination is monocular, a more complete examination of the turbinates, meatuses, choana, and septum can be performed. Following endoscopic sinus surgery direct visualization into the ethmoid, maxillary, frontal, and sphenoid sinuses is often possible.

27. Are nasal cultures efficacious?
Yes. However, the cultures are highly technique-dependent and they must be properly obtained. Cultures taken blindly or with anterior rhinoscopy are unreliable and often contaminated by flora from the nasal vestibule. Accurate cultures require endoscopic placement of a Culturette swab directly into the middle meatus without touching other areas of the nasal mucosa.

IMAGING

28. Are plain sinus radiographs efficacious?
Sometimes. A thorough history and physical examination can usually make the diagnosis of acute sinusitis. Plain radiographs are usually not required. Plain films can be ordered to confirm a diagnosis that is in question, but once the diagnosis has

been made, the x-rays rarely change the treatment plan. The maxillary sinuses can be evaluated on a Waters view, and the frontal sinus can be visualized on a lateral skull film. Evaluation of the ethmoid sinuses, sphenoid sinus, and osteomeatal complex is difficult. Classic radiographic findings indicative of sinusitis include mucosal thickening, air-fluid levels, and sinus opacification. While plain radiographs were once considered the gold standard for diagnosing chronic sinusitis, computed tomography (CT) has now become the standard of care.

29. When should a CT scan of the sinuses be obtained?

Computed tomography is considered the gold standard for diagnosing sinusitis. It is generally reserved for patients with chronic sinusitis due to its cost and the amount of radiation exposure. Sinus CT scans provide both diagnostic and therapeutic information about the sinuses. Diagnostically, the CT scan precisely documents the degree of mucosal thickening, sinus opacification, and polypoid disease. Therapeutically, preoperative CT scans document the anatomy of the skull base, orbital wall, and osteomeatal complex.

The timing of a sinus CT scan should be considered carefully. A limited sinus CT scan is often ordered to initially document chronic sinus disease. A repeat CT scan after "maximal medical management" (i.e., an aggressive attempt to treat the chronic sinus symptoms) will reveal whether the patient responds to medical therapy or is a surgical candidate. Persistent sinus disease in the face of maximal medical management is an indication for surgical intervention. Maximal medical management generally entails 4 to 6 weeks of oral antibiotics, a nasal steroid spray, brief treatment with a topical decongestant, oral steroids, and antihistamines when indicated.

Maximal medical management prior to a follow-up CT scan simplify the treatment algorithm for chronic sinusitis. There are four options:
- If the patient remains symptomatic and has significant sinus disease on the follow-up CT scan, then the patient is a likely candidate for sinus surgery.
- If the CT scan is normal and the patient's symptoms are improved, no further intervention is necessary.
- If symptoms persist despite a normal CT scan, then the diagnosis of sinusitis must be questioned.
- If there is significant disease on the CT scan, but the patient is asymptomatic, observation is generally indicated.

30. What CT scan findings are indicative of sinus disease?
- Obstruction of the osteomeatal complex
- Circumferential sinus mucosal thickening
- Complete sinus opacification
- Nasal polyps or masses
- Anatomic abnormalities (e.g., concha bullosa, paradoxical turbinate, septal deviation)

31. What radiographic findings are suggestive of chronic indolent fungal sinusitis or fungus ball?

A sinus cavity with peripheral mucosal edema and central radiopacity (metallic appearing).

TREATMENT

Antibiotics

32. When should antibiotics be prescribed for acute sinusitis?

Antibiotic treatment of acute sinusitis is controversial. Some studies conclude that oral antibiotics reduce the severity and duration of symptoms, while other studies show no effect. Consequently, some authors advocate supportive treatment with decongestants, mucolytics, nasal irrigations, and hydration. Other authors advocate first-line antibiotic therapy. A conservative approach is to treat routine sinusitis patients symptomatically for 7 to 10 days. If there is no improvement, or if the symptoms worsen, the patient should be started on antibiotic therapy. Commonly used first-line agents include amoxicillin, trimethoprim-sulfamethoxazole, and erythromycin plus a sulfonamide.

33. What is the most appropriate length of antibiotic treatment for acute sinusitis?

The duration of antibiotic therapy for acute bacterial sinusitis is also controversial. Historically, patients have been treated for 10 to 14 days. There is little clinical data to refute or support this approach. Recently, several studies have shown that a 3-day course of oral antibiotics is as efficacious as 10 days of therapy. Unfortunately, the literature remains unclear and the majority of clinicians continue to treat for 10 to 14 days.

34. Which antibiotics are most appropriate for chronic sinusitis?

Patients with chronic sinusitis have had symptoms for greater than 3 months and have usually failed multiple courses of first-line antibiotic agents. There is a greater incidence of Gram-positive cocci and beta-lactamase–producing organisms with chronic sinusitis. Therefore, second-line antibiotics, such as amoxicillin clavulanate, cefuroxime, levofloxacin, and clindamycin, are indicated.

35. What is the most appropriate length of antibiotic treatment for chronic sinusitis?

Chronic sinusitis requires prolonged treatment for complete eradication of the disease. Short courses of antibiotics often provide only temporary symptomatic relief. A prolonged course of therapy lasting 4 to 6 weeks in combination with steroids and decongestants is often required to completely clear the infection.

36. Explain the term *maximal medical management* of chronic sinusitis.

The term *maximal medical management* implies the maximal *medical* treatment short of surgical intervention. For patients with refractory sinus disease, this often consists of (a) 4 to 6 weeks of a second-line antibiotics; (b) 4 to 6 weeks of topical nasal steroids; (c) 2 weeks of a topical decongestant (with brief breaks to avoid rebound nasal congestion); (d) 2 weeks of oral prednisone; and (e) antihistamines as indicated. If symptoms persist despite maximal medical management, surgical intervention should be considered.

Ancillary Treatment

37. List the risks associated with topical and systemic decongestants.
- Prolonged use of topical decongestants (oxymetazoline, phenylephrine) results in rebound nasal congestion and rhinitis medicamentosa.
- Systemic sympathomimetic agents (pseudoephedrine, phenylephrine, and phenylpropanolamine) can significantly increase the heart rate and blood pressure. Caution must be used when prescribing these agents to patients with hypertension and coronary artery disease.

38. Are antihistamines efficacious for nonallergic bacterial sinusitis?
No. Antihistamines, particularly the first-generation agents, can thicken mucosal secretions and reduce mucociliary transport. Antihistamines are primarily indicated when there is an allergic component to the sinusitis.

39. What role do topical nasal steroids play in the treatment of acute and chronic sinusitis?
Topical nasal steroids reduce mucosal edema, open the natural sinus ostia, and increase mucociliary drainage in chronic sinusitis. Nasal steroids have a slow onset of action and therefore may be less efficacious for acute sinusitis.

40. What role do systemic steroids play in the treatment of chronic sinusitis?
Chronic sinusitis patients treated with short courses of antibiotics (1–2 weeks) may have persistent infection and mucosal edema despite therapy. Short-term antibiotic therapy may briefly reduce the bacterial load, but the infection "rebounds" after the antibiotics are discontinued. Systemic steroids act to reduce mucosal edema in the paranasal sinuses. The combination of systemic steroids, prolonged antibiotic administration (4–6 weeks), and topical therapy (nasal steroids and decongestants) gives the patient the greatest opportunity to clear a chronic infection.

41. List some relative contraindications to the use of systemic steroids for treatment of chronic sinusitis.
- Diabetes mellitus
- Psychiatric history
- Active tuberculosis
- Pregnancy
- Seizure disorder
- Osteoporosis
- Congestive heart failure

Surgery

42. What are the common sinus indications for otolaryngologic referral?
- Sinusitis refractory to maximal medical management.
- Impending complications of sinusitis (orbital cellulitis, meningitis, or brain abscess).

• Fixed nasal obstruction (septal deviation, polyp, tumor).
• Sinusitis associated with an underlying systemic disease.

43. What are the common indications for functional endoscopic sinus surgery?
• Recurrent acute sinusitis with a defined site of obstruction
• Chronic sinusitis refractory to medical management
• Nasal polyposis
• Nasal obstruction
• Fungal sinusitis
• Sinus mucocele
• Complications of sinusitis

COMPLICATIONS

44. What are the most common complications of sinusitis?
• Facial cellulitis
• Osteomyelitis (Potts' puffy tumor)
• Mucopyocele
• Orbital cellulitis/abscess/blindness—particularly in the pediatric population
• Meningitis
• Cavernous sinus thrombosis
• Brain abscess
Pediatric sinusitis patients are at an increased risk for orbital and intracranial complications. Symptoms suggestive of impending complications include periorbital swelling, progressive headache, meningeal signs, and mental status changes. An urgent workup that includes a contrast-enhanced CT scan of the brain and sinuses should be performed if there is any suggestion of potential complications.

SINUSITIS AND ASTHMA

45. How does sinusitis affect asthma?
Bronchial asthma can be exacerbated by a variety of stimuli including allergens, exercise, temperature changes, chemical irritants, stress, and infection. Sinusitis results in an increased upper respiratory tract bacterial load. Purulent postnasal drainage may result in bronchial irritation and exacerbation of asthma.

46. What is Samter's syndrome?
Samter's syndrome is a triad of symptoms including nasal polyposis, bronchial asthma, and aspirin sensitivity. Aspirin blocks the cyclooxygenase pathway and preferentially shunts arachidonic acid into the lipoxygenase pathway. This results in an overproduction of leukotrienes, bronchoconstriction, and asthma exacerbations. It may also promote polyp formation. The nasal polyps are often refractory to medical management and may require multiple polypectomies.

BIBLIOGRAPHY

1. Benninger MS, Anon J, Mabry RL: The medical management of rhinosinusitis. Otolaryngol Head Neck Surg 117(suppl):S41–S49, 1997.
2. Hadley JA, Schaefer SD: Clinical evaluation of rhinosinusitis: History and physical examination. Otolaryngol Head Neck Surg 117(suppl):S8–S11, 1997.
3. Kennedy DW: Medical management of sinusitis: Educational goals and management guidelines. Ann Otol Rhinol Laryngol 104(suppl 167):22–30, 1995.
4. Lanza DC, Kennedy DW: Adult rhinosinusitis defined. Otolaryngol Head Neck Surg 117(suppl): S1–S7, 1997.
5. Osguthorpe JD, Hadley JA: Rhinosinusitis. Current concepts in evaluation and management. Med Clin North Am 83:27–41, 1999.

8. URTICARIA AND ANGIOEDEMA

Massoud Mahmoudi, D.O., Ph.D., and Stanley M. Naguwa, M.D.

1. What are urticaria and angioedema? Could they occur together?

Urticaria, or hive, is characterized as an erythematous, circumscribed, and pruritic skin lesion that blanches with pressure. Urticaria develops as a result of mast cell degranulation. Urticaria can develop in different parts of the body. It's diameter ranges from several millimeters to as much as several centimeters. When the lesion occurs in the deeper dermis, it is called angioedema and usually involves extremities, genitalia, and lips, tongue, or larynx. Angioedema is associated with pain or a burning sensation. The etiology of urticaria/angioedema may be of a single etiology or it may be multifactorial or idiopathic.

Urticaria and angioedema affect approximately 20% of the population and can occur together or can present as one entity. Fifty percent of patients have simultaneous urticaria and angioedema, whereas 40% have only urticaria and 10% only have angioedema. One example in which angioedema develops in absence of urticaria is hereditary angioedema.

2. What are acute and chronic urticaria/angioedema reactions?

Acute urticarial/angioedema reactions are those that resolve on their own, by medication, or by identification and treatment of the underlying cause. Acute urticaria/angioedema lesions usually develop rapidly and resolve in a few hours. Although the lesions might recur, the duration of the reactions is less than 6 weeks. If recurrences persist beyond 6 weeks, it is labeled chronic urticaria, which have nonnecrotizing perivascular lymphatic infiltrates, mast cells, and monocytes.

3. List the etiologies of urticaria and angioedema.

The Table lists some of the etiologies.

Potential Causes of Urticaria and Angioedema

Idiopathic

Food allergy

Food additives and preservatives—benzoic acid derivatives, dyes (especially tartrazine), etc.

Drug reactions
    Antibiotics—penicillin, cephalosporins, sulfa derivatives, vancomycin, etc.
    Cyclooxygenase inhibitors—aspirin, NSAIDs
    Over-the-counter medications—vitamins, cold formulas, etc.
    Antihypertensive agents—angiotensin-converting enzyme inhibitors, beta-blockers, diuretics, etc.
    Psychotropics—sedatives, tranquilizers, etc.
    Hyperosmolar radiocontrast media
    Opiates—morphine-sulfate, codeine
    Muscle relaxants—d-tubocuraine
    Hormonal—birth control pills, thyroid replacement, synthetic ACTH, insulin
    Chemotherapeutic medications—doxorubicin (Adriamycin)
    Intravenous gamma globulin

(Table continued on next page.)

Potential Causes of Urticaria and Angioedema (cont.)

Drug reactions (cont.)
- Protamine
- Enzymes—papain
- Vaccines
- Antisera

Immunotherapy injections

Insect bites and stings
- Hymenoptera—wasp, honey bee, yellow jacket, hornet, fire ant
- Others—caterpillar, spider

Physical
- Dermatographism
- Cholinergic
- Localized heat
- Cold
- Delayed pressure
- Exercise-induced anaphylaxis
- Solar
- Vibratory
- Aquagenic

Endocrine disorders
- Thyroid disease—hypo-thyroidism or hyperthyroidism, thyroiditis
- Diabetes mellitus
- Progesterone hypersensitivity
- Hyperparathyroidism

Collagen vascular diseases—particularly systemic lupus erythematosus, rheumatoid arthritis, Sjögren's syndrome

Infection
- Viral—hepatitis B, infectious mononucleosis
- Bacterial
- Parasitic—invasive helminths, giardiasis
- Fungal

Malignancy—lymphoma, solid tumors, myeloproliferative disorders

Vasculitis
- Idiopathic hypocomplementemic
- Idiopathic normocomplementemic
- Associated with systemic diseases
- Serum sickness—heterologous protein administration, drugs
- Schnitzler's syndrome

C_1 esterase inhibitor deficiency syndromes (angioedema only)
- Hereditary angioedema
- Acquired angioedema

Contact—latex, animals, food, plants, sea nettles

Inhalant atopy

Transfusion reaction

Rare miscellaneous
- C_3b inactivator deficiency
- Familial cold urticaria
- Amyloidosis with nerve deafness
- Episodic angioedema with eosinophilia
- Carboxypeptidase N deficiency

From Huston PH, Bressler RB: Urticaria and angioedema. Med Clin North Am 76:805–840, 1992, with permission.

Multiple causes of urticaria and angioedema have been reported. Clinicians need to investigate all the potential causes. An entity is called idiopathic when no obvious etiology has been identified.

4. What is physical urticaria?

Physical urticaria is a form of urticaria that results from an external stimulus to the skin or a physical activity. Environmental exposure, such as heat, cold, solar irradiation, or water, or stimuli, such as trauma, vibration, pressure, exercise, and dermographism, can cause its development.

5. Define cold urticaria.

Cold urticaria is a form of physical urticaria that is induced by exposure of body parts to cold or icy objects or by exposure of the whole body to a cold environment. A few minutes after exposure of the body part (immediate reaction), urticaria develops at the site of exposure (local reaction). The urticaria can also occur adjacent to the exposed area. Such urticarial reactions can also be delayed (delayed reaction).

6. Briefly review the different types of cold urticaria.

Idiopathic cold urticaria: (also known as **primary cold urticaria**). A type of urticaria in which no known disease is found.

Secondary cold urticaria: Cold urticaria which is associated with systemic diseases such as cryoglobulinemia, cryofibrinogenemia, leukocytoclastic vasculitis, cold agglutinins and hemolysins, and collagen vascular disease or infectious causes such as mononucleosis, syphilis, rubeola, parasitic infections, or hypothyroidism. Griseofulvin and oral contraceptives have also been reported in association with this type of urticaria.   — vc i Ce cure k-

Cold reflex urticaria: A type of urticaria that develops near the area exposed to cold.

Cold-induced cholinergic urticaria: The lesions formed in this type of urticaria resemble cholinergic urticarial lesions. The occurrence of the urticarial lesions is dependent on exercise in a cold environment.

Cold-dependent dermographism: The formation of dermographism occurs on cooled skin (stroking the skin and chilling the area are both required for the reaction to occur).

7. What is cholinergic/heat-induced urticaria?

Heat-induced urticarias are form of physical urticarias and are divided into generalized heat urticaria (cholinergic) or localized heat urticaria. Generalized heat urticaria (cholinergic) comprises up to 7% of all urticaria. The reaction can occur as a result of a hot shower, exercise, sweating, or anxiety. Systemic symptoms, such as wheezing, abdominal cramp, or syncope, can occur. Urticarial lesions of this entity are unique in shape, small, punctate, 1 to 5 mm in diameter with surrounding flare. Localized heat urticaria is either immediate type or delayed type. In immediate type, urticaria lesions develop within 5 minutes of heat exposure and last up to 1 hour. In delayed type, urticaria lesions develop within 6 to 18 hours of heat exposure.

8. What is a solar urticaria?

Solar urticaria is a form of physical urticaria that occurs within 1 to 3 minutes of exposure to light and that disappears within 1 to 3 hours. It has been classified into six types (see Table). Patients in each category are sensitive to a specific range of wavelengths. The lesions may be transferred passively with serum. The classification includes the wavelengths of:

Type	Wavelength
1	2850 to 3200Å
2	3200 to 4000Å
3	4000 to 5000Å
4	4000 to 5000Å
5	2800 to 5000Å
6	4000Å

✓ porphyra

Types 1 and 4 can be transferred passively with serum. Mechanism of Type 1 is reported to be allergic.

9. Describe dermographism.

It is the appearance of the wheal area of patient's skin, after the area is stroked with a blunt object (positive test).

10. Explain aquagenic urticaria.

Aquagenic urticaria is a rare form of physical urticaria. Hives develop upon exposure to water, regardless of the temperature. The aquagenic urticarial lesions resemble cholinergic urticaria. Diagnosis of aquagenic urticaria can be accomplished by water-exposure challenge.

11. What is a vibratory angioedema?

This rare form of physical angioedema can be hereditary or acquired. The acquired form is either idiopathic or occupational. Some examples of the occupational form occur after using a jackhammer or after horseback riding. The edema develops locally, or it can be generalized. Within minutes, pruritus and swelling occurs, peaking 4 to 6 hours later. The pruritus and swelling can last as long as 24 hours.

12. Explain the cause of pressure urticaria/angioedema.

This physical urticaria/angioedema develops as a result of 4 to 8 hours of direct pressure such as walking, sitting, or use of hand tools.

13. What is urticarial vasculitis?

Urticarial vasculitis is unique lesions that have features of both urticaria and vasculitis. The wheals are erythematous, circumscribed, and have foci of purpura. The urticarias usually last longer than 24 hours. Some systemic manifestations have been reported, such as arthralgias, arthritis, pulmonary disease, renal diseases, gastrointestinal disease, and fever. Some of the factors/diseases associated with urticarial vasculitis include: connective tissue diseases, such as systemic lupus erythematosus (SLE); Sjögren's syndrome; serum sickness; infectious diseases, such as hepatitis B and lyme disease; and drugs, such as cimetidine, diltiazem, and procarbazine.

14. Describe Schnitzler's syndrome.

It is a rare syndrome consisting of urticaria, fever, bone pain with osteoconden-sation and IgM gammopathy. The majority of reported cases have an erythrocyte sedimentation rate (ESR) of over 60 mm/hour, a leukocyte count greater than 10,000, and arthralgias.

15. What is papular urticaria?

Papular urticaria is a form of urticaria that results from various insect bites, such as from mosquitoes, chiggers, and fleas. The resulting lesions are pruritic, and can be crusted or excoriated. Management of this type of urticaria includes identification of the source of bites, for example, animal fleas, and removal of the source or avoid-ance. Symptomatic relief using antihistamines is recommended.

16. Which drugs can cause urticaria/angioedema?

The most common drug known to cause urticaria/angioedema is penicillin via an IgE-mediated reaction. Urticarial reaction caused by penicillin can occur within a few minutes or after 10 days. Other antibiotics, such as the cephalosporins and sulfa drugs, have also been reported to cause IgE-mediated reactions.

Drug-induced urticaria/angioedema can also occur as a result of a non-IgE me-diated reaction. Vancomycin-associated "red man syndrome" is a result of a non-IgE–mediated mast cell degranulation. Cyclooxygenase inhibitors, such as aspirin and NSAIDs, are another class of drugs that cause non-IgE–mediated urticaria/an-gioedema. Other classes of medication causing urticaria/angioedema include antihy-pertensive agents, such as angiotensin-converting enzyme inhibitors (angioedema), beta-blockers, diuretics, muscle relaxants, and hyperosmolar radiocontrast media reagents. Over-the-counter medications (such as vitamins and cold remedies) and medications such as psychotropics, sedative tranquilizers, opiates (such as morphine sulfate and codeine), and hormonal preparations (such as birth control pills, thyroid replacement medications, synthetic ACTH, insulins, and chemotherapeutic reagents), have been reported to cause urticaria. Intravenous gamma-globulin prepa-rations, enzymes such as papain, vaccines, and antisera have been shown to cause reactions, as well. Use of intravenous gamma-globulin has also been associated with urticaria/angioedema in certain individuals. Such reactions develop when individu-als with IgA antibody receive intravenous gamma-globulin preparation containing IgA.

17. Can food cause urticaria/angioedema?

Urticaria/angioedema may develop after ingestion of food. Identification of the offending food is at times difficult. If possible, additives to the food items should be identified, because some, such as tartrazine (yellow dye number 5) and benzoic acid derivatives, can be a cause of the reactions.

18. Are there endocrine causes of urticaria and angioedema?

Autoimmune thyroiditis is a known endocrine cause. It has a reported preva-lence of 17%. Hyperthyroidism, hyperparathyroidism, progesterone hypersensitiv-ity, and diabetes mellitus are also associated with urticaria.

19. What is contact urticaria?

Urticarial lesions are produced as a result of contact with a variety of substances such as food, chemicals, drugs, latex, and animal products. The mechanism leading to the urticaria can be allergic, nonallergic, or both. One of the most publicized and common allergic types of contact urticaria is a reaction to latex. Healthcare workers who use rubber gloves are in danger of developing latex hypersensitivity. Chemical additives to rubber during the manufacturing process can also cause contact dermatitis. Contact urticaria and contact dermatitis reportedly coexist in some latex-allergic individuals.

20. Describe hereditary angioedema and acquired C1-INH deficiency. ← *levels* *functional*

Hereditary angioedema is an autosomal dominant disorder in which patients are deficient in C1 inhibitor (C1-INH) and develop angioedema in absence of urticaria. There are two types of C1-INH deficiency, Type 1 and Type 2. Both types have reduced C1-INH functions. Type 1 has reduced levels of C1-INH, whereas Type 2 has normal levels of C1-INH. Therefore, it is important to order a C1-INH functional assay to determine which type is causing angioedema. During the asymptomatic period, C2 level is normal and C4 is reduced. During the symptomatic period, C2 is reduced and C4 is further reduced (see the Table). There is also an acquired form of the disorder in which C1 is reduced. Recommended tests for a workup of hereditary angioedema should include C1, C2, C4, C1-INH, and C1-INH functional assay.

PRESENCE OF SYMPTOMS	C2	C4
−	normal	reduced
+	reduced	further reduced

21. Describe the episodic (and nonepisodic) angioedema that is associated with eosinophilia.

In the early 1980s, four cases of an entity named episodic angioedema associated with eosinophilia were reported. The patients had recurrent angioedema associated with urticaria, weight gain of up to 18%, leukocytosis, and eosinophilia. All patients also had elevated IgM. Glucocorticoid therapy was effective in those who used it. In the late 1990s, several similar cases from Japan were reported although these had a few unique differences from the cases reported earlier, as well as features similar to some of the previously reported "episodic angioedema associated with eosinophilia" cases. The authors proposed the term *nonepisodic angioedema associated with eosinophilia* to describe this unique group. This all-female group had an absence of recurrent attacks and angioedema was localized to the extremities. They also had normal IgM levels. The duration of symptoms was 1 to 2 months, and not all cases had associated urticaria. Thirteen of 33 cases had spontaneous remission, and effective therapy with prednisone in 8 cases and antihistamine in 1 case was reported.

22. What is the possible pathophysiology of urticaria and angioedema?

The pathophysiology of urticaria/angioedema involves degranulation of mast cells. Induction and release of mediators may be a result of IgE-mediated phenomenon when antigen-specific IgE binds to a high-affinity IgE receptor, FcεR1, on the mast cell surface, such as most antibiotics, causing activation and degranulation of

mast cells. Mast cell degranulation may also be a result of non-IgE–mediated phenomenon, such as with vancomycin or polymyxin B which cause direct mast cell degranulation, or agents such as opiates and ionic contrast dyes. The other mechanism of mast cell degranulation is complement mediated, as in acquired angioedema and serum sickness. Regardless of the induction pathways, a variety of mast cell mediators are released. Histamine is a major mediator. Histamine causes the triple reaction of Lewis, which includes erythema (capillary dilatation), flare (arteriolar dilatation), and wheal (extravasation of fluid because of increased vascular permeability). The Figure depicts mast cell inducers and mediators.

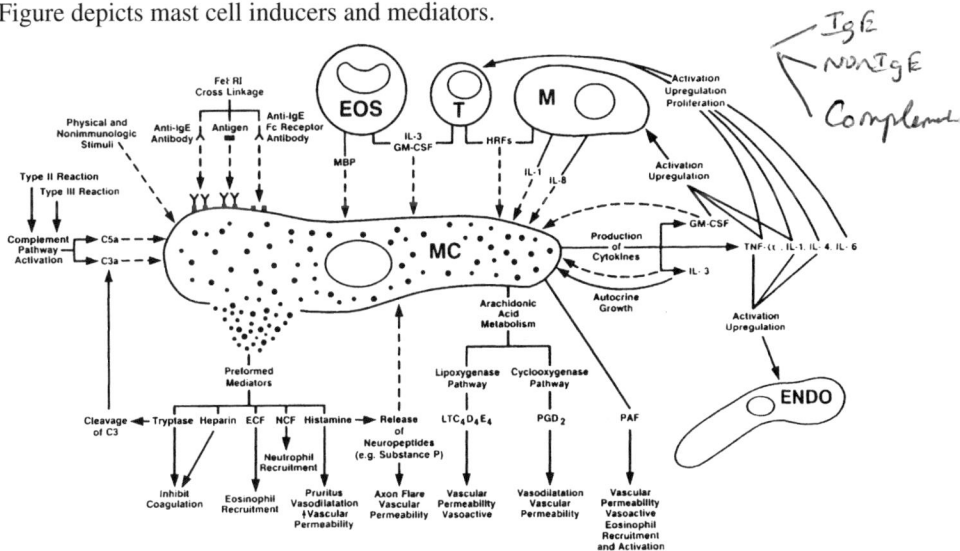

Mast cell activation and degranulation in urticaria and angioedema. MC = mast cell; T = T cell; M = monocyte; EOS = eosinophil; ENDO = endothelial cell; MBP = major basic protein; HRF = histamine-releasing factor; GM-CSF = granulocyte macrophage-colony stimulating factor; PAF = platelet-activating factor; LT = leukotriene; IL = interleuken; NCF = neutrophil chemotactic factor; ECF = eosinophil chemotactic factor; λ = antibody; ■ = antigen; ---→ = degranulation stimulus. (From Huston PH, Bressler RB: Urticaria and angioedema. Med Clin North Am 76:805–840, 1992, with permission.)

23. How should one approach a patient with urticaria and angioedema?

History—Investigation of urticaria/angioedema should be systematic. To start, it is important to acquire a list of medications. Such inquiry should include over-the-counter medications, as well as cold formulas, vitamins, and herbs. It is important to discover whether any new medication(s) have been added or added and stopped in the last several months. At times, patients forget to include over-the-counter, immunotherapy, and injectable medications on their medication lists.

The next step of the history taking is to investigate the onset of symptoms. Physicians should investigate when, how, and where the symptoms started and what the environment was like; that is, cold, hot, icy, and so on. Environmental questions can help physicians, who may be suspicious of cold-, heat-, or solar-induced causes.

The other pertinent question determines what the patient was doing at the time of the onset of the lesions. Examples include the occurrence of the symptoms at the

start of a new job in which the patient used a jackhammer (vibratory urticaria) or when coming from school and noticing the lesions in the areas where a new and heavy backpack was worn (pressure urticaria). When the symptoms started is also a clue in the investigation of the cause of urticaria. Were the symptoms noticed after ingestion of food items, after starting a new medication, or after an insect sting? It is important to find out the sequence of symptoms involved, as well as the areas of the body involved. How long do the reactions usually last and how frequent are the reaction intervals? Were the reactions urticaria, or angioedema, or both? Was pruritus involved? Were the reactions local or systemic? Were life-threatening symptoms such as laryngoedema or hypotension involved?

At times, the patients' complaints are indicative of the type of urticaria/angioedema. For example, a patient's report of developing hives when holding a car's steering wheel in cold weather or when placing hands under cold tap water or in icy water should lead to suspicion of cold-induced urticaria. Sometimes patients report developing hives after local exposure to heat or heated water (local heat-induced) or after a hot shower or after sunbathing (generalized heat-induced or cholinergic urticaria).

The remaining history includes obtaining information on past medical/surgical history. Inquiry should include investigation of recent illness or infections such as viral hepatitis or infectious mononucleosis. Patients should be asked if they have a history of chronic medical conditions such as endocrinopathies (i.e., diabetes, thyroid disease, or malignancies) or atopy. If the past medical/surgical history is benign, then does a review of the system suggest any medical conditions? For example, constipations, cold intolerance, and/or weight gain could be a sign of hypothyroidism.

Family history at times helps to elucidate the etiology of urticaria/angioedema, indicating the presence of the patient's suspected angioedema in family members (hereditary angioedema). Unfortunately, in many cases, the results of investigations are frustrating and there is no obvious etiology (idiopathic urticaria/angioedema).

History key questions

a. *When* did the symptoms start? *What* time of the day was it? Did the symptoms start after ingestion of food or medication? Was it after an insect sting?

b. *What* was the environment like? Did the reaction develop after a cold, heat, or solar exposure?

c. *What* were you doing when the reaction developed? Exercising (if yes, was it outdoor or indoor activity)? Were you swimming? What was the water temperature like? Did the reaction develop while you were doing something involving vibration or pressure? Were you exposed to latex products?

Physical examination—Unfortunately, at the time of presentation to an allergist's office, patients are usually asymptomatic. When the patients present with urticaria and/or angioedema, physicians need to have a focused examination; that is, they need to check for location of hives and angioedema, noting the morphology of the lesions (size; erythema; whether the lesions are sporadic or diffused; whether they are blanchable by pressure). Is dermographism present?

Based on history and suspicion, several tests can be done in office settings: ice cube test; heat-induced test; water exposure test; allergen-induced test (latex); vibratory; pressure; dermographism test; exercise-induced test; skin challenge test. Laboratory tests that help to identify the urticaria/angioedema etiology are summarized in the Table. The last step is management/treatment of the symptoms.

Food and drug reactions	Elimination of offending agent, challenge with suspected foods, lamb and rice diet, special diets eliminating natural salicylates and food additives
Inhalant allergens	Skin tests, in vitro histamine release from human basophils, radioallergosorbent test
Collagen vascular diseases and cutaneous vasculitis	Skin biopsy, CH_{50}, C4, C3, factor B, immuno-fluorescence of tissue
Malignancy with angioedema	CH_{50}, C1q, C4, C1-INH determinations
Cold urticaria	Ice cube test
Solar urticaria	Exposure to defined wavelengths of light, red cell protoporphyrin, fecal protoporphyrin, and coproporphyrin
Demographism	Stroking with narrow object (e.g., tongue blade, fingernail)
Pressure urticaria	Application of pressure for defined time and intensity
Vibratory angioedema	Vibration with laboratory vortex for 4 minutes
Aquagenic urticaria	Challenge with tap water at various temperatures
Urticaria pigmentosa	Skin biopsy, test for dermographism
Hereditary angioedema	C4, C2, C1-INH by protein and function
Familial cold urticaria	Challenge by cold exposure, measurement of temperature, white blood cell count, sedimentation rate, and skin biopsy
C3b inactivator deficiency	C3, factor B, C3b inactivator determinations
Idiopathic	Skin biopsy, immunofluorescence (negative), autologous skin test

Adapted from Kaplan AP: Urticaria and angioedema. In Middleton E, et al (eds): Allergy Principles and Practice, 5th ed. St. Louis, Mosby, 1998, pp 1104–1122.

Physical examination key notes
a. Observe the location of the lesions and their morphology. (Are the lesions sporadic, coalesced, or diffused? Is there erythema?)

b. Press the reaction area. Is the reaction site blanchable on pressure?

c. Perform office tests such as an ice cube test, pressure/vibration/exercise test, latex test, or cold or heat exposure test as suspected by history and if indicated.

24. Describe the ice cube test.
It is a simple test that is done when the physician suspects cold-induced urticaria. The test simply involves placing an ice cube on the volar aspect of the patient's forearm for about 5 minutes. The patient usually feels pruritus within a few minutes of exposure. After removal of the ice, the patient develops a hive in the area of exposure as well as erythema (positive test). Erythema without pruritus or hives, or absence of a reaction is considered a negative test. Hives can also occur in the vicinity of ice exposure (cold-reflex urticaria).

25. How is a dermographism test done?
Dermographism involves a graphic appearance on the skin. The test is performed by striking the volar aspect of the skin with a blunt object. In about 5 minutes, a hivelike reaction develops in the area of stroked skin. At times, the patient

may have cold-induced dermographism, which is defined as the occurrence of dermographism dependent upon cold exposure. Skin is stroked with a blunt object and is then chilled.

26. What is a challenge test?

It is the production of lesions or symptoms by the suspected stimuli. The test needs to be done in an office setting with necessary resuscitation tools. The simplest form of the challenge test is a skin prick/puncture test. Suspicious items, such as food or latex allergens, are introduced to the skin in the presence of positive and negative controls, and the wheal and flares are compared with the controls for interpretation.

27. What is a use test?

This challenge test is used to investigate latex allergies. The patient wears a trimmed latex glove on one digit. After 15 minutes of exposure, the latex glove is removed and the area is inspected for the presence of hives. If hives are not noted where the glove is worn, then the whole glove is worn for the same amount of time. If no reaction is noted after removal of the glove, then the test is considered negative. The glove can also be worn on a damp hand. When performing this challenge test, one has to be cautious about laryngeal edema and systemic symptoms and anaphylaxis.

28. Which test is used for pressure urticaria (angioedema)?

The test is performed by applying a 5- to 15-lb weight on forearm for 10 to 20 minutes. If urticaria or angioedema develop after 4 to 6 hours, then the test is positive.

29. Describe the test for heat-induced urticaria.

Diagnosis of localized heat-induced urticaria involves placing a container with warm water (50 to 55°C) for 5 minutes on the patient's extremity and observing the reactions. Immediate reactions occur within 5 to 10 minutes; delayed reactions develop within 6 to 18 hours. Generalized heat-induced urticaria (cholinergic urticaria) can develop either by intradermal injection of methacholine or by exercise, such as running for 5 to 15 minutes.

30. How are urticaria/angioedema treated and managed?

The goal of management of patients with urticaria/angioedema is to identify the etiology of the reaction and to treat the underlying cause or to avoid the precipitating factor, if possible. For example, in suspected food allergy, patients are encouraged to keep a diary of food items that have been ingested before the reactions. If the food item is not identified, the patient is placed on a simple diet, such as rice and lamb, for 5 days. If the underlying cause of the urticaria/angioedema is food related, then the urticaria/angioedema should resolve on this diet. After urticaria/angioedema resolves, food items can be added to the diet one at a time, every 2 to 3 days, and the patient is checked for reactions. If the cause is not easily identified, an investigation for a systemic disease such as autoimmune thyroiditis, dermatitis herpetiform, erythema multiforme, papular urticaria, or hypersensitivity vasculitis should be performed.

If the underlying cause cannot be identified, then management should focus on symptomatic relief. Oral antihistamines are the mainstay of management, traditional

antihistamines or the second generations of antihistamines. Hydroxyzine, an older-generation antihistamine, is a good choice and can be used to a maximum dose of 200 mg in divided doses. Newer-generation antihistamines such as loratadine (Claritin) 10 mg daily or cetirizine (Zyrtec) 10 mg daily can be used as well. As a note, older-generation antihistamines are sedating and have an anticholinergic effect. Newer antihistamines have none to minimal sedating effect and have no anticholinergic effects. Therefore, patients should be warned not to take a first-generation antihistamine before driving or engaging in any hazardous activity due to the possibility of sedation and impaired judgment. In cold-induced urticaria, cyproheptadine, an H1-receptor antagonist, is the drug of choice. Doxepin is another choice due to its H1 and H2 blockage properties. Antihistamines should be used regularly to prevent reoccurrence of the lesions. If there is no response to antihistamines, a steroid course can be administered. The decision to use a steroid burst or a taper depends on the duration and persistence of hives. Calcium channel blockers are reported to be helpful in patients with chronic idiopathic urticaria. Androgens, such as stanozolol (1–4 mg/day) or danazol (50–400 mg/day), or fibrinolytic agents, such as aminocaproic acid, and tranexamic acid, have been used in hereditary angioedema.

Treatment and management of urticaria/angioedema (summary/key points)

a. Identify the precipitating factor(s) and avoid them if possible.

b. Implement precautionary measures if avoidance is not possible. For example:
  • If underlying urticaria/angioedema is due to bee stings, do not wear shirts/clothing with flowers or bright or dark colors, especially outdoors.
  • Do not wear perfume or colognes when outdoors, as they attract bees.
  • Watch for open containers when outdoors, due to the risk of hidden bees.

c. Treat associated diseases such as hypothyroidism; this might improve the urticaria, although it has not been well studied.

d. Provide symptomatic relief with medications if the precipitating causes are not identified. Carry epinephrine to self-inject in anaphylaxis situations, as in those resulting from bee stings or latex exposures.

BIBLIOGRAPHY

1. Bressler RB, Sowell K, Huston DP: Therapy of chronic idiopathic urticaria with nifedipine: Demonstration of beneficial effect in a double-blinded, placebo-controlled, crossover trial. J Allergy Clin Immunol 83:756–763, 1989.
2. Chikama R, Hosokawa M, Miyazawa T, et al: Nonepisodic angioedema associated with eosinophilia: Report of 4 cases and review of 33 young female patients reported in Japan. Dermatology 197:321–325, 1998.
3. Gleich GJ, Schroeter AL, Marcoux JP, et al: Episodic angioedema associated with eosinophilia. N Engl J Med 310:1621–1626, 1984.
4. Harber LC, Holloway RM, Whealty VR, et al: Immunologic and biophysical studies in solar urticaria. J Invest Dermatol 41:439–443, 1963.
5. Howard R, Frieden IJ: Papular urticaria in children. Pediatr Dermatol 13:246–249, 1996.
6. Huston PH, Bressler RB: Urticaria and angioedema. In Bush RK (ed): Clinical Allergy: The Medical Clinics of North America. Philadelphia, WB Saunders, 1992.
7. Kaplan AP: Urticaria and angioedema. In Middleton E Jr, Reed CE, Ellis EF, et al (eds): Allergy Principles and Practice, vol. 2, 5th ed. St. Louis, Mosby, 1998, pp 1104–1122.
8. Kontou-Fili K, Borici-Mazi R, Kapp A, et al: Physical urticaria: Classification and diagnostic guidelines, an EAACI position paper. Allergy 52:504–513, 1997.
9. Leznoff A: Chronic urticaria. Can Fam Physician 44:2170–2176, 1998.
10. O'Donnell B, Black AK: Urticarial vasculitis. Int Angiol 14:166–174, 1995.

11. Mahmoudi M, Dinneen AM, Hunt LW: Simultaneous IgE-mediated urticaria and contact dermatitis from latex. Allergy 53:1009–1010, 1998.
12. Mydlarski PR, Katz AM, Sauder DN: Contact dermatitis. In Middleton E Jr, Reed CE, Ellis EF, et al (eds): Allergy Principles and Practice, vol. 2, 5th ed. St. Louis, Mosby 1998, pp 1135–1147.
13. Puddu P, Cianchini G, Girardelli CR, et al: Schnitzler's syndrome: Report of a new case and a review of the literature. Clin Exp Rheumatol 15:91–95, 1997.
14. Sharma JK, Miller R. Chronic urticaria: Review of the literature. J Cutan Med Surg 3:221–228, 1999.
15. Wanderer AA, Grandel KE, Wasserman SI, et al: Clinical characteristics of cold-induced systemic reactions in acquired cold urticaria syndromes: Recommendations for prevention of this complication and a proposal for a diagnostic classification of cold urticaria. J Allergy Clin Immunol 78:417–423, 1986.

9. ATOPIC DERMATITIS

Rosemary Hallett, M.D.

1. What is atopic dermatitis?

Atopic dermatitis is a chronic, relapsing inflammatory skin condition character-ized by extreme pruritus, edema, exudation, crusting, and scaling. It has been termed "the itch that rashes" because there is no primary skin lesion. The rash is caused by scratching and excoriation in response to the pruritus. Atopic dermatitis has a chronic, relapsing course. Irritation and rubbing lead to lichenification in chronic lesions. All of the skin is prone to generalized dryness, even uninvolved areas.

2. What diseases make up the allergic triad?

Asthma, allergic rhinitis, and atopic dermatitis. Children with atopic dermatitis tend to experience allergic rhinitis and asthma subsequently. These three diseases affect 8–25% percent of the worldwide population. The incidence is higher in de-veloped countries and urban areas, particularly western societies, but they may occur in any race or geographic location. Children with atopic dermatitis tend to have more severe asthma than asthmatic children without atopic dermatitis. The al-lergen sensitization through the skin may cause a more severe and persistent respi-ratory disease.

3. Is there a genetic basis for atopic dermatitis?

Almost 50% of patients with atopic dermatitis have a family history of atopy. Of interest, the trait for atopy may be inherited via a maternal gene located on chromosome 11, and clinical studies have demonstrated a higher risk of atopy if there is a history on the maternal side as opposed to the paternal side. Other inter-est has been in chromosome 5q31-33, which contains genes for cytokines inter-leukin (IL)-3, IL-4, IL-5, IL-13, and granulocyte-macrophage colony-stimulating factor (GM-CSF)

4. Has the incidence of atopic dermatitis changed?

The incidence has increased, paralleling the increase in asthma and allergic rhinitis.

5. What are the specific anatomic distributions of atopic dermatitis? How do they vary with age?

The infantile form is characterized by lesions on the face, trunk, neck, and ex-tensor surfaces of the extremities. The anatomic distribution changes as patients age, and lesions occur on the flexor surfaces—antecubital fossa, popliteal fossa, neck, hands, and feet. Adults may have more hand involvement associated with occupa-tional work (e.g., wet, frictional work or exposure to chemicals). Any area of the body can be involved in severe cases, although it is uncommon to see lesions in some flexor surfaces, such as the axillary, gluteal, or groin area. If such lesions are present, another diagnosis should be considered.

6. At what age does atopic dermatitis start?

It usually begins in infancy; 49–75% of patients present by 6 months of age, usually within the first 2–3 months. By the age of 5 years there is a tendency to remission, but the dermatitis may persist in the adult form with lesions in the antecubital and popliteal fossae, on the wrists, behind the ears. and on the face and neck. By 5 years, 80–90% of patients have the disease. Patients tend to grow out of their disease, and the incidence drops to 10–15% by age 14. However, if an adolescent has moderate-to-severe atopic dermatitis, it is likely to persist into adulthood in more than 80% of patients. Characteristics for a poorer prognosis include severe childhood disease, family histories of atopic dermatitis, associated asthma or allergic rhinitis, onset before the age of 1 year, and female gender. Adult onset should raise a higher index of suspicion for other diseases.

7. What are the different stages of atopic dermatitis?

Acute lesions are characterized by erythema and scaling. Tiny erythematous vesicles may rupture and weep. Intraepidermal vesiculation (spongiosis) is present. Subacute lesions develop mild scaling and lichenification. As the lesions become more chronic, scaling and lichenification are more prominent, with minimal skin erythema. Chronic lesions may be hyper- or hypopigmented.

8. How is the diagnosis of atopic dermatitis made?

The diagnosis is clinical; there are no definitive lab tests. The main feature is pruritus. Other key findings include a chronic, relapsing course, family history of atopy, and early age of onset. Distribution of skin findings is more important than the actual appearance of the individual lesions. Other characteristics include accentuated lines or grooves below the margin of the lower eyelids (atopic pleat, Dennie's line, or Morgan's fold), periorbital darkening, palmar hyperlinearity, and keratosis pilaris (rough sandpaper texture from follicular accentuation to lateral aspects of the arms and thighs). Guidelines devised in 1980 require all three major criteria and three or more minor criteria.

Major criteria
- Pruritus
- Dermatitis affecting flexural surfaces in adults and face and extensor surfaces in infants
- Chronic or relapsing dermatitis

Minor criteria

Features of the so-called "atopic facies"
- Facial pallor or erythema
- Hypopigmented patches
- Infraorbital darkening
- Infraorbital folds or wrinkles
- Cheilitis
- Recurrent conjunctivitis
- Anterior neck folds

Triggers of atopic dermatitis
- Foods
- Emotional factors
- Environmental factors
- Skin irritants (e.g., wool, solvents, sweat)
- Complications of atopic dermatitis
- Susceptibility to cutaneous viral and bacterial infections
- Impaired cell-mediated immunity
- Immediate skin test reactivity
- Raised serum IgE
- Keratoconus
- Anterior subcapsular cataracts

Others
- Early age of onset
- Dry skin
- Ichthyosis
- Hyperlinear palms
- Keratosis pilaris
- Hand and foot dermatitis
- Nipple eczema
- White dermatographism
- Perifollicular accentuation

Although no lab test is definitive, in about 80% of patients with atopic dermatitis serum IgE concentrations are increased 5–10-fold above normal. IgE levels fluctuate with the stage of the disease and return to normal when the disease is inactive. However, IgE levels are not used routinely in the evaluation of patients with suspected atopic dermatitis. Allergy testing may be indicated in patients with reactions to aeroallergens, such as asthma and rhinitis, and in children with food sensitivity.

9. **What other diagnoses need to be considered?**
- Other eczematous and dermatitis conditions, including nummular eczema, dyshidrotic eczema, and seborrheic dermatitis.
- Allergic and irritant contact dermatitis, which can mimic and be associated with atopic dermatitis.
- Stasis dermatitis
- Systemic diseases
- Immunodeficiency diseases
- Certain malignancies
- Infectious agents

10. **Describe the typical features of nummular and dyshidrotic eczema.**

Nummular eczema is characterized by circular or oval, coinlike lesions. The most common locations are on the trunk or the extensor surfaces of the extremities, particularly on the pretibial areas or dorsum of the hands. Dyshidrotic eczema is located on the palmar and plantar sides of the palms, fingers and soles.

11. **What are the typical features of seborrheic dermatitis?**

Seborrheic dermatitis describes greasy, brownish scales usually seen on the scalp and often beginning as "cradle cap." It also may involve the ear and contiguous skin, sides of the nose, eyebrows, and eyelids. Sometimes in infancy it is difficult to distinguish seborrheic dermatitis from atopic dermatitis, particularly when the face is primarily involved. Seborrhea in infancy has a shorter course than atopic dermatitis and responds much more rapidly to treatment.

12. **Describe the characteristics of allergic contact dermatitis. What are the most common causes?**

Allergic contact dermatitis first requires sensitization to an antigen, which takes approximately 1 week. On re-exposure to the antigen, an eczematous reaction may become clinically apparent in 1–2 days. The lesions may be linear, arcuate, or well-demarcated patches in the configuration of contact with the offending agent. It is usually not seen in the flexural areas. Common causes include neomycin; preservatives used in topical ointments; poison ivy, oak, and sumac; nickel; cosmetics; and latex.

13. How is irritant contact dermatitis characterized?

Irritant dermatitis is a nonallergic reaction caused by various compounds; it is an extremely common form of eczema. It also has a sharply demarcated morphologic configuration in the area of the applied irritant. It is commonly seen in infancy in the perioral area (due to fruit juices) and diaper areas.

14. What do allergic and irritant contact dermatitis have in common?

Both allergic and irritant contact dermatitis can have acute, subacute, and chronic forms. Patients with atopic dermatitis are particularly prone to both allergic and irritant contact dermatitis in addition to atopic dermatitis lesions. Patients with atopic dermatitis use numerous creams and medications. Patients with active or inactive atopic dermatitis have a greater skin response to an irritant compared with healthy controls. The mechanism is unclear but may be secondary to an intrinsic hyperreactivity in inflammatory cells. Allergic and irritant contact dermatitis may result from numerous creams and medications applied to the skin.

15. What is stasis dermatitis? What other lesions may be mistaken for atopic dermatitis?

Stasis dermatitis develops on the lower extremities secondary to venous incompetence and chronic edema. Early findings may consist of mild erythema and scaling associated with pruritus with pigmented hemosiderin deposits.

Psoriasis has scaly, silvery patches that may be mistaken for atopic dermatitis. The lesions are variably pruritic. Common areas for psoriasis are the elbows, knees, gluteal cleft, and scalp; lesions usually are symmetrical.

Ichthyosis vulgaris causes scales that are larger than those of atopic dermatitis. The pruritus is usually milder.

Children with **untreated phenylketonuria** acquire an eczematous dermatitis often confused with atopic eczema. It is responsive to a diet low in phenylalanine.

16. Which systemic diseases may cause skin lesions resembling atopic dermatitis?

Histiocytosis X (Letterer-Siwe disease, Langerhan cell histiocytosis) and **acrodermatitis enteropathica** are serious systemic diseases occurring early in life. They usually present with failure to thrive. Hemorrhagic manifestations are common in the eczematous eruption of histiocytosis X. In acrodermatitis, the skin around the oral, nasal, genitourinary, and rectal areas usually is involved.

17. What immunodeficiency diseases may be associated with skin lesions resembling atopic dermatitis?

- Wiskott-Aldrich syndrome
- X-linked agammaglobulinemia
- Ataxia-telangiectasia
- Job's syndrome
- Hyper IgE syndrome
- Biotinidase deficiency

18. What malignancies need to be considered in the differential diagnosis?

Cutaneous T-cell lymphoma is usually asymmetric and pruritic with no scales. Sezary syndrome may involve the whole body. Both malignancies need to be considered, particularly in adults and nonresponsive patients.

19. What infectious agents may be confused with atopic dermatitis?

Candida spp., herpes simplex, *Staphylococcus aureus*, and scabies need to be considered. Scabies lesions are located on the palms and soles with vesicles and commonly start with large papules on the upper back. The mite of scabies or its ova can be seen in scrapings from the vesicles.

20. Describe the immunologic abnormalities behind atopic dermatitis.

Atopy is characterized immunologically by reduced cell-mediated immunity, defective antibody-dependent cellular cytotoxicity, decreased numbers of immunoregulatory T cells, high concentrations of serum IgE, and a high incidence of IgE-mediated responses on skin testing to common inhaled antigens. Patients with atopic dermatitis have elevated numbers of circulating eosinophils and increased serum IgE levels.

21. Explain the chronic inflammatory process associated with atopic dermatitis.

Atopic dermatitis is caused by a chronic inflammatory process that is similar to the inflammatory cascade in the airways of asthmatics. Atopic patients have a genetic tendency toward the expression of allergen-specific CD4 lymphocytes that induce T_H2 cytokines, resulting in a cascade of cytokines IL-4, IL-5, and IL-13 and a reduced ability to produce interferon-γ. These cytokines induce migration of eosinophils, release of mast cells, and a change in the immunoglobulin isotype to IgE. An abnormally high level of macrophage migration inhibitory factor is needed for T-cell activation and is expressed primarily in activated T_H2 cells. Peripheral blood monocytes from patients with atopic dermatitis also have a lower incidence of spontaneous apoptosis and are unresponsive to IL-4–induced apoptosis after stimulation. Cytokines IL-4 and IL-13 are responsible for promoting isotype switching to IgE. They also inhibit T_H1 cytokines and upregulate CD23 on monocytes and B cells. IL-4 and IL-13 stimulate RANTES (regulated on activation normally T-cell expressed and secreted), eotaxin, and monocyte chemotactic protein (MCP)-1 expression in fibroblasts, probably leading to a local eosinophil infiltration.

22. What determines the location of allergic disease?

The location of allergic disease is thought to be determined by the route of allergen sensitization, tissue chemokine expression, and tissue compartmentalization of immune responses. Memory T cells have the ability to migrate to different tissues. In atopic dermatitis, the T cells that infiltrate the skin contain a cell adhesion molecule called cutaneous lymphocyte-associated (CLA) antigen. T cells migrating into the skin express significantly higher levels of CLA than T cells isolated from the airway of asthmatics. Thus the inflammatory process moves to the skin as opposed to the airways in asthmatics. Patients with atopic dermatitis have an increased number of CLA-positive T cells in the circulation. CLA-positive T cells secrete IL-5 and IL-13, prolong eosinophil survival, and induce IgE synthesis.

Local tissue expression of chemokines probably plays a major role in the localization of sites of inflammation, especially for eosinophils, which are not known to have specific tissue homing receptors. A chemokine (CTACK/CCL27) may cause CLA antigen to be induced on T cells. Other chemoattractants, such as IL-16, attract CD4-positive T cells in acute lesions vs. chronic lesions. The C-C chemokines,

RANTES, MCP-4, and eotaxin also are found in higher concentrations in the skin of patients with atopic dermatitis. These higher concentrations probably attract eosinophils and T_H2 lymphocytes into the skin. The chemokine receptor CCR3 also may be involved in mediating chemokines to attract inflammatory cells. Leukotriene B4 also is released on exposure to allergens and may act as a chemoattractant for the initial influx of inflammatory cells.

23. What promotes the chronicity of atopic dermatitis on an immunologic basis?
   Eosinophils and monocyte macrophages have a prolonged survival in atopic skin, perhaps secondary to the expression of IL-5, which promotes eosinophil survival and function. Epidermal keratinocytes and infiltrating macrophages also cause an increase in GM-CSF, which maintains survival and function of monocytes, Langerhan cells, and eosinophils. Epidermal keratinocytes, when stimulated with interferon-γ and tumor necrosing factor alpha (TNF-α) were found to produce increased levels of RANTES, which enhance the chemotaxis of eosinophils. Mechanical trauma also can induce the release of TNF-α and other cytokines.

24. Explain the immunologic basis for the pruritus.
   The cause of pruritis is not completely understood, but proinflammatory mediators and cytokines are thought to play a role. Histamine injected into the skin demonstrates a lower itch threshold in atopic skin. Histamine levels are increased in all areas of skin in patients with atopic dermatitis, not simply areas that are affected directly. Lichenified areas are characterized by an increase in mast cells. Substance P, a neuropeptide that induces mast cell degranulation, also is increased in the skin of patients with atopic dermatitis, along with increased releasability of histamine from basophils. Of interest, the injection of acetylcholine into the skin increases pruritus, possibly indicating that the mechanism is not completely dependent on histamine. Blocking the cytokines also reduces the pruritus. Other mediators, such as leukotrienes, neuropeptides, and proteases, also can induce pruritus. Nonantigenic mechanisms may play a role in pruritus and inflammatory response. Patients with atopic dermatitis have a lower threshold of itch and cutaneous hyperreactivity. Mechanical trauma to the keratinocytes results in a cytokine and proinflammatory cascade, possibly causing the pruritus.

25. What cells are seen in the skin of patients with atopic dermatitis?
   Acute skin lesions have intercellular edema of the epidermis called **spongiosis**. Antigen-presenting cells in the skin, such as Langerhan cells and macrophages, have surface-bound IgE molecules. Acute lesions have an infiltrate of perivenular T cells. The infiltrate usually is activated memory T cells with CD3, CD4, and CD45 RO, indicating prior sensitization. Mast cells are present in various stages of degranulation. Chronic lesions have minimal spongiosis. IgE-bearing Langerhan cells and eosinophils are increased, and macrophages are abundant. Hyperplastic epidermis is present, and hyperkeratosis is prominent in areas of lichenification. Mast cells are usually fully granulated. Eosinophil proteins are found in the elastic fibers throughout the upper dermis. Eosinophil major basic protein, eosinophil cationic protein, and eosinophil-derived neutrotoxin are elevated in atopic dermatitis sera and correlated with disease severity.

26. What pathologic mechanisms other than immunologic abnormalities are associated with atopic dermatitis?

Defective skin barrier function, decreased water content in the skin, reduced water-binding capacity, and higher transepidermal water loss.

27. What are the common triggers for a flare of atopic dermatitis?

Irritants, allergens, soaps, detergents, fabric softeners, and physical environment. Flares also can be triggered by infectious agents, emotional stressors, and abrasive or occlusive clothing. In adolescent patients, these triggers may be reason to avoid certain occupations (e.g., those with excessive exposures).

28. What recommendations should be made about altering the physical environment?

Extremes of heat and humidity should be avoided. A warm climate with moderate humidity is optimal for most patients. Exposure to sunlight and salt water is of benefit to many patients, but sunburns should be avoided with nonirritating sunblock. In humid conditions, care should be taken to avoid sweat retention, which can lead to "prickly heat" rash or miliaria rubra and miliaria pustulosa. Clothing should be light and nonocclusive. Cotton is less irritating than polyester or wool.

29. How do food allergies manifest in children with atopic dermatitis?

Food allergies have a greater significance in childhood. The onset of dermatitis frequently coincides with the introduction of certain foods into the infant's diet. Cutaneous symptoms develop after food challenges in 50–90% of patients. Common food allergies and possible triggers for atopic dermatitis in children include egg, milk, peanut, soybean, and wheat. Overall, about 20–30% of children with eczema have food hypersensitivity to one or more of the six common allergens. Even continued ingestion of small amounts can provoke chronic inflammation.

Children tend to outgrow food allergies, which are not common triggers for atopic dermatitis in adults. Arbitrary exclusion of numerous foods from the diets of infants without clear evidence that they are involved in the disease can lead to malnutrition, and the causative agent should be identified through double-blinded food challenges. In pediatric patients, food allergen sensitization can be reduced by breastfeeding and by delaying the introduction of solid foods until after 6 months of age. Breast-feeding mothers should avoid ingestion of high-risk foods in atopic-prone infants to reduce sensitization.

30. What is the significance of food allergies in adults?

Adults should be evaluated for food allergies if they have a relevant history. Skin testing and evaluation of IgE have a high incidence of false-positive results. Immediate skin tests to specific allergens do not always indicate clinical sensitivity, and patients who outgrow atopic dermatitis frequently continue to have positive skin tests. This finding suggests that the relationship is not exclusively dependent on IgE-mediated mast cell degranulation. If food is believed to be a possible cause in patients with serious atopic dermatitis, an elemental diet may be followed with reintroductions of foods one at a time and observation for flares.

31. Describe the role of aeroallergens and household allergens in atopic dermatitis.

Aeroallergens play more of a role as the atopic child grows older. Studies have shown worsening of symptoms with patch testing of aeroallergens. Inhalation of aeroallergens may exacerbate the skin disease. Sera from 95% of patients with atopic dermatitis had IgE to house dust mites compared with 42% of asthmatic patients. House dust mite-specific lymphocyte stimulation is greatly elevated in infants with atopic dermatitis. Recommendations of empiric avoidance of dust mite and animal danders may be warranted because avoidance improves symptoms.

32. Immunotherapy improves symptoms of allergic rhinitis and asthma. Can it be used for atopic dermatitis?

There is no role for immunotherapy in patients with atopic dermatitis. Anecdotally it has been associated with both aggravation and improvement of dermatitis. Immunotherapy may help other atopic diseases in the patient.

33. What role do infectious agents play in flares of atopic dermatitis?

Dry, xerotic skin creates small fissures that can serve as an entry to skin pathogens. Patients with atopic dermatitis have an increased tendency for development of bacterial and fungal skin infections. The most common pathogens are *Staphylococcus aureus* and herpes simplex. *S. aureus* is colonized on the skin of 90% of patients with atopic dermatitis compared with only 5% of healthy people. Empiric treatment with oral antibiotics often results in improvement, even if no active infection is seen. Observation of pustules within areas of dermatitis indicates that *S. aureus* may be present.

34. How are bacterial and fungal skin infections treated?

An antibiotic with good staphylococcal coverage, such as cephalexin or dicloxacillin, should be administered for 3–4 weeks. Some patients may require longer treatment (6–12 weeks). Bactroban can be used for early topical treatment and also can be applied to the nares of staphylococcal carriers who experience frequent relapses when antibiotics are discontinued. However, other topical antibiotics are of little therapeutic value and can lead to sensitization to the agents, particularly neomycin.

35. Describe the immunologic mechanism of a flare caused by *S. aureus*.

S. aureus secretes exotoxins that act as superantigens. These superantigens activate T cells and macrophages. Cultures of *S. aureus* on the skin of atopic patients show that one-half of the organisms secrete enterotoxins A and B and toxic shock syndrome toxin-1 (TSST-1). The enterotoxins act as superantigens and inhibit monocyte apoptosis by stimulating GM-CSF. Most patients with atopic dermatitis make specific IgE antibodies directed against the staphylococcal toxins found on skin. Basophils then release histamine when exposed to the IgE-specific toxin.

36. What other infections can contribute to atopic dermatitis?

Malassezia furfur (Pityrosporum ovale) is a saprophytic yeast that can be found as part of normal skin flora. It is commonly present in the seborrheic areas of the

skin. Patients with atopic dermatitis may have IgE antibodies to *M. furfur*; such antibodies are more common in patients with head and neck dermatitis. Healthy controls
or asthmatic patients rarely have IgE sensitization to *M. furfur*. Treatment involves
antimycotic therapy. Other skin lesions include common warts and molluscum con-
tagiosum, which probably result not from an immunologic mechanism but from decreased inherent resistance and increased autoinoculation.

37. How does herpes simplex manifest in atopic dermatitis?
Herpes simplex may begin as a cold sore and then become generalized and
complicated by ocular involvement. It may present as umbilicated vesicles or
grouped erosions. Systemic dissemination associated with generalized vesicular and
pustular lesions, fever, and constitutional symptoms has a 20% mortality rate.

38. Is atopic dermatitis associated with an autoimmune component?
Early studies showing sensitivity to human skin dander and an increase in cell
proliferation with human skin extracts in patients with atopic dermatitis suggested
that an autoallergen component may be involved. Recently, IgE to human proteins
has been seen in patients with severe disease. The involved autoallergens are intracellular proteins and have been identified in IgE immune complexes. These antibodies were not seen in patients with other autoimmune diseases, such as chronic
urticaria and systemic lupus erythematosus, or in healthy controls.

39. Describe the role of emotional stressors in atopic dermatitis.
Emotional stressors induce flares of atopic dermatitis. Patients should be advised to seek psychological counseling or behavior modification and to reduce stress
at school and home.

40. What ocular symptoms may be seen?
Keratoconus is occasionally seen in children with atopic dermatitis, possibly
secondary to chronic rubbing of the eyelids. Cataracts, rarely seen in children, occur
in 5–10% of adults with severe disease.

41. How is atopic dermatitis treated?
Standard treatment for atopic dermatitis is focused on topical anti-inflammatory
preparations and lubrication of the skin. Advances in treatment have focused on
immune regulation; however, standard modalities are the starting point.

42. What measures should be taken to protect the skin?
Treatment should be aimed at controlling the itch-scratch cycle and hydration of
the skin. The keys are avoidance of triggers and good skin care. The general principles of skin care include hydration and emollients. Hydration involves short baths
(15–20 minutes) in tepid water. Patients should avoid excessively hot water and extended submersions. Mild, moisturizing soaps should be used (e.g., Dove, Cetaphil).
Bubble bath can cause excessive irritation. Colloidal oatmeal or baking soda can be
added to the bath for an antipruritic effect. Bath oils, however, are not effective because they coat the outer layer of the skin and may seal out the moisture in the hy-
drated skin. Patients should pat dry and avoid excessive toweling and rubbing.

Creams should be applied immediately after bathing to retain hydration. Lotions have a high water and low oil content and may contain alcohol, which can worsen xerosis via evaporation and trigger a flare of the disease. In contrast, thick creams (e.g., Eucerin, Cetaphil, Nutraderm), which have a low water content, or ointments (e.g., petroleum jelly, Aquaphor, Petrolatum), which have zero water content, offer better protection against xerosis. Emollients are less expensive than corticosteroids, control the itch, and have no side effects. Emollients containing alcohol should be avoided. The cheaper alternatives, including petroleum jelly, mineral oil, and Crisco, can be just as effective. Another cheap but highly effective alternative is udder cream (Bag Balm). Care should be taken to avoid irritating ingredients such as methylsalicylate. Nails should be trimmed short to avoid excessive trauma to the skin. Cotton gloves can be worn at night to decrease scratching during sleep.

43. What medication is recommended for treatment of atopic dermatitis?

The backbone of topical medication for atopic dermatitis is corticosteroids. The goal of therapy should be low-potency corticosteroids and emollients for maintenance therapy and mid- and high-potency corticosteroids for exacerbations. Hydrocortisone (1–2.5%) is useful for patients with mild disease. A medium-potency corticosteroid ointment (triamcinolone 0.1%) can be used for more severe disease. Higher-potency topical steroids can be used for a short period in some patients with acute flares, then reduced to a lower potency when the lesions improve. Areas of lichenified skin may require stronger steroids in a thicker form for prolonged periods. Topical steroids should be applied twice daily and may be mixed with an emollient base. Ointments and creams have a thicker consistency and may increase the potency of a steroid compared with lotions. They are preferred but may not be as well tolerated. Occlusive bandages further increase the potency of the steroid.

44. What are the common side effects of topical steroids?

Topical steroids are divided into groups based on potency. The ultra-high-potency steroids have more a pronounced side-effect profile and must be prescribed judiciously. Patients must be educated about duration of usage and areas to avoid. High-potency corticosteroids should be avoided on the face, genitalia, and intertriginous areas. Side effects include skin atrophy, telangiectasia, striae, and suppression of the hypothalamic-pituitary-adrenal axis. High-potency corticosteroids should be used only for a short period and in areas that are lichenified and not easily treated with mid-potency steroids.

45. When should systemic steroids be used?

Oral steroids may be used for severe flares (e.g., prednisone, 40–60 mg/day for 3–4 days, then 20–30 mg/day for 3–4 days). Dramatic rebound flares may be seen on discontinuation. Short courses can be used in conjunction with an intensified topical program.

46. Describe the role of antihistamines.

Histamines play a minor role in pruritus. No large randomized, placebo-controlled trials support their use. Many patients experience relief with antihistamines, but it is unclear whether it is due to the antipruritic or sedating effect. Nighttime

dosing can provide antihistaminic effect without daytime sedation. The H_1 blockers hydroxyzine and cetirizine are particularly effective because they block some IgE-mediated late-phase response. Hydroxyzine can be used in large doses (75–100 mg) at bedtime. Because topical antihistamines can be sensitizing, direct application to the skin is not recommended.

47. What about other drugs with antihistaminic effects?
Doxepin is a tricyclic antidepressant with antihistamine effects. A single dose at bedtime can be effective. H_2 blockers may be a helpful adjunct for refractory pruritus.

48. What effect do dressings have on atopic dermatitis?
Wet dressings are highly effective as an adjunct to therapy and for acute flares. Ointment is applied directly after bathing, followed by wet dressings with a dry cover. One option is a 1:20 Burow's solution. Wet pajamas can be applied over lotions if the extremities are involved and covered with a dry pair of pajamas or sweat suit. This technique, which also can be applied to the face and hands, is best suited for overnight use.

49. Describe the use of coal tar extracts for severe disease.
Coal tar extracts may applied during bathing if the above measures are not effective. Acute use can cause stinging and irritation and is not well tolerated because of odor.

50. Discuss the role of phototherapy.
Phototherapy combined with PUVA (psoralens plus ultraviolet A radiation) or combinations of ultraviolet A (UVA) and ultraviolet B (UVB) help to control the disease. The combination of UVA and UVB is better than either therapy alone. Disadvantages include an increased risk of skin cancer and expense. This modality is best used by a dermatologist familiar with both atopic dermatitis and phototherapy.

51. How is cyclosporine used? What are its side effects?
Oral cyclosporine (3–6 mg/kg/day) has been shown to be beneficial for severe atopic dermatitis unresponsive to topical corticosteroids, but its use is limited by side effects, including nausea, hypertrichosis, hypertension, paresthesias, and hepatic and renal toxicity. Serum should be monitored monthly with blood pressure and renal function. Cyclosporine typically is used for 6 weeks, and the disease may flare on discontinuation. Topical cyclosporine has not been shown to be effective.

52. What other drugs have been used?
Azathioprine and methotrexate may be helpful. Topical tacrolimus (FK 506) reduces clinical symptoms. Its action is similar to that of cyclosporine with a better safety profile.

53. What alternative modalities may be promising for the future?
Recombinant interferon-γ has been shown to be safe and effective in a randomized, controlled trial. Studies with interferon-α have had equivocal results. These modalities are expensive and require patient education. They have not been in the

forefront of research. Intravenous immunoglobulin dosed at 2 gm/kg showed clinical improvement, decreased steroid usage, and reduced skin-test reactivity to allergens. It also reduces IL-4 protein expression in patients with atopic dermatitis. At this time further research is needed. Leukotriene antagonists may have a role in treatment of atopic dermatitis, as demonstrated in a study of 4 patients. Chinese herbal medicines have been reported to be helpful, but they are associated with liver toxicity. The herbal content has not been well characterized, and many formulations have been shown to contain corticosteroids.

54. When are the indications for referral to a dermatologist or an allergist?
- Severe or persistent disease with 20% general skin involvement
- Severe or persistent disease with 10% skin involvement affecting eyelids, hands, or intertriginous areas
- Disease unresponsive to first-line therapy
- Erythroderma or extensive exfoliation
- Disease that requires more than one course of systemic corticosteroids
- Disease that requires admission to hospital for atopic dermatitis
- Identification of allergen and triggers
- Intensive education
- Associated asthma or rhinitis
- Impaired quality of life
- Infection
- Ocular complications
- Psychosocial complications
- Uncertainty of diagnosis

55. What is the prognosis of atopic dermatitis?
Dermatitis usually can be controlled with control of triggers, local treatments, and counseling of patients (including the fact that no immediate cure is available). Quality of life can be severely impaired because of disruption of school, family, and social interactions. Poor sleep due to intense pruritus can also impair quality of life. Of interest, when parents of patients with atopic dermatitis and asthma were asked which disease was more difficult to deal with, most of them chose atopic dermatitis. Atopic dermatitisis a chronic, relapsing disease that can be highly frustrating for families. Education and support are vital. For additional information the patient can contact the National Eczema Association for Science and Education (1-800-818-7456; website: http://eczema-assn.org).

BIBLIOGRAPHY

1. Behrman RE, et al (eds): Nelson Textbook of Pediatrics, 16th ed. Philadelphia, W.B. Saunders, 2000.
2. Bratton DL, et al: GM-CSF inhibition of monocyte apoptosis contributes to the chronic monocyte activation in atopic dermatitis. J Clin Invest 95:211–218, 1995.
3. Bratton DL, et al: Staphylococcal toxic shock syndrome toxin-1 inhibits monocyte apoptosis. J Allergy Clin Immunol 103:895–900, 1999.
4. Bunikawskin R, et al: Prevalence and role of serum IgE antibodies to the *Staphylococcus aureus*-derived superantigens. J Allergy Clin Immunol 103:119–124, 1999.
5. Callen JP: Current Practice of Dermatology. New York, McGraw-Hill, 1996.

6. Carucci JA, et al: The leukotriene antagonist zafirlukast as a therapeutic agent for atopic dermatitis. Arch Dermatol 134:785–786, 1998.
7. Cookson,WO, Young RP, Sanford AJ, et al: Maternal inheritance of atopic IgE responsiveness on chromosome 11q. Lancet 340:381, 1992.
8. Forrest S, et al: Identifying genes predisposing to atopic dermatitis. J Allergy Clin Immunol 105:1066–1070, 1999.
9. Hanifin JM, Rajka G: Diagnostic features of atopic dermatitis. Acta Dermatol Venereol 92(Suppl):44, 1980.
10. Hashem N, et al: Infantile eczema: Evidence of autoimmunity to human skin. Lancet 2:269–270, 1963.
11. Jolles S, et al: Intracellular interleukin-4 profiles during high-dose intravenous immunoglobulin treatment of therapy-resistant atopic dermatitis. J Am Acad Dermatol 40:121–123, 1999.
12. Keane FM: Analysis of Chinese herbal creams prescribed for dermatological conditions. BMJ 318:563–564, 1999.
13. Klein PA, Clark RA: An evidence-based review of the efficacy of antihistamines in relieving pruritus in atopic dermatitis. Arch Dermatol 135:1522, 1999.
14. Koro OF, et al: Chemical mediators in atopic dermatitis: Involvement of leukotriene B4 released by a type I allergic reaction in the pathogenesis of atopic dermatitis. J Allergy Clin Immunol 103:663–670, 1999.
15. Kuster W, Peterson M, Christophers E, et al: A family study of atopic dermatitis: Clinical and genetic characteristics of 188 patients and 2,151 family members. Arch Dermatol Res 282:98, 1990.
16. Leung DYM, et al: Atopic dermatitis: New insights and opportunities for therapeutic intervention. J Allergy Clin Immunol 105: 860–876, 2000.
17. Leung DYM, et al: The presence of IgE on macrophages and dendritic cells infiltrating into the skin lesion of atopic dermatitis. Clin Immunol Immunopathol 42:328–337, 1987.
18. Mazer BD, et al: An open-label study of high-dose intravenous immunoglobulin in severe childhood asthma. J Allergy Clin Immunol 87:976–983, 1991.
19. Morale J, et al: CTACK, a skin-associated chemokine that preferentially attracts skin-homing memory to T cell. Proc Natl Acad Sci USA 96:14470–14475, 1999.
20. Nickel RB, et al: Chemokines and allergic disease. J Allergy Clin Immunol 104:723–742, 1999.
21. Picker LJ, et al: Differential expression of lymphocyte homing receptors by human memory/effector T cells in pulmonary versus cutaneous immune effector sites. Eur J Immonol 24:1269–1277, 1994.
22. Pincelli CF, et al: Neuropeptides in skin from patients with atopic dermatitis: An immunohistochemical study. Br J Dermatol 122:745–750, 1990.
23. Shaw JC: Atopic dermatitis. UptoDate, Version 8.3, 2000.
24. Shimizu EA, et al: Increased production of macrophage migration inhibitory factor by PBMCs of atopic dermatitis. J Allergy Clin Immunol 104:659–664, 1999.
25. Sicherer SH, et al: Food hypersensitivity and atopic dermatitis: Pathophysiology, epidemiology, diagnosis and management. J Allergy Clin Immunol 104(Suppl):S11–S22, 1999.
26. Taha RA, et al: Eotaxin and monocyte chemoattractant protein (MCP-4) mRNA expression in acute versus chronic atopic dermatitis. J Allergy Clin Immunol 10(Suppl):946A, 1998
27. Trepka MJ, Heinrich J, Wichmann HE: The epidemiology of atopic diseases in Germany: An east-west comparison. Rev Environ Health 11:119, 1996.
28. Yawalkar N, et al: Enhanced expression of eotaxin and CCR3 in atopic dermatitis. J Invest Dermatol 113:43–48, 1999.

10. OCULAR ALLERGY

Mark Zlotlow, M.D.

1. What diseases are being discussed?

The terms *ocular allergy* and *allergic conjunctivitis* are often used interchangeably. There are several types of ocular allergic disease.

   a. Allergic conjunctivitis
   b. Allergic keratoconjunctivitis
   c. Vernal conjunctivitis
   d. Giant papillary conjunctivitis
   e. Contact allergy

The importance of these diseases, especially allergic conjunctivitis, lies in their frequency. Both allergic keratoconjunctivitis and vernal conjunctivitis can produce corneal lesions and visual impairment. In general, however, these disorders do not permanently impair vision.

Dry eye syndrome and blepharitis are also discussed because of the frequency they present in an allergist's office. They are not, however, allergic diseases.

Lastly, there is a discussion of the differential diagnosis of red eyes and conjunctival inflammation. For an allergist, a major question is treatment versus referral to an ophthalmologist for treatment.

2. Why is the conjunctiva an active immunologic organ?

Because the conjunctiva forms a barrier to exogenous substances, it is expected to have a sophisticated immunologic repertoire. Under normal circumstances, a variety of cells active in phagocytosis and in the processing and elimination of antigen, such as lymphocytes, neutrophils, and plasma cells, are present. Specific structures are involved in some of these functions. The papillae of the palpebral conjunctiva contain collections of nonspecific inflammatory cells and tissue elements. In the normal conjunctiva, follicles are found, especially in the lower fornix. These follicles are filled with lymphocytes in various stages of development.

There are two types of mast cells in the conjunctiva, MC_t and MC_{tc}. The former contains only tryptase in its granules. It predominates at mucosal surfaces and increases markedly in aeroallergen sensitivity. Its function is dependent on the presence of T lymphocytes. MC_{tc} contains both tryptase and chymase in its granules. It is T-cell independent and found in fibrotic processes. In normal conjunctiva, the mast cells are predominantly of the MC_{tc} subtype.

3. How do you examine the conjunctiva?

To examine the bulbar conjunctiva, gently retract the opposite lid, and then ask the patient to look up or down as appropriate. The lower palpebral conjunctiva can be everted for examination by placing a finger by the lid margins and drawing downward. The upper palpebral conjunctiva is examined by everting the lid. While the patient is looking down, the upper lid is grasped at its base with a cotton swab. It is then pulled out and up. To return the lid to its normal position, ask the patient to look up.

4. How do you do a conjunctiva scraping for eosinophils and why is it useful?

The lower conjunctival sac is anesthestized with a topical anesthetic eyedrop. After a sufficient interval, the inner surface of the lower lid is gently scraped with a platinum spatula several times. The material is spread on a glass slide and stained with an appropriate stain such as Hansel stain. The slides are examined for the presence of eosinophils or eosinophil granules.

Nonallergic individuals do not have eosinophils. Therefore, the presence of eosinophils or granules strongly supports a diagnosis of allergic conjunctivitis. The rate of positive scrapings is variable depending on the patient population and the chronicity of the disease.

5. List the symptoms of allergic conjunctivitis (AC).
    a. Itching, both ocular and periocular
    b. Redness
    c. Tearing
    d. Burning
    e. Stinging
    f. Watery discharge
    g. Photophobia

6. Which of these symptoms is most characteristic of AC?

Itching of the eye is the most characteristic and often the predominant symptom. In contact dermatitis, it is itching of the lid. Itching occurs in other disorders, such as dry eyes, but it is not usually the predominant symptom.

7. Describe the signs of AC.
    a. Redness is usually mild to moderate in severity. Severe redness suggests another diagnosis.

    b. Swelling (chemosis) is usually subtle and visualized with a slitlamp. Occasionally it is marked and disproportionate to the redness.

    c. Milky appearance of the palpebral conjunctiva, caused by edema, obscures the blood vessels. A velvety, beefy-red appearance suggests a bacterial cause.

    d. A white exudate can occur in the acute stage. It can become stringy in the chronic stage.

    e. Lid edema and ecchymoses, the "allergic shiner," are frequent. The latter phenomenon has been attributed to impaired venous return from the skin and subcutaneous tissue. However, proof of this is lacking.

    f. As AC usually occurs with allergic rhinitis, symptoms of the latter disorder are present.

8. What are the differences between seasonal and perennial AC?

Seasonal AC occurs much more frequently. It usually occurs with allergic rhinitis, but can occur without it. The symptoms are caused by seasonal aeroallergens, usually specific pollens. In 78% of patients, there is increased specific IgE. There is also elevated specific tear fluid IgE in 96% of the affected patients. The length of the season correlates with the pollinating seasons of the specific aeroallergens.

Perennial AC occurs less frequently. Dust mites, animal dander, and feather sensitivity are the usual causative aeroallergens. Although, as the name implies, the symptoms are perennial, seasonal exacerbations may occur in these patients. As with seasonal AC, it usually occurs with perennial allergic rhinitis. There is also a high rate of both specific serum and tear fluid IgE to the causative agent.

Both disorders share the same pathophysiology. The differences are primarily in the length of symptoms and the aeroallergens that provoke symptoms.

9. Describe the conjunctival provocation test and state why is it useful.
An offending pollen is instilled into the conjunctival sac. In sensitive individuals, the typical symptoms and signs of AC are produced. Scoring of the reactions is through a scoring system that includes such objective and subjective factors as conjunctival erythema, chemosis, tearing, and pruritis.

This is one of the original methods used to establish specific sensitivity. It is particularly useful in the evaluation of antiallergic medication, immunotherapy and the pathophysiology of the disorder. As a diagnostic test, it may reveal specific eye sensitivities that do not provoke nasal symptoms. In one study, it correlated with RAST in 71% of the cases. In 6% of the uncorrelated cases, the provocation test was positive but the RAST was negative.

10. In conjunctival challenges, there are early and late phase reactions. In addition to time of onset, how do these reactions differ?
In both reactions, mast cells are central to the process. Administration of grass pollen extract to a sensitized individual results in marked symptoms within 20 minutes. They subside in 40 minutes. During this time, there is a marked increase in tryptase and histamine presumably from mast cells.

At 6 hours there is a second reaction with another peak of histamine and an increase in eosinophilic cationic protein. There is no increase in tryptase and few basophils. At this point, the cellular infiltrate contains mast cells, neutrophils, eosinophils, and macrophages. There are few CD4+ and CD8+ T cells. There is an increase in the adhesion molecules, E-selectin, and ICAM-1. This explains the increase in both eosinophils and granulocytes in the late phase reaction. With the increase of eosinophils, there is a consequent increase in eosinophil cationic protein.

11. Which mast cell subtypes are increased in AC?
MC_t mast cells are modestly increased in both the epithelium and the subepithelium in both seasonal and perennial AC. Many proinflammatory mediators— including histamine, leukotriene, prostaglandin (PGD_2), tryptase, carboxypeptidase A, cathepsin G, platelet-activating factor, and other chemoattractants—are increased in AC.

12. Name some of the functions of the soluble factors that are released.

Factor	Function
IL-4	1. Switches B cells to IgE production from IgM production
	2. Promotes T helper cell growth and differentiation
IL-5	1. Promotes growth and differentiation of eosinophils
	2. Chemoattractant and priming agent for eosinophils

IL-6	1. Augments T and B-Cell function
	2. Potentiates effects of other cytokines
Stem cell factor	1. Regulates mast cell growth and differentiation
	2. Enhances IgE-dependent mast cell-mediator release
	3. Cytokine generation and release
	4. Chemoattractant for mast cells
TNFα	1. Primary agent for mediator secreting cells
	2. Up-regulation of adhesion molecules

13. Eosinophils are characteristically found in large numbers in AC. List the factors that they release that contribute to the pathology.

Major basic protein
Eosinophil cationic protein
Eosinophil-derived neurotoxin

14. What are the available classes of drugs for treatment? What are their advantages and disadvantages?

DRUG CLASS	ADVANTAGES	DISADVANTAGES
Oral antihistamines	Ease of administration Particularly useful with coexisting allergic rhinitis. Some of the drugs are available OTC or as generics, and they are less expensive	Often need to be supplemented with topical agents May have systemic side effects May increase dry eyes
Topical antihistamine–decongestants (e.g., Opcon-A or Naphcon-A)	Available over the counter Few side effects May be considered first-line	Overuse results in conjunctivitis medicamentosa, an increase in conjunctival injection and rebound hyperemia that may persist after discontinuing the drops Usually only effective in mild cases
Topical antihistamines (e.g., levocabastine and emedastine)	Proven potency as a topical antihistamine in laboratory and clinical studies	Requires a prescription
Topical antihistamine and mast cell stabilizer (e.g., olopatadine and ketotifen)	Dual mode of action as antihistamine and mast cell stabilizer	Requires prescription Usually only requires b.i.d. dosage
Mast cell stabilizer (e.g., cromolyn and lodoxamide)	Inhibits both early and late phase reactions Safe	Effect not present until used 2–5 days; maximum benefit in 15 days Needs to be used regularly 4–6 times a day; this decreases compliance
Nonsteroidal anti-inflammatory such as ketorolac	Specifically indicated to relieve itching Analgesic properties	Safety in aspirin-allergic patients not yet demonstrated

(*Table continued on next page.*)

DRUG CLASS	ADVANTAGES	DISADVANTAGES
Topical corticosteroids	Effective for short-term use	Raises intraocular pressure Risks of incurring infection of the cornea and conjunctiva Risks of cataract formation

15. Name the available OTC antihistamine-decongestant combinations.

Trade Name	Composition	Concentration (%)
Vasocon-A	Antazoline phosphate	0.5
	Naphazoline	0.05
Naphcon-A	Pheniramine maleate	0.3
	Naphazoline	0.025
Ocuhist	Pheniramine maleate	0.3
	Naphazoline	0.025
Opcon-A	Pheniramine maleate	0.315
	Naphazoline	0.027

16. Why this combination of antihistamine and decongestant?

In several clinical studies, the combination proved to be more effective than either agent singly or than a placebo. These studies employed conjunctival challenge with allergen. Both itching and redness were the clinical symptoms evaluated.

17. What are the advantages of levocabastine, which is only an antihistamine, over the combination products and mast cell stabilizers?

Levocabastine was specifically developed as an H1-receptor antagonist for ocular use. In animal studies, it has been a potent and specific agent with little affinity for H2, serotonin, and muscarinic receptor sites In human clinical studies, it had an onset of action within 15 minutes and a duration of approximately 16 hours. In one study, it proved slightly more effective than antazoline/naphazoline. It had the advantage of requiring less frequent dosing and had less reported irritation. It also proved more effective than oral terfenadine. Several studies showed it to be comparable to or superior to sodium cromolyn. The clinical criteria included redness, itching, lacrimation, photophobia, and lid and conjunctival edema. In one study, it proved to be equally effective as lodoxamide.

18. Is emedastine, which is also an antihistamine, any better than levocabastine?

It is a particularly selective H1-receptor antagonist. In both challenge and environmental studies, it was superior to placebo in relieving the signs and symptoms of allergic conjunctivitis. There are no studies comparing it to levocabastine.

19. What is the role of oral antihistamines?

All oral antihistamines have some efficacy in allergic conjunctivitis, because AC is frequently associated with allergic rhinitis. Thus, the oral preparations may be useful monotherapy for both disorders. It may reduce the need for topical therapy

to an as needed basis. The newer nonsedating antihistamines have not been proven any more efficacious for AC. They also share the anticholinergic side effects of the older preparations. Dryness of the mucosal membranes, both conjunctival and oropharyngeal, may occur. The conjunctival dryness may precipitate symptoms of dry eye syndrome.

Oral decongestants, which are frequently used in combination with antihistamines, can produce mydriasis. In a predisposed individual, it could precipitate an attack of acute closed-angle glaucoma.

20. How do mast cell stabilizers work? Is one product superior to the other?

The exact mechanism of action of both cromolyn and lodoxamide is unknown. In studies, lodoxamide prevented the release of histamine, leukotrienes, and slow-reacting substance of anaphylaxis (SRS-A). It also inhibits eosinophil chemotaxis.

Both drugs have negligible systemic absorption. Thus, side effects are topical. They include burning or stinging, hyperemia, tearing, itching, and dry eye symptoms. Both drugs use benzalkonium chloride as the preservative and thus concomitant use with contact lenses is proscribed.

In vitro, lodoxamide is much more potent than cromolyn in preventing mediator release from mast cells. However in clinical studies, neither product is superior for AC.

These products have their main utility as prophylactic agents. For maximal efficacy, they need to be used on a daily q.i.d. schedule. In the case of seasonal AC, they should be started several weeks before the onset of the season.

21. Why is the nonsteroidal anti-inflammatory drug (NSAID) ketorolac effective for AC?

Ketorolac tromethamine (Acular) 0.5% has been effective in relieving the itching in AC. It is a highly potent NSAID that inhibits prostaglandin synthetase. It has been shown to reduce prostaglandin E2 in tears. Both PGE2 and PGI2 have been demonstrated to induce pruritus. In two separate seasonal environmental studies, it was superior to placebo in reducing symptoms of inflammation, itching, swollen eyes, burning and stinging. Some burning on administration is the most common side effect. Safety in aspirin-sensitive individuals has not been established.

22. What is the efficacy of drugs with combined antihistamine and mast cell stabilizing properties?

Olopatadine (Patanol) is a highly selective and potent H1 blocker. It is also a potent inhibitor of mast cell degranulation. It has the advantage of two to three times a day dosing. It has an 8-hour duration of action. In a comparison with ketorolac in an allergen challenge study, it proved to be more effective in reducing both hyperemia and ocular itching. It was also significantly more comfortable

Ketotifen fumarate 0.025% is a newly released preparation for allergic conjunctivitis. It has both antihistamine and mast cell stabilizing properties. In clinical studies, it has proven to be more effective than placebo. There is only sparse data comparing its efficacy with olopatadine. The parent compound, ketotifen, has been available for many years in many parts of the world for treatment of asthma and allergic rhinitis.

Given the dual mechanisms of action, this class of drugs may be the most effective for treatment of allergic conjunctivitis with the exception of topical steroids. However, the clinical trials are insufficient to prove this point.

23. Describe the benefits and risks of topical corticosteroids.

Corticosteroids are potent anti-inflammatory drugs that are very effective in relieving the symptoms of allergic conjunctivitis. Their efficacy as a group exceeds that of the other classes of drugs previously discussed. Phosphate preparations are highly soluble in aqueous vehicles and are therefore available as solutions. Acetate and alcohol preparations are suspensions. Ointments are also available. In the case of dexamethasone, the ointment is less-well-absorbed in the cornea and anterior chamber, although contact time between the eye surface and the drug is increased.

There are multiple serious complications associated with the use of corticosteroids. Both topical and systemic preparations are associated with the development of subcapsular cataracts. Although the pathogenesis of this complication is not fully understood, both total dosage and duration of treatment are associated with its development. Discontinuation of the drug does not alter the opacity.

Increased ocular pressure has been demonstrated with the use of both systemic and topical preparations. The effect is reversible with the discontinuation of the drug. However, the increase in pressure can cause optic nerve damage and visual field changes similar to open-angle glaucoma. The ability to produce this effect varies amongst the various preparations. Genetic differences, age, and coexistent diabetes are also contributing factors.

As a class of medications, steroids suppress the activation and migration of leukocytes. This decreases resistance to microbial infection. Both conjunctivitis and keratitis, bacterial and viral, can occur. Vision-threatening infections, such as fungal keratitis, fungal endophthalmitis, and toxoplasmic chorioretinitis, are potential risks of treatment.

Acute anterior uveitis with associated mydriasis, ptosis, and loss of accommodation has been reported. Refractive changes, blurring vision, increased corneal thickening and pseudotumor cerebri are complications that also have been reported.

Systemic absorption can also occur. For example, decreased serum cortisol levels were found after 6-week of treatment with topical 0.1% dexamethasone sodium phosphate.

Of the available preparations, two drugs, fluorometholone (FML) and medrysone (HMS), are favored for the treatment of allergic conjunctivitis. Although less potent than other preparations, they also have less risk of side effects. FML is mildly hydrophobic and concentrates in the epithelial layer of the cornea before passing through to the hydrophobic layers of the stroma. It is inactivated in the anterior chamber. HMS, available in a 1.0% suspension, also has a weak effect on the cornea.

Two newer preparations, loprednol etalionate (Alrex) and rimexolone (Vexol) may offer an even better safety profile for allergic conjunctivitis. Lopredenol is a modification of prednisolone that is rapidly hydrolyzed in the anterior chamber to an inactive metabolite. Rimexolone is currently approved for postsurgical inflammation and uveitis. It is also rapidly inactivated in the anterior chamber. In a number of studies, it showed less increase in intraocular pressure as compared to 1% prednisolone

and 0.1% dexamethasone, while having similar potency as an anti-inflammatory agent.

The efficacy of corticosteroids for allergic conjunctivitis is more than matched by the potential for serious complications. They should be used only for a short period of time and only if other agents have failed. Given the required caution monitoring by an ophthalmologist is certainly a wise choice. Prescribing this class of medicine without examination and *ad lib* refills are definitely unwise.

VERNAL KERATOCONJUNCTIVITIS

24. What are the symptoms of vernal keratoconjunctivitis (VKC)?

The most common symptom is itching of the eye, which often is quite intense. A thick, ropy discharge is present. The discharge consists of mucus, eosinophils, epithelial cells, and neutrophils. Photophobia, burning, and a foreign body sensation are other symptoms.

25. Describe the signs of VKC.

The principal findings are giant papillae on the superior tarsal and, sometimes, limbal conjunctiva. These papillae give the surface a cobblestone appearance. A stringy mucus coats the cobblestones.

Translucent globular deposits at the limbus in the form of an arc, or even a complete circle, characterize the limbal form of the disease. Within these deposits Horner-Trantas dots can be found. These chalk-white infiltrates are composed of clumps of degenerating epithelial cells, eosinophils, and neutrophils. These dots are virtually pathognomonic of the disease.

In more severe cases, there can be a diffuse epithelial keratitis. A shield ulcer may rarely be present. This is a well-defined, centrally located epithelial defect of the cornea.

26. What is the epidemiology of VKC?

Worldwide it is said to account for 0.1% to 0.5% of all ocular disorders. It is particularly prevalent in hot, dry environments. It is primarily a disease of childhood, with a majority of the patients being between 5 and 25 years of age. Until puberty there is a male predominance between 2:1 and 3:1. By age 20 years, the distribution is even between the sexes. There may be recurrent episodes over a 2 to 10-year period before resolving.

In more temperate climates, the disorder has a seasonal predilection for spring and summer. Hence, the term vernal in the name. There is usually a family and personal history of atopy. There is also a high frequency of positive skin tests to relevant inhalant allergens, particularly pollens. However, immunotherapy has not been particularly effective for VKC.

27. Describe the cellular-level changes involved in the pathogenesis of VKC.

Mast cells play an important role in VKC. The predominant cell, MC$_{tc}$ is found in high numbers in both epithelial and subepithelial levels of the conjunctiva. Approximately 80% of the mast cells are degranulated. Histamine levels are 10-fold higher than in normals. This is partly due to a decrease in histaminase levels.

↑ M BP
↑ ECP
↑ M E TC *Th
↑ eos.
C D4 T cells only

Eosinophils are also found in increased numbers within the epithelial and subepithelial layers. Only in VKC may more than two eosinophils per high-powered field be found on light microscopy. Because many of the eosinophils are degranulated, there is a marked increase in major basic protein. This protein has been recovered on the mucoid plaque overlying the shield ulcer and from elution from the ulcer itself. It is thought to be integral to the formation of the ulcer. Eosinophil cationic protein has also found to be elevated in the tears.

In VKC, 70% of the eosinophils expressed estrogen and progesterone receptors. This may partly explain the predominance of the disorder in prepubertal children and the decline in incidence with age.

The lymphocyte population shows an increase in CD4+ T cells but not CD8+ T cells. The T cells are predominantly of the TH-2 phenotype and appear to be produced locally. With cytokine profiles showing the TH-2 phenotype, there is a suggestion that VKC results from a maturation shift of CD4+ T cells to a pattern stimulating a mast cell and eosinophil response.

Bonini and associates hypothesize that the data taken together suggests that the pathogenesis of VKC lies in the up-regulation of the "cytokine gene clusters." This cluster is located on chromosome 5q. It includes the genes for IL-3, IL-4, IL-5, IL-13, and granulocyte/macrophage colony-stimulating factor (GM-CSF). These products lead ultimately to the TH-2 prevalence, increased polyclonal IgE production, and marked increase in mast cells and eosinophils. Thus, VKC is a TH-2–driven disorder.

28. Name some nonpharmacologic treatments for VKC.

Cool compresses and ice packs are often helpful, perhaps due to a vasoconstricting effect. Sleeping in an air-conditioned room may provide increased comfort. Artificial tears used frequently may dilute mediators and act as a barrier. Rubbing the eyes should be discouraged as the trauma may increase mediator release.

For some patients, patching the eye provides some relief from photophobia. Both patches and goggles may reduce allergen exposure. Such general allergen control measures such as dust mite controls and avoiding the outdoors on windy days and peak pollination times offer some benefit.

Although immunotherapy is not specifically effective for VKC, it may be useful if there is coexisting allergic rhinoconjunctivitis.

29. What pharmacologic treatments are available?

The drugs used for allergic conjunctivitis are useful for this disorder. Both systemic and topical antihistamines may reduce itching.

Both cromolyn and lodoxamide have specific indications for VKC. Lodoxamide has been shown to prevent keratitis and shield ulcers. It may also reverse some corneal changes. In one controlled study, it proved superior to cromolyn in providing relief from both the symptoms and signs of VKC.

Ketorolac has not been specifically approved for use in VKC. However 1% suprofen, a NSAID indicated for inhibition of intraoperative miosis, has demonstrated activity for VKC.

Olopatadine and ketotifen are not specifically indicated for VKC. Their modes of action as mast cell stabilizers and antihistamines make some benefit a logical inference.

Topical corticosteroids should be reserved for severe cases and used only for short-term treatment. This is particularly true with the self-limited nature of the disorder and the numerous side effects of corticosteroids.

30. Are there any surgical treatments available?

Cryotherapy of the tarsal conjunctiva often provides temporary relief. Conjunctival autografts have been performed with limited benefit. Superficial keratectomy of plaques may aid reepithelization. Excimer laser phototherapeutic keratectomy has been used to treat central corneal lesions. It may prove useful for superficial corneal scars. Corneal shield ulcers may also respond to soft contact lenses, patching, and tarsorrhaphy.

ATOPIC KERATOCONJUNCTIVITIS (AKC)

31. What is the epidemiology of AKC?

The disease is strongly associated with atopic dermatitis. However, some patients who have other atopic diseases such as asthma, have AKC without skin involvement. The disorder starts in late adolescence and early adulthood. Spontaneous resolution is rare. There is a male predominance.

32. List the symptoms of AKC.

The principal symptoms, as with VKC, are tearing, itching, and photophobia. The involvement is bilateral.

33. Describe the findings in AKC.

In a study of 37 patients with AKC, there was significant lid involvement. Eczematous changes of the skin of the lids occurred in 81%. Clinical blepharitis and meibomitis was found in almost 90%. *Staphylococcus aureus* was frequently recovered with the blepharitis. About half of the patients had maceration of the inner and outer canthi. Punctal ectropion, ptosis, and loss of lashes were also seen in about 50% of the patients.

All of the patients had papillae greater than 0.9 mm in diameter on both the upper and lower lids. In 10 of 37 patients, these papillae were greater than 1.0 mm in the upper eyelid. Reticular scarring was found in 28 of 37 patients. Symblepharon was found in 10 of 37 patients.

There are multiple corneal lesions in AKC. Punctate erosions were found in all patients. Neovascularization was found in 65% of the patients. Shield ulcers and sheets of mucus adherent to the ulcers were found in about one-half of patients; keratoconus occurred in about one-third of patients.

Infections with staphylococcus auras or herpes simplex are relatively frequent.

Cataracts can develop in severe chronic forms of the disease, especially the young. These cataracts are frequently bilateral and may progress quickly to complete opacification. As the cataract is frequently a posterior capsular one, identical to that produced by corticosteroids, it is difficult to determine whether the etiology is the disease or the treatment.

34. How can AKC be differentiated from allergic conjunctivitis and vernal keratoconjunctivitis when many of the symptoms are the same?

Allergic conjunctivitis usually occurs with allergic rhinitis. Usually lid changes do not occur with allergic conjunctivitis, but they are frequent in AKC. Lesions of atopic dermatitis usually occur on other skin surfaces.

VKC is usually a disease of prepubertal children, whereas AKC begins in young adults. Lid and blepharal involvement do not occur with VKC, but are characteristic of AKC. The palpebral involvement of VKC is large papillae on the upper lid. In AKC, both lower and upper palpebral conjunctiva are involved.

35. What are some of the immunologic findings in this disorder?

As with atopic dermatitis there is elevated serum IgE. This also occurs in tear fluid but with less frequency. Although positive RAST and skin tests are frequent, they are not always of clinical significance as exacerbates of the disease.

There is an increase in mast cells, but they are of the MC_{tc} subtype. This subtype appears to be T-cell independent and is characteristic of fibrotic processes.

As in VKC, the number of CD4+, but not CD8+, T cells is increased. Most of the CD4+ cells are memory cells. In VKC and giant papillary conjunctivitis (GPC), about 50% of the cells coexpressed CD45RO and CD4RA. This was not found in AKC. This suggests that the T cells found in the conjunctiva in AKC may be recruited from circulating memory T cells. In VKC and GPC, the T cells are produced locally.

36. How is AKC treated?

For patients with specific sensitivities, avoidance measures are indicated. Mast cell stabilizing agents are regularly administered. Ocular itching may be controlled with oral antihistamines or topical nonsteroidal anti-inflammatory drugs. Thus far, there is little evidence of a role for combined topical mast cell-stabilizing antihistamine agents.

Topical steroids in bursts are often required to reduce both conjunctival and eyelid inflammation, as well as keratitis. Blepharitis requires assiduous attention to lid scrubs and occasional antibiotics.

Some of the complications may require surgical intervention. Lid surgery may be necessary for correction of ectropion or entropion. The development of cataracts often leads to surgical removal and replacement with a posterior chamber intraocular lens. Although keratoconus can frequently be managed with contact lenses, it may require corneal transplantation.

GIANT PAPILLARY CONJUNCTIVITIS (GPC)

37. What is GPC?

The disease is named for the large papillae that are found on the upper tarsal surface. These papillae resemble the findings in VKC. GPC is associated most frequently with the wearing of soft contact lenses. No one particular soft lens has a higher incidence. It has also been reported with the following entities: rigid contact lenses; ocular prosthesis; exposed sutures in ocular surgery; limbal dermoid tumors; and cyanoacrylate tissue adhesive.

38. Describe the symptoms of GPC.
There is a decreased tolerance to the wearing of lenses. Irritation, redness, burning, and itching occur with the intolerance. Mucus production occurs with these symptoms.

39. What are the signs of GPC?
During the early stages of the disease, there is increased awareness of the lens, mild itching, and mucus in the inner canthus upon arising. Mucus coating of the lens may blur vision. Papillae may be found on the upper tarsal conjunctiva.

With increased disease progression, the symptoms, lens coating, and mucus production increase. The papillae increase in both size and number. There is marked injection of the conjunctiva and a loss of the normal vascular pattern.

In the most advanced cases, there is a complete intolerance to lens wear. The mucus production is much increased and the lids can be stuck together in the morning. The upper tarsal surface is thickened and the vasculature is totally obscured. The papillae are large and may have flattened apices.

40. Why mention GPC in a book on allergy?
There is significant usage of contact lenses, particularly soft contact lenses, in the general population. In the early stages of this disorder, there is itching, irritation, and a minimal mucoid discharge. Either the patient or the referring physician may attribute these symptoms to allergic conjunctivitis. Given the frequency of allergic conjunctivitis it is important to differentiate between the two disorders.

In the more advanced stages, the symptoms and the appearance of giant papillae mimic vernal keratoconjunctivitis.

41. Describe some of the histopathologic changes.
In GPC, mast cells, eosinophils, and basophils are found in both the epithelium and substantia propria. The concentration of inflammatory cells per mm^3 is similar to normal tissue. Because there is an increase in the total mass of tissue, the number of cells is increased. The histologic appearance is very similar to VKC. However, the histamine levels are about 25% less. In both GPC and VKC, mast cells are found in both the epithelium and the substantia propria. In both normals and normal contact lens wearers, mast cells are found only in the substantia propria. In GPC, the mast cells are of the MC$_{tc}$ subtype, whereas in VKC, the mast cells are of the MC$_t$ subtype.

There is an increase in immunoglobulins and complement in the tear fluid. The level of neutrophil chemotactic factor is 15 times that of normal levels.

42. What is the pathophysiology of this disorder?
There is still debate on this matter. It may be a primarily immunologic disorder. However it may be that mechanical trauma or irritation initiates the immunologic changes that are found.

43. How is GPC treated?
The most obvious treatment, discontinuing contact lens wear, does not meet with the universal approval of patients. The lens itself can be made less irritating by reducing the coating. Improved cleaning, decreased time wearing the lenses, or a

change in design or material may be sufficient. The use of a daily use disposable lens may improve or solve the problem.

The use of mast cell stabilizers and NSAID topically has been reported to be of some benefit. While topical steroids are effective, long-term use would involve the substantial risk of side effects.

KERATOCONJUNCTIVITIS SICCA AND DRY EYE SYNDROME

44. State the difference between dry eye syndrome (DES) and keratoconjunctivitis sicca (KCS).

Dry eye syndrome is a constellation of symptoms and signs caused by a decrease in the quantity or abnormal quality of the tear-film layer. KCS is a specific disorder that is caused by a quantitative or qualitative abnormality of lacrimal gland secretion.

45. What are the components of the tear-film layer?

The tear film consists of three layers: the outer, middle, and inner layers. The meibomian glands secrete the outer layer of lipids. These glands secrete a phospholipid that stabilizes the tear-film layer and reduces the rate of evaporative loss. This layer is 1.0 μm thick.

The main and accessory lacrimal glands secrete the middle aqueous layer, which is 7.0 μm thick. It contains the water-soluble components of the tear film such as immunoglobulins, lysozyme, and complement.

The inner mucin layer is derived from the goblet cells of the conjunctiva. It adheres the hydrophilic aqueous layer to the hydrophobic corneal epithelium. This helps to make the tear film a smooth, even layer over the entire conjunctiva. The tears are spread by blinking.

46. What are the symptoms of DES?

The most common complaint is a foreign-body sensation described by many as a feeling of sand in the eye. Tearing, pain, photophobia, and redness also occur. There may be a decrease in vision from an irregular tear film on the cornea. A reduction of the aqueous component may lead to eyelid crusting in the morning. Dry windy weather can exacerbate these symptoms.

Several conditions including AC, GPC, and blepharitis can mimic these symptoms. Patients with borderline dryness may develop the symptoms only when wearing contact lenses. This possibility is increased with the use of extended-wear soft lenses that have a higher water content, which is drawn from the tear layer.

47. What are the signs of DES?

A slitlamp examination with minimal manipulation can show a continuous tear meniscus. In normal individuals, it is 0.3 to 0.5 mm in height. It is decreased in DES. Redundant conjunctiva, injection of the conjunctiva, and mild chemosis may be seen. In severe cases, the epithelium may be keratinized. A stringy mucous may form in the inferior fornix.

48. Describe some objective tests of the tear film.

Staining the tear film with fluorescein stain demonstrates any denuded areas of epithelium. It also demonstrates the tear meniscus.

Tear film breakup time quantitatively measures a mucus deficiency in the tear layer. After instillation of fluorescein, the patient is asked to blink and then keep the eye open for at least 5 to 10 seconds. The time from the link to the appearance of a dry spot is the tear breakup time. Any time less than 10 seconds indicates a mucin deficiency or meibomian gland dysfunction.

Rose bengal staining can also be used to evaluate the ocular surface. The Schirmer test quantitatively measures tear secretions by the lacrimal gland. The Jones test evaluates the patency of the nasolacrimal apparatus. Both of these latter tests are used for objective evaluation of dry eyes.

49. How is DES treated?

The initial treatment is the frequent use of tear substitutes. Most patients use them on a p.r.n. basis. However, with the occurrence of symptoms there is a degree of damage to the ocular surface. Therefore, regular treatment four times a day for several days to weeks enables healing. Then reduction of dosage to as low as two times a day may be sufficient. Dry, windy weather necessitates more frequent treatment. The hypotonic, nonviscous solutions will last up to 2 hours. The more viscous solutions, which generally have cellulose as a base, last longer but may cause some blurring of vision by creating a nonuniform tear layer. Ointments are useful for bedtime use and as adjuncts for severe dryness.

Surgical treatment involves anccicular occlusion, which decreases tear drainage. The occlusion may be done with temporary or permanent plugs. Cautery, diathermy, or argon laser can be used to create permanent occlusions.

50. List the connective tissue diseases that cause KCS.

Sjögren's disease
Rheumatoid arthritis
Sarcoidosis
Amyloidosis
Systemic lupus erythematosus

CONTACT DERMATITIS OF THE EYE AND EYELID

51. Why is contact dermatitis of the eye important?

Contact dermatitis is the most common eruption of the eyelid. The eyelid, with its thin soft skin, is particularly vulnerable to delayed sensitivity reactions. With its location and cosmetic implications, affected individuals will frequently seek medical attention.

52. Name the most common contactants.

Cosmetics applied to the hair, face, and fingernails are the most frequent sensitizers. Often they cause no problems at the site of application, but for reasons mentioned previously affect the eyelid. Irritant reactions may also occur from cosmetics

applied around the eye. Although tolerance to an irritant may develop, an irritant contact dermatitis can develop. Clinically, it cannot be differentiated from an allergic contact dermatitis.

53. What are some common sensitizers?

Water-based mascara contains emulsifiers that can be irritating. However, for some individuals it is the waterproof mascara itself that is not tolerated. A cake-type mascara or eyeliner can be a suitable alternative.

Products for eye and periorbital use contain antimicrobial preservatives to prevent contamination. Parabens, which are esters of parahydroxybenzoic acid, are the most commonly used. Although they may cause reactions when placed in the eye, they are usually tolerated topically on the lid. Quarternum 15 and imidazolidnyl urea are preservatives that generate formaldehyde. They may be antigenic in their own right or cause irritation from the formaldehyde they release. Other preservatives that are sensitizers include potassium sorbate, di-isopropanolamine, and ditertiarybutyl hydroquinone.

Some nail polish contains a toluene-sulfonamide formaldehyde resin that is a sensitizer when dry. Rubbing the eyes with the hands places the sensitizer on the lid. Paradoxically, the nail beds and paronychial areas are not involved. Dubbed "ectopic dermatitis," it is a phenomenon that extends to hair products. Hypoallergenic nail polishes substitute a polyester resin.

Eyeliners, eyeshadows, and artificial lashes may also be sources of sensitizers for the lid and conjunctiva. Eyelash liners and tweezers that contain nickel can also be sensitizers.

54. What are the causes of contact dermatitis of the conjunctiva?

"Conjunctivitis medicamentosa" typically arises from the repeated use of a topical ocular medication. After an initial improvement of the problem, a red eye returns. This prompts the use of multiple medications with no relief. Often the treatment is the cessation of all topical medications for several days. The patient returns for relevant scrapings and cultures to diagnose the original problem.

Pronounced vasodilatation, chemosis and a watery discharge mark the conjunctival response to this entity. In severe cases, there may even be keratitis. The skin of the lids becomes edematous, erythematous, and even ulcerated.

Topical anesthetics and glaucoma medications have been causative agents. However, preservatives are by far the most common cause. Benzalkonium and thimerosal are the most commonly used preservatives, and thus the most common culprits. All multiple-dose preparations require some preservatives. In liquid preparations, chlorbutanol, a rare sensitizer, can be an alternative. In lubricants, sodium perborate, which generates hydrogen peroxide, can be an alternative preservative.

55. How can these reactions be diagnosed?

For lid involvement, patch testing is utilized. Interpretation is difficult because of frequent false-positive irritant reaction. Also, in the case of eye cosmetics the typical vesicular eruption often does not occur in the positive test.

56. What are the other causes of conjunctivitis?

In all of the diseases mentioned below there is both irritation and discharge. In all of the cases, the pupils are normal and there is normal intraocular pressure.

1. Bacterial

A. Symptoms: 1. Redness. 2. Irritation. 3. Foreign body sensation. 4. Copious mucopurulent discharge. 5. Lids stuck together in the morning. 6. Recent respiratory tract infection or blepharitis.

B. Objective findings: 1. Papillary reaction of palebral conjunctiva. 2. Mild to pronounced hyperemia of conjunctiva. 3. Mild edema of the lids. 4. Lashes matted. 5. After fluorescein staining, punctate stain on inferior one-third of corneal conjunctiva.

C. Common organisms and some unique features:

1. *Neisseria gonnorhea* and *Neisseria meningitidis.* These organisms can cause a hyperacute reaction characterized by a marked mucopurulent discharge, eyelid edema, and chemosis. It can cause ulceration, scarring, and even perforation leading to blindness. Inoculation from infected genitalia is the usual mode of transmission.

2. *Streptococcus* and *Hemophilus.* These organisms are most commonly seen in children and institutional settings. These organisms can cause petechial hemorrhages.

3. *Staphylococcus.* The most common organism causing conjunctivitis in adults. Although usually an acute problem, the existence of chronic blepharitis can lead to a chronic conjunctivitis.

2. Chlamydia

A. Symptoms: 1. Foreign body sensation. 2. Lacrimation. 3. Redness. 4. Photophobia. 5. Lid swelling. 6. Mucopurulent discharge. 7. Incubation period 2–10 days. 8. Untreated can last for months.

B. Objective findings: 1. Palpebral conjunctiva has initial papillary hypertrophy. 2. Chronic follicular response. 3. Painless preauricular adenopathy may be present. 4. Concomitant otitis media may occur. 5. Corneal involvement may occur with epithelial keratitis, subepithelial opacities, phlyctenular lesions, or micropannus.

C. Epidemiology: 1. Generally found in young adults. 2. Transmission usually from infected genitalia.

3. Viral

A. Symptoms: 1. Clear watery discharge. 2. Soreness or pain. 3. Foreign-body sensation. 4. Photophobia. 5. Glare. 6. Slight blurring of vision.

B. Objective Findings: 1. Follicles more prominent in the lower lid. 2. Tender preauricular lymph nodes. 3. Both epithelial and subepithelial keratitis can occur. 4. Subepithelial opacities can occur.

C. Common organisms and some unique features:

1. *Adenovirus:* These viruses cause four different clinical syndromes: (a) epidemic keratoconjunctivitis; (b) pharyngoconjunctival fever; (c) a nonspecific acute sporadic conjunctivitis; (d) a chronic papillary conjunctivitis.

Epidemic keratoconjunctivitis has an incubation period of 2 to 14 days and a self-limited course of 2 to 14 days. Several diagnostic signs are tender preauricular nodes, diffuse subepithelial infiltrates, formation of a membrane on the upper or lower conjunctiva, and petechial hemorrhage. Malaise, slight fever, and headache may precede the onset of symptoms.

Pharyngoconjunctival fever is more common in children. Antecedent symptoms of sore throat and fever may precede the illness. Malaise, myalgia, headache, and

gastrointestinal disturbance may accompany the eye disease. As the disease is shed for up to 30 days in feces, a recent history of swimming in a pool or contact with a previously infected individual may be obtained.

2. *Herpes simplex:* The key differentiating sign are small vesicles around the lid, particularly the lid margins. Other signs include: (a) a follicular conjunctivitis; (b) preauricular or submandibular lymphadenopathy; (c) lid edema; (d) a superficial punctate keratitis which may occur 1 to 2 weeks after the conjunctivitis. The causative organism, HSV-1, can remain latent in the trigeminal ganglion and cause recurrent ocular infection in up to 25% of the cases.

3. *Varicella-Zoster:* Patients have other features of either varicella or zoster. Mild to severe ocular complications may occur in over 50% with the involvement of the trigeminal nerve.

57. What are the other causes of an acute red eye?

1. Acute Angle Closure Glaucoma

It usually occurs in older female patients. The symptoms stem from the sudden rise in intraocular pressure. Symptoms include (a) blurred vision; (b) ocular pain; (c) frontal headache; (d) colored haloes; (e) nausea and emesis. The prominent findings are fixed and dilated pupil and a dull corneal reflex from the edematous cornea. **This is an ocular emergency and requires immediate care by an ophthalmologist.**

2. Ruptured Globe

There is usually a history of penetrating trauma to the globe. A sharp pain is present. Ocular complaints can vary. The most important diagnostic findings are hypotony, shallow anterior chamber and a sluggish pupillary response to light. Subconjunctival hemorrhages and periocular abrasions may be seen. **This is an ocular emergency and requires urgent consultation with an ophthalmologist.**

3. Episcleritis

The patients are usually adults between the ages of 20 and 50 years with a female predominance. The presenting symptoms are rapid onset of pain and irritation in one or both eyes. There may be tenderness over the area of redness. There is no circumlimbal injection or visual disturbance. The cornea and anterior chamber are normal. The symptoms usually progress over 3 to 5 days and resolve in 10 days. It is found in these systemic diseases: (a) SLE; (b) polyarteritis; (c) Lyme disease; (d) rheumatoid arthritis; (e) Crohn's disease; (f) hepatitis B infection; (g) gout; and (h) syphilis.

4. Idiopathic Anterior Uveitis

There is sudden onset of pain, redness of the eye and photophobia without a history of trauma. The disease is usually unilateral occurring in adults between the ages of 20 and 50 years. The affected pupil is miotic. The vasculature of the limbal area is engorged and reddened. Ptosis may occur secondary to blepharospasm.

5. Iritis

There is pain, photophobia, and a circumlimbal injection. The pupil is miotic and the intraocular pressure is decreased. The anterior chamber is abnormal. This disorder is usually found with these systemic diseases: (a) ankylosing spondylitis; (b) Reiter's syndrome; (c) ulcerative colitis; (d) sarcoidosis; (e) Behçet's disease.

6. Subconjunctival Hemorrhage

This common but benign problem presents suddenly without symptoms such as pain, discharge, or visual disturbance. The pupils, anterior chamber, and cornea are

all normal. There is no history of discharge. Although usually idiopathic, it can occur with hypertension and bleeding disorders.

BIBLIOGRAPHY

1. Abelson MB: Evolution of olopatadine, a new ophthalmic antiallergic agent with dual activity, using the conjunctival allergen challenge model. Ann Allergy Asthma Immunol 81(3):211–218, 1998.
2. Abelson MB, McGarr PJ, Richard KP: Anti-allergic therapies. In Zimmerman T, Kooner, et al: Textbook of Ocular Pharmacology, 1997, pp.609–633.
3. Bielory L: Contact dermatitis of the eye. Allergy Clin N Am 17(1);131–138, 1997.
4. Bielory L, Friedlaender M, Fujishima H: Allergic conjunctivitis. Allergy Clin N Am 17(1):19–3, 1997.
5. Bonini S, Bonini S, Lambiase A, et al: Vernal keratoconjunctivitis: A model of 5q cytokine gene cluster disease. Int Arch Allergy Immunol 107:95–98, 1995.
6. Caldwell DR, Verin P, Hartwich-Young R, et al: Efficacy and safety of lodoxamide 0.1% and cromolyn sodium 4% in patients with vernal keratoconjunctivitis. Am J Ophthalmol 113:632–637, 1992.
7. Constad WH, Bhagat N: Keratitis sicca and dry eye syndrome. Allergy Clin N Am 17(1):53–73, 1997.
8. Donshik PC, Ehlers WH: Giant papillary conjunctivitis. Allergy Clin N Am 17(1):53–73, 1997.
9. Friedlaender MH: Ocular allergy. In Middleton E, Reed CE, et al. (eds): Allergy: Principles and Practice, 4th ed, St. Louis: CV Mosby, 1993, p 1651.
10. Irani A: Ocular mast cells and mediators. Allergy Clin N Am 17(1):1–13, 1997.
11. Jackson BW: Differentiating conjunctivitis of diverse origins. Surv Ophthalmol 38:91–104, 1993.
12. Leonardi A, Briggs RM, Bloch KJ, et al: Correlation between conjunctival provocation test (CPT) and systemic allergometric tests in allergic conjunctivitis. Eye 4:760–764, 1990.
13. Lee Y, Raizman MB: Vernal conjunctivitis. Allergy Clin N Am 17(1): 33–51, 1997.
14. McGill JI, Holgate ST, Church MK, et al: Allergic eye disease mechanisms. Br J Ophthalmol 82:1203–1214, 1998.
15. Richard C, Triquand C, Bloch-Michel E: Comparison of topical 0.05% levocabastine and 0.1% lodoxamide in patients with allergic conjunctivitis. Eur J Ophthalmol 8(4):207–216, 1998.
16. Sendrowski DP: Acute conjunctival inflammation. In Bezan D, LaRussa F, Nishimoto J, et al. (eds.): Differential Diagnosis in Primary Eye Care. Butterworth-Heinemann, 1999, pp 107–113.
17. Sendowski DP: Acute red eye. In Bezan D, LaRussa F, Nishimoto J, et al. (eds.): Differential Diagnosis in Primary Eye Care. Butterworth-Heinemann, 1999, pp 97–105.
18. Siret DJ: Oral and topical antihistamines: Pharmacologic properties and therapeutic potential in ocular allergic disease. J Am Optom Assoc 69(2):77–87, 1998.
19. Tuft SJ, Kemeny DM, Dart JK, Buckley RJ: Clinical features of atopic keratoconjunctivitis. Ophthalmology 98:150–158, 1991.

11. ANAPHYLAXIS

Arif M. Seyal, M.D.

1. What is anaphylaxis and how does it differ from anaphylactoid reaction?
Anaphylaxis is a potentially life-threatening clinical syndrome that is characterized by the sudden onset of generalized, often unanticipated symptoms, affecting multiple organ systems in the body. Clinical features in anaphylaxis result from IgE-mediated antigen-induced release of mediators from previously sensitized mast cells and basophils. Anaphylactoid reaction is a systemic reaction that is clinically similar to anaphylaxis but is not caused by IgE-mediated immune response. Anaphylaxis and anaphylactoid reactions are usually immediate in nature and occur within 30 minutes after exposure to the causative agent, but in some cases, onset may be delayed an hour or longer.

2. What are the factors that influence the incidence of anaphylaxis?
Several factors may influence the incidence of anaphylaxis. These factors include history of underlying atopy, route of administration of antigen/causative agent, age and gender of the patient.
- **Atopy.** Approximately 50% of the individuals who experience exercise-induced anaphylaxis have an underlying history of atopy. There also appears to be a higher incidence of anaphylaxis due to food, radiocontrast material, and latex in atopic individuals.
- **Route of administration of antigen**. There is a higher incidence of anaphylactic reactions after parenteral administration of antibiotics and biologic agents. Oral administration of antibiotics appears to be considerably safer.
- **Age and gender**. Anaphylactic reactions are more common in adults than in children. Women appear to be affected twice as often by food-associated exercised-induced anaphylaxis. Approximately 60% of the cases of anaphylaxis tend to occur in individuals younger than 30 years. A higher incidence of systemic allergic reactions due to hymenoptera sting in males may be secondary to increased exposure.

3. What is the role of H1 and H2 histamine receptors in the pathogenesis of anaphylaxis and anaphylactoid reaction?
Most of the clinical features of anaphylaxis can be produced by intravenous infusion of small doses of histamine, which, by acting through both H1 and H2 receptor subtypes, can cause vasodilatation, increased mucus gland secretions, and hypotension.

H1 receptor-mediated effects include increased vascular permeability, smooth muscle contraction, and enhanced bronchial mucus production. It also causes the stimulation of sensory nerve endings leading to the release of neuropeptides. Cardiac effects include increased rate of depolararization of sinoatrial node and coronary vasospasm.

H2 receptors mediate coronary artery vasodilatation, and have positive inotropic and chronotropic effects on cardiac muscles. H2 receptors also increase mucus secretion from goblet and cells bronchial glands (see Table).

Granule-Associated Preformed Mediators of Anaphylaxis

MEDIATORS	PATHOPHYSIOLOGIC EFFECT	CLINICAL EFFECT
Histamine		
(Vasoactive and Spasmogen) H1 Receptors Mediated Effects	Increased capillary permeability; vasodilatation; contraction of smooth muscles (bronchial and intestinal)	Flushing; pruritus; urticaria; ngioedema; hypotension; wheezing and abdominal cramps; tachycardia; and myocardial ischemia.
ach/ation of T Suppress Cell	Coronary vasoconstriction; increased rate of depolarization of SA node; irritation of the nerve endings; and neuropeptide release. Increased mucus gland secretion.	Increased mucus gland secretions.
H2 Receptors Mediated Effects	Peripheral vasodilatation; coronary artery vasodilatation; positive inotropic and positive chronotropic effects on cardiac smooth muscle. Decreased fibrillation threshold. Increased glandular secretions.	Hypotension; tachycardia; atrial and ventricular arrythmias. Increased goblet cells and bronchial gland secretions.
Enzymes		
Tryptase	Neutral protease. Activates complement C3 and generates C3a. Enhances contractile effect of histamine.	Plasma half-life ~2 hours. May be a useful marker of mast-cell activation.
Chymase	Acts as potent angiotensin-converting enzyme.	May play an important role in cardiovascular homeostasis.
Chemotactic Factors		
Eosinophilic chemotactic factor (ECFA) Neutrophilic chemotactic factors of anaphylaxis (NCFA)	Chemotactic factors for inflammatory cells (eosinophils and neutrophils)	Important for the late-phase reaction.
Heparin	Anticoagulant, complement inhibitor, and binds Heparin	Probable anti-inflammatory effect.

4. List the most common clinical features of anaphylaxis and their order of relative frequency.

Clinical features of anaphylaxis are frequently sudden in onset, and may range from mild to very severe, and occasionally to fatal. Following are the clinical features of anaphylaxis listed according to their relative frequency (see Table).

CLINICAL FEATURES	PERCENT OF PATIENTS
Urticaria and angioedema	> 90
Dyspnea and wheezing	47–60
Dizziness, near syncope, syncope and hypotension	30–33

(Table continued on next page.)

CLINICAL FEATURES	PERCENT OF PATIENTS
Flushing of skin	> 28
Nausea, vomiting, and abdominal cramps	25–30
Laryngeal edema, tongue swelling, choking, and dysphonia	24
Rhinitis and nasal congestion	16
Substernal chest discomfort	6
Headache	>5
Pruritus without rash	4
Seizure	1.5–2

See references 10, 11, and 22.

5. What are the pathophysiologic effects and clinical manifestations related to the newly synthesized mediators that are released by the mast cells and basophils?

Newly Generated Mediators of Mast Cells and Basophils that Play a Role in Anaphylaxis and Anaphylactoid Reactions

Arachidonic Acid Metabolites		
Lipoxygenase Pathway		
Leukotriens • LTC4 • LTD4 • LTB4	Contraction of airway smooth muscles, increased vascular permeability, chemotactic activity	Wheezing, hypotension and possible late phase reaction
Cyclooxygenase Pathway • Prostaglandins (PG D2 and PG F2) • Thrombaxane A2	Bronchoconstriction, peripheral vasodilatation, coronary artery vasoconstriction	Hypotension; wheezing, and myocardial ischemia
Platelet-Activating Factor (PAF)	Bronchoconstriction, vasodilatation, increased vascular permeability, and decreased myocardial contractility	Wheezing, hypotension, and cardiac arrhythmias, and pump failure probably in the late-phase reaction

6. Describe the mechanism of radiocontrast material (RCM)-associated anaphylaxis. Is skin testing an aid in its diagnosis?

The exact mechanism of anaphylactoid reaction to RCM is unknown. IgE does not appear to be involved in this reaction. Possible mechanisms of RCM-induced anaphylactoid reaction include the direct release of mediators from mast cells and basophils, complement activation, inhibition of cholinestrase, recruitment of inflammatory mediators, and indirect release of the prostacyclin by vascular endothelial cells.

Skin testing has no value in the diagnosis of RCM-associated anaphylaxis.

7. How can you reduce the risk of recurrent anaphylactoid reaction to hyperosmolar (HOS) radiocontrast material?

The risk of recurrent anaphylactoid reaction to high-osmolality contrast material can be reduced to < 1% by use of low-osmolality contrast material and a pretreatment regimen.

8. What are the most common foods implicated in fatal anaphylactic reactions?

Although any food can cause a fatal anaphylactic reaction, certain foods have been implicated more frequently than other foods. The more frequently implicated foods include peanuts, tree nuts (walnut, cashew, hazelnut, pistachio, and brazil nuts), fish, shellfish (shrimp, crab, oyster, and lobster), certain fruits (e.g., kiwifruit), and seeds (psyllium, cottonseed, and sesame seed).

9. How can exercise-induced anaphylaxis be differentiated from cholinergic urticaria?

Exercise-induced anaphylaxis is a form of physical allergy that usually occurs after prolonged exercise, and is manifested by the symptoms of generalized warmth, pruritus, urticaria, angioedema, nausea, vomiting, abdominal cramps, diarrhea, and vascular collapse.

Cholinergic urticaria is characterized by the small punctate (1–4 mm), extremely pruritic wheals (microhives) surrounded by prominent erythema. Exercise, hot showers, sweating, and anxiety can trigger cholinergic urticaria. Some patients may also experience the systemic symptoms. Passive heat challenge (by using hyperthermic blanket or submersion in hot water) appears to be a valuable diagnostic test in the differentiation of cholinergic urticaria from exercise-induced anaphylaxis. One must, however, exercise extreme caution in performing this test. Patients with cholinergic urticaria develop punctate hives and occasionally systemic symptoms, whereas patients with EIA anaphylaxis remain asymptomatic.

10. Define the role of antihistamines in prevention of exercise-induced anaphylaxis (EIA).

Prophylactic treatment with H1 and H2 antihistamines has not been proven effective in preventing EIA. In selected patients, use of prophylactic antihistamines may blunt the severity or reduce the frequency of attacks. Cholinergic urticaria, on the other hand, is responsive to the prophylactic hydroxyzine.

11. Describe the probable mechanism of ASA and other nonsteroidal anti-inflammatory drug (NSAID)-induced anaphylaxis, and how you can confirm the diagnosis.

The mechanism by which non-steroidal anti-inflammatory drugs cause development of an anaphylactic syndrome is not well defined. It is likely that inhibition of cyclooxygenase by aspirin and other nonsteroidal anti-inflammatory drugs may result in a shift of arachidonic acid metabolism from the cyclooxygenase to the lipoxygenase pathway, thus leading to increased peptidoleukotriens productions. Increased levels of peptidoleukotriens may result in the symptoms of hypotension, bronchoconstriction, and increased mucus production, urticaria, and angioedema.

There is no reliable skin test or in vitro study to confirm the diagnosis. The ASA/NSAIDs challenge can be performed in an intensive-care setting.

12. What are the various mechanisms of anaphylaxis/anaphylactoid reactions?
I. IgE mediated
    A. Native proteins (complete antigens)
        1. Foods

Fish, shellfish, crustaceans, eggs, milk, peanuts, nuts, fruits such as kiwifruit, and seeds (cottonseed, sesame, and psyllium) are the most common foods implicated.

2. **Animal and Human Proteins**

   Stinging insects (hymenoptera, fire ants), biting insects (kissing bug or triatoma)

   Antilymphocyte globulin (ALG)

   Avian-based vaccine (measles, mumps, influenza, and yellow fever)

   Murine-derived monoclonal antibodies

   Seminal fluid

3. **Hormones**

   Insulin, corticotropin (ACTH)

4. **Enzymes**

   Streptokinase, chymopapain

5. **Aeroallergens**

   Skin test or Immunotherapy for pollens, house dust mites, and molds

6. **Others**

   Latex (gloves and other medical devices), protamine

B. **Haptens (IgE-mediated reactions against the protein hapten conjugate)**

1. **Antibiotics**

   Penicillin, cephalosporins, sulfonamides, and streptomycin

2. **Disinfectants**

   Ethylene oxide

3. **Smooth muscle relaxants such as succinylcholine**

II. **Non-IgE mediated**

A. **Complement activation** and generation of anaphylotoxins (C3a, C4a, C5a)

   Human plasma and blood products, gamma globulin

B. **Direct activation of mast cell or basophil** mediators

   Opiates, tubucurare, dextran, radiocontrast materials, fluorescein dye for angiography, and some chemotherapeutic agents.

C. **Modulators of arachidonic acid metabolism**

   Nonsteroidal anti-inflammatory drugs such aspirin, ibuprofen, and indomethacin.

III. **Unknown Mechanism**

A. **Sulfites**

   Food additives

B. **Steroids**

   Progesterone and hydrocortisone

C. **Physical triggers**

   (Exercise-induced anaphylaxis, food-dependent exercise-induced anaphylaxis, systemic cold-induced urticaria, and systemic heat-induced urticaria)

D. **Systemic mastocytosis**

E. **Idiopathic anaphylaxis**

13. Name the common clinical conditions that may mimic anaphylaxis/ana-phylactoid reaction.

Anaphylaxis should be differentiated from a variety of other clinical syndromes or symptom complexes that may mimic or be easily confused with anaphylaxis/ana-phylactoid reactions.

1. Shock
   a. Hemorrhagic (massive gastrointestinal blood loss)
   b. Cardiogenic (acute myocardial infarction)
   c. Septic
2. Vasovagal reaction
3. Carcinoid syndrome
4. Systemic mastocytosis
5. Pheochromocytoma
6. Hereditary angioedema
7. Nonorganic causes
   a. Panic disorder
   b. Vocal cord dysfunction
   c. Globus hystericus

14. How is a vasovagal reaction differentiated from a true anaphylaxis/anaphy-lactoid response? What is the most appropriate treatment of vasovagal reaction?

Vasovagal reaction may occur after any injection and the usual clinical manifes-tations include dizziness, diaphoresis, pallor, weakness, sweating, nausea, hypoten-sion, and bradycardia. Patients lack pruritis, urticaria, angioedema, tachycardia, and bronchospasm.

Administration of atropine sulfate (.3–1 mg) intramuscularly or intravenously usually reverses a vasovagal reaction.

15. Describe carcinoid syndrome and the effect of epinephrine on carcinoid flush.

Carcinoid syndrome is usually associated with flushing, abdominal cramps, di-arrhea, and, occasionally, bronchospasm. This condition is caused by the release of vasoactive substances such as serotonin, bradykinin, and histamine, by the slow-growing tumors. These tumors are usually located in the bronchi, stomach, pancreas, and small intestine. Effected patients have elevated plasma level of 5-hydroxyindol acetic acid (5HIAA). An elevated level of the 5HIAA in 24-hour urine collection is diagnostic of carcinoid syndrome.

Epinephrine is contraindicated because it may provoke carcinoid flush.

16. What is systemic mastocytosis?

Systemic mastocytosis is a clinical syndrome caused by the accumulation of mast cells in multiple organs including skin, bone marrow, liver, and gastrointesti-nal tract. Clinical features of flushing, pruritis and anaphylactic response may be associated with urticaria pigmentosa and may develop spontaneously or after taking nonsteroidal anti-inflammatory drugs, opiates, or alcohol. Other common features are osteoporosis, bone demineralization, and anemia due to bone marrow involvement.

17. How is systemic mastocytosis distinguished from anaphylaxis/anaphylactoid reaction?

In systemic mastocytosis, baseline α-protryptase level is markedly elevated (> 20 ng/mL). In all probability, this reflects the total mast cell burden and can be used to assess the response to treatment directed to lower total mast cell load. In systemic anaphylaxis, serum β-tryptase is level is > 5 ng/mL.

18. What is the significance of anemia and thrombocytopenia in systemic mastocytosis?

Extensive bone marrow infiltration by mast cells in systemic mastocytosis is associated with hematologic abnormalities such as anemia, thrombocytopenia, eosinophilia, and lymphopenia. Anemia (specially hemoglobin < 11 g/dL), thrombocytopenia, decreased bone marrow fat cell (< 20%), constitutional symptoms, and liver function abnormalities are all associated with poor prognosis.

19. What is the importance of serum tryptase as a diagnostic marker of anaphylaxis?

Tryptase is a neutral protease present in the human mast cells and may be an important marker for mast cell involvement in anaphylaxis. More than 99% of total body tryptase is present in mast cells. During anaphylaxis, when mast cells degranulate, tryptase is slowly released into the blood. In the normal blood, tryptase level is less than 1 ng/mL. Tryptase levels peak 1 hour after the experimental insect-sting induced-anaphylaxis and then decline with a half-life of 2 hours. Recent evidence suggests that β-tryptase is the primary form that is stored in the mast cells granules, and is released upon mast cell activation. Therefore, β-tryptase level in serum correlates best with clinical events causing the degranulation of mast cells through an IgE-mediated (anaphylactic) or a non-IgE–mediated (anaphylactoid) reaction. By using the G5 capture assay, normal serum β-tryptase level is < 1 ng/mL and is elevated to > 5 ng/mL during systemic anaphylaxis with hypotension. In general, the greater the severity of anaphylactic reaction, the higher the level of β-tryptase in the serum. An elevated level of β-tryptase within several hours of the clinical event would confirm the diagnosis of systemic anaphylaxis. The level of β-tryptase drops back to within normal range within 24 hours after the anaphylactic event.

α-Tryptase is not stored in the granules and is constantly released from the mast cells in small amounts. In systemic mastocytosis, serum level of α-tryptase is elevated to > 20 ng/mL.

20. Does a normal plasma histamine level 4 hours after the insect sting-induced anaphylaxis have any diagnostic value?

Histamine is stored in the granules of human mast cell and basophills. During systemic anaphylaxis, histamine is released from the mast cells into the circulation and surrounding tissues where it is rapidly metabolized.

Plasma histamine level peaks at 10 to 15 minutes after the insect sting-induced anaphylaxis, and returns to baseline within 30 minutes. In addition, during the blood clotting and specimen handling, basophils can release a significant amount of histamine, which may make it difficult to interpret an elevated level of histamine that

may have occurred in vivo or in vitro. Therefore, a normal plasma histamine level 4 hours after the anaphylactic reaction has no clinical significance.

21. What is idiopathic anaphylaxis?

Idiopathic anaphylaxis is the diagnosis of exclusion. Diagnosis of idiopathic anaphylaxis can be made after a meticulous history is taken and a review of emergency room records, patient's records, and laboratory studies have excluded any underlying causative factor. The mechanism of idiopathic anaphylaxis (IA) is not known.

Two possibilities have been considered to explain this phenomenon. IA is a mast cell activation syndrome that is precipitated by the unrestrained release of the of the histamine-releasing factors (HRF) from T lymphocytes. Alternatively, IA may be an autoimmune disease in which B lymphocytes produce IgG antibodies against IgE, which is fixed to the mast cells. IgG antibody against IgE activates the mast cells causing release of histamine and other mediators.

22. How is a patient with greater than six episodes per year of anaphylactic reaction that are characterized by urticaria and massive tongue swelling treated?

Frequent (> 6) episodes of severe idiopathic anaphylaxis are treated with 60 to 100 mg of prednisone daily for 1 week followed by slow tapering (no more than 5–10 mg per month). In addition, daily antihistamine (hydroxyzine) and beta2 agonists (e.g., albuterol) are given. Overall, patients have good prognosis for achieving a remission. Many patients are ultimately able to go off the steroids.

23. A 38-year-old hypertensive female who is being treated with atenolol is stung by a honeybee and develops symptoms of anaphylaxis within 5 minutes. Upon arrival in the emergency department, she has hypotension, generalized urticaria, and wheezing. She is treated with epinephrine but remains hypotensive. How would you further treat this patient?

Patients being treated with beta-blocking agents generally respond poorly to epinephrine. In such patients, hypotension should be treated with vigorous intravascular volume repletion. Atropine may be administered 0.2 to 0.5 mg subcutaneously every 10 minutes to a maximum of 2 mg. Atropine is helpful in reversing bradycardia. Glucagon exerts its inotropic and chronoprotic effect on heart muscles independent of beta-receptors. This can be given intravenously as a bolus of 1 to 5 mg followed by continuous infusion at the rate of 5 to 15 mcg per minute. Occasionally, intravenous dopamine or isoproterenol is needed to treat protracted hypotension.

24. What is the late-phase systemic anaphylactic reaction?

Most anaphylactic reactions begin within 30 minutes after exposure to the causative agent. In most patients, the anaphylactic reaction is uniphasic, and does not reoccur after complete resolution of the early phase. In some patients, however, a second episode of symptoms is seen approximately 3 to 4 hours (sometimes up to 8 hours) later without any reexposure to the offending agent. It is estimated that approximately 7 to 20 percent of the patients will have biphasic anaphylactic reaction. The exact mechanism of the late-phase systemic anaphylactic reaction is unclear. It is possible that this response is initiated by the release of newly formed mast cell

mediators, specifically chemoattractant (eosinophilic chemotactic factor and neu-trophil chemotactic factor), and further release of cytokines, but thus far no correla-tion between the symptoms of late anaphylaxis and mediators release have been found.

25. What is the role of glucocorticoids in prevention of late-phase systemic anaphylactic reaction?

Glucocorticoid and other treatment (antihistamine and epinephrine) of anaphy-lactic reaction have not been shown to prevent late-phase anaphylactic response. Glucocorticoids can, however, be administered to blunt the late-phase anaphylactic response as they have proven to be efficacious in other clinical situations associated with the late-phase reaction.

26. How long after the successful treatment of acute anaphylaxis should a patient be kept under observation in a medical facility?

There are generally no clinical features that allow identification of patients likely to experience biphasic anaphylactic reaction. Therefore, it is important that patients presenting with severe anaphylaxis be observed closely in the emergency department for at least 12 hours following the resolution of the acute phase of ana-phylactic reaction. Patients with mild reactions may be observed at home and in-structed to return immediately should there be the slightest hint of recurrent symptoms. Instruction in self-administration of epinephrine may be necessary in some patients.

27. What is progesterone-induced anaphylaxis and how is it treated?

Unexplained episodes of anaphylactic syndrome resembling idiopathic anaphy-laxis can occur in young females during pregnancy, or in the premenstrual period, evidently exacerbated by the cyclical changes in progesterone. These patients usu-ally undergo remission during lactation. Episodes of anaphylaxis can also be pro-voked by administration of progesterone and luteinizing hormone-releasing hormone (LH-RH). Treatment includes administration of LH-RH analog. Sometimes bilateral oophorectomy is necessary.

28. Describe the cardiovascular effects of the mediators released by the mast cell and basophils.

Vasoactive mediators released by mast cells during an anaphylaxis or anaphy-lactoid reaction can affect the human cardiovascular system. Histamine causes a re-duction in the systemic vascular resistance. This leads to a fall in systolic, diastolic, and mean aortic pressure, and to an increase in the heart rate. This effect of hista-mine is mediated through both the H1 and H2 receptors. In addition to the peripheral vasodilatation, H2 receptors cause an increase in the heart rate and cardiac muscle contractility, as well as coronary vasodilatation. H1 receptors mediate chronotropic effects and coronary vasoconstriction. Histamine administration, after H2-receptor blockade alone with cimetidine, may intensify coronary vasoconstriction.

Platelet-activating factor (PAF) causes cardiac arrhythmias and myocardial pump failure. PAF may be responsible for the late or protracted phase of anaphy-laxis. Arachidonic acid metabolites, peptide-leukotrienes (LTC4, LTD4, and LTE4),

are powerful coronary vasoconstrictors in guinea pigs, rats, and monkeys. In humans, peptide-leukotrienes can induce transient hypotension, increased heart rate, and coronary artery vasoconstriction.

The antigens and a variety of other agents, such as protamine, general anesthetics, and intravenous contrast media, can be involved in the anaphylactoid reaction. They can directly activate cardiac mast cells, thus leading to the release of vasoactive mediators. Clinically, anaphylaxis has been associated with myocardial ischemia and infarction, ST-T wave abnormalities on the EKG, and atrial and ventricular arrythmias, as well as conduction abnormalities.

29. Why is the detection of anaphylaxis during general anesthesia usually delayed?

Detection of anaphylaxis during general anesthesia may be delayed due to the patient's inability to verbalize initial symptoms. Clinical features of urticaria and erythema can be masked by the drapes used during the surgical procedure. Furthermore, anesthetics can directly produce hemodynamic instability without causing anaphylactic or anaphylactoid response. Often the early appreciable clinical features of anaphylaxis during general anesthesia may include sudden onset of hypotension, bronchospasm, and sudden oxygen desaturation. An increase in airway pressure may also be seen. Elevated serum β-tryptase is helpful in diagnosis of anaphylactic reaction during general anesthesia.

30. List the probable causes of anaphylaxis during general anesthesia.

The following commonly used drugs have been implicated in anaphylactic reactions. Because many drugs are administered over a very short period of time, it may be difficult to pinpoint a causative agent.

1. Incidence of anaphylaxis secondary to thiopental is 1:400 to 1:30,000; other intravenous hypnotics, such as ketamine and etomidate, are rarely the cause of systemic allergic reaction

2. Muscle relaxants such as succinylcholine may produce dose dependent non-IgE–mediated release of the mediators; in some cases, there is evidence for the IgE–mediated mechanism

3. Systemic reactions to the opioids are also due to the direct (non-IgE–mediated) mediator release

4. Intravenous antibiotics

5. Hypertonic intravenous solutions such as mannitol

6. Blood products

7. Intravenous radiocontrast material (RCM)

8. Latex

9. Ethylene oxide used for gas sterilization of the medical and surgical equipment

10. Topical antibiotics

11. Bone cement (methylmethacrylate) has been known to cause hypotension, hypoxia, and noncardiogenic pulmonary edema; mechanism is unknown

31. Describe the pretreatment regimen for prevention of anaphylactoid reaction to the radiocontrast material.

In patients with a history of anaphylactoid reactions to radiocontrast material (RCM), prophylactic pretreatment is necessary. Oral glucorticoids, H1 and H2

antihistamines, and ephedrine have been recommended for prevention of recurrent reaction.

Prednisone 50 mg is given orally 13, 7, and 1 hour before RCM administration.

Diphenhydramine 50 mg is given orally or intramuscularly 1 hour before the procedure.

Ephedrine 25 mg (when not contraindicated) is given orally, 1 hour before the administration of RCM.

Modification of this regimen has been recommended to include additional use of H2 antihistamine, lower-dose corticosteroids, and to exclude ephedrine.

In an emergency situation, 200 mg of hydrocortisone every 4 hours and 50 mg of diphenhydramine intramuscularly 1 hour before the procedure have proven successful.

Use of radiocontrast material with low osmolality is highly recommended.

If possible, beta-adrenergic blocking agents and angiotensin-converting enzyme (ACE) inhibitors should be discontinued.

32. How should an episode of acute anaphylaxis/anaphylactoid reaction be treated in the emergency department?

Early recognition, prompt treatment, and close observation are the keys to the successful management of anaphylaxis. Severity of anaphylactic reactions may vary from mild localized urticaria and pruritus to severe hypotension, airway obstruction, and cardiovascular collapse. The clinical features on presentation should determine initial treatment. The following treatment strategy can be used and modified as necessary.

- Quickly assess the patient's airway, vital signs, and level of consciousness.
- Administer oxygen.
- Establish and maintain oropharyngeal airway.
- Epinephrine: Aqueous epinephrine is the most important drug for the treatment of anaphylaxis and should be administered promptly. An adult dosage is 0.3 mL to 0.5 mL (of 1:1000 aqueous solution) and for children 0.01 mL/kg body weight given subcutaneously or intramuscularly. This dosage can be repeated every 15 minutes for two doses and continued every 4 hours as needed. In life-threatening anaphylaxis, epinephrine can be administered intravenously in 1:10,000 or higher dilutions at a slow rate.
- If anaphylaxis is due to an injection, place the tourniquet above the injection site and infiltrate the site with 0.10 to 0.20 mL of epinephrine (1:1000) to slow further absorption of injected medication.
- Administer 25 to 50 mg of diphenhydramine (for children 1–2 mg/kg body weight); it is usually given intravenously. In mild cases, it may be given orally.
- Ranitidine administered intravenously.
- Hydrocortisone 250 to 500 mg given intravenously. Mild cases can be treated with prednisone orally.
- Treat hypotension with intravenous fluids and vasopressors. Dopamine is the vasopressor of choice.
- Treat bronchospasm with β2 agonists (albuterol administered via nebulizer).
- Patients receiving beta-adrenergic–blocking drugs may not respond to epinephrine. In addition to intravenous fluids, they may be treated with 1 mg of glucagon administered intravenously, followed by continuous infusion at the

rate of 1 to 5 mg/hour. Atropine may be needed for the treatment of reflex bradycardia.

33. What are cold-induced urticaria and anaphylaxis? How can they be differentiated from familial cold urticaria?

Cold-induced urticaria is characterized by the onset of pruritus, erythema, and swelling occurring immediately after the skin has been exposed to the cold stimulus. Urticarial lesions are usually localized to the exposed parts of the skin. Hives may also be brought on by a direct contact with the cold objects. Eating cold foods may cause lip or tongue swelling, but pharyngeal and laryngeal edema is rare. Total body exposure to the cold such as during swimming may cause massive mediator release resulting in generalized urticaria, hypotension, and syncope. Drowning due to severe hypotension while swimming has been reported. A cold challenge or an ice test can confirm diagnosis. An ice cube is placed on the forearm for 5 minutes and the area observed for another 10 minutes. Hives actually appear as the skin temperature is returning to normal. This disease may begin at any age and tends to remit spontaneously in a few months to 2 years.

Familial cold urticaria is a rare syndrome, which is inherited as an autosomal dominant trait. Chills, fever, myalgias, arthralgias, headache, leukocytosis, and burning erythematous maculopapular rash that appears within 30 minutes to 3 hours after systemic cold exposure characterize it. Skin lesions in this disorder are not true urticarias because biopsy of such lesions reveals intense inflammatory reaction consisting mostly of polymorphonuclear cells, occasional eosinophils around the dilated blood vessels and edema. Cold water and ice cube tests are negative.

BIBLIOGRAPHY

1. Burstein M, Rubinow A, Shalit M: Cyclic anaphylaxis associated with menstruation. Ann Allergy 66:36–38, 1991.
2. Douglas DM, Sukenick E, Andrade WP, Brown JS: Biphasic anaphylaxis: An inpatient and outpatient study. J Allergy Clin Immunol 93(6):977–985, 1994.
3. Felix SB, Bauman G, Hashemi T, Neimczyk M, Ahmad Z, Bardel WE: Characterization of cardiovascular events mediated by the platelet-activating factor during systemic anaphylaxis. J Cardiovasc Pharmacol 6:987–997, 1990.
4. Felix SB, Baumann G, Helmus S, Sattelberger U: Role of histamine in the cardiac anaphylaxis: Characterization of histaminergic H1 and H2 receptor effects. Basic Res Cardiol 5:531–539, 1988.
5. Fisher MM: Clinical observation on the pathophysiology and treatment of anaphylactic cardiovascular collapse. Anesth Intensive Care 14:14–21, 1986.
6. Hogan AD, Schwartz LB: Markers of mast cell degranulation. Methods 13(1):43–52, 1997.
7. Horan RF, Austen KF: Systemic mastocytosis: Retrospective review of a decade clinical experience at the Bringham and Women Hospital. J Invest Dermatol 96:5S–14S, 1991.
8. Horan RF, Pennoyer DS, Sheffer AL: Immunol Allergy Clin North Am 11(1):117–141, 1991.
9. Horan RF, Sheffer AL: Food-dependent, exercise-induced anaphylaxis. Immunol Allergy Clin North Am 11:757, 1991.
10. Kemp SF, Lockey RF, Wolf BL, Lieberman P: Anaphylaxis: A review of 266 cases. Arch Intern Med 155:1749–1754, 1995.
11. Lieberman P: Anaphylaxis and anaphylactoid reactions. In Middleton E, Ellis EF, Yunginger JW, et al. (eds): Allergy Principles and Practice, vol. 2, 5th ed. St. Louis, Mosby Year Book, 1998, pp 1079–1902.
12. Marshal CP, Pearson FC, Sagona MA, et al: Reaction during hemodialysis caused by allergy to ethylene oxide gas sterilization. J Allergy Clin Immunol 75:285–290, 1985.
13. Moscicki RA, Sockin SM, Corsello BF, Ostro MG, Block KJ: Anaphylaxis during induction of general anesthesia: Subsequent evaluation and management. J Allergy Clin Immunol 86:325–332, 1990.

14. Nicklas RA, et al. (eds): Diagnosis and management of anaphylaxis. J Allergy Clin Immunol 101(6):Part 2, 1998.
15. Patterson R, Clayton DE, et al: Fatal and near fatal idiopathic anaphylaxis. Allergy Proc 16(3):103–108, 1995.
16. Sampson HA: Fatal food-induced anaphylaxis. Allergy 53(suppl 46):125–130, 1998.
17. Schwartz LB: Tryptase: A clinical indicator of mast cell-dependent events. Allergy Proc 15(3):119–123, 1994.
18. Sheffer AL, Austen KF: Exercise-induced anaphylaxis. J Allergy Clin Immunol 66:106–111, 1980.
19. Slater JE, Kaliner M: Effects of sex hormones on the histamine release in the recurrent idiopathic anaphylaxis. J Allergy Clin Immunol 80:285–290, 1987.
20. Stark BJ, Sullivan TJ: Biphasic and protracted anaphylaxis. J Allergy Clin Immunol 78:76, 1986.
21. Stevenson DD: Diagnosis, prevention, and treatment of adverse reactions to aspirin and nonsteroidal anti-inflammatory drugs. J Allergy Clin Immunol 74:617–622, 1984.
22. Yocum MW, Butterfield JH, Klien JS, et al: Epidemiology of anaphylaxis in Olmsted County: A population-based study. J Allergy Clin Immunol 104:452–456, 1999.

12. SERUM SICKNESS

James C. Leek, M.D.

1. Describe classic serum sickness.

Serum sickness was described in the early twentieth century in patients who received equine hyperimmune serum for the treatment of diphtheria and other infectious diseases. Fever, skin rash, arthralgias, and lymphadenopathy began 8–12 days *after the administration of horse serum. The frequency of serum sickness correlated with the dose of heterologous serum given. Repeated administration produced an accelerated reaction.

2. In what current clinical settings is serum sickness seen?

In addition to the use of heterologous antisera for the treatment of botulism and venomous snake or black widow spider bites, serum sickness is frequently seen in antithymocyte globulin therapy and in monoclonal antibody immunotherapy. Serum sickness syndrome also is occasionally seen in the use of homologous hyperimmune sera or in the administration of high-dose intravenous immunoglobulin therapy. It is an uncommon side effect of thrombolytic therapy with streptokinase. The most common circumstance in which a serum-sicknesslike reaction is seen today is in drug reactions to a variety of drugs. Among these are penicillins, cephalosporins (particularly cefaclor), sulfonamides, minocyclines, thiazides, hydantoins, beta-blockers, and various nonsteroidal anti-inflammatory agents.

3. What is the pathophysiology of serum sickness?

Serum sickness is mediated by the formation of immune complexes to an external antigen. Patients develop high levels of immune complexes that peak concurrently with maximal clinical disease activity. Complement activation occurs, triggering an inflammatory response. Serum C3 and C4 levels fall at the onset of clinical symptoms and correlate with clinical activity. Immunoglobulin and complement deposition is found in the small blood vessels in lesional skin biopsies.

4. Describe the clinical presentation of serum sickness.

One to 2 weeks after antigen exposure, fever and an urticarial or morbilliform rash develop. Symmetric arthralgias are usual with frank arthritis, particularly involving the large joints, somewhat less common. Generalized lymphadenopathy and sometimes splenomegaly are seen. Peripheral edema, abdominal pain, nausea, and vomiting are often present. Most cases are relatively mild and resolve spontaneously within several weeks. Occasionally more severe manifestations, including pericarditis, vasculitis, glomerulonephritis, or neurologic manifestations, occur.

5. What clinical laboratory findings are seen?

Elevated white blood count is common sometimes with eosinophilia. Peripheral plasmacytosis may be seen. The urinalysis may show mild proteinuria or hematuria. The serum complement levels of C3 and C4 are often low in serum sickness due to

heterologous, but proteins may be less commonly depressed in drug-induced serum sicknesslike syndromes.

6. Describe the cutaneous findings of serum sickness.

Urticarial or morbilliform rashes are the most commonly seen. Significant pruritus is usually present. A linear serpiginous erythematous lesion of the borders of the palms, soles, and digits may be the earliest cutaneous finding and is highly characteristic of serum sickness. The palpable purpuric lesions of cutaneous leukocytoclastic vasculitis may also be seen, but are less common than urticarial or morbilliform rashes.

7. What ocular findings may be present?

Visual blurring is a common symptom. Retinal hemorrhages may be seen. Anterior uveitis occasionally occurs and may be a presenting sign.

8. Describe the hepatitis-associated serum sicknesslike syndrome.

This is a prodromal syndrome that occurs in 20–30% of patients with hepatitis B prior to the icteric phase. It is associated with high levels of hepatitis B antigens in the serum and circulating immune complexes. An urticarial skin rash is the most frequent finding with arthralgias and arthritis commonly seen, and proteinuria and hematuria sometimes present. Hepatitis B surface-antigen hemoglobin and C3 have been identified in dermal blood vessels on skin biopsy. This syndrome is self-limited and resolves when jaundice develops.

9. What are the neurologic complications of serum sickness?

Headaches are common; peripheral neuropathies occur occasionally. A brachial plexopathy is a characteristic finding but is seen infrequently. A rare occurrence of the Guillain-Barré syndrome has been reported.

10. How is serum sickness syndrome managed?

A suspected inciting drug or antigen should be withdrawn. Most serum sickness syndromes are relatively mild and are self-limited. Mild cases may be managed with antihistamines, analgesics, and topical corticosteroids. With more severe involvement, a course of systemic corticosteroid tapering over several weeks is indicated. Because readministration of the inciting antigen causes a serum sickness reaction, which appears after several days of exposure and is often more severe, readministration of the suspected drug or closely related agents should be avoided.

BIBLIOGRAPHY

1. Bielory L, Gascon P, Lawley TJ, et al: Human serum sickness: A prospective analysis of 35 patients treated with equine anti-thymocyte globulin for bone marrow failure. Medicine 67:40–57, 1988.
2. Calabrese LH, Duna GF: Drug-induced vasculitis. Curr Opin Rheumatol 8:34–40, 1996.
3. Chan G, Kowdley KV: Extrahepatic manifestations of chronic viral hepatitis. Compr Ther 21:200–205, 1995.
4. Creamer JD, McGrath JA, Webb-Peploe M, Smith NP: Serum sickness-like illness following streptokinase therapy. A case report. Clin Exp Dermatol 20:468-470, 1995.
5. Erffmeyer JE: Serum sickness. Ann Allergy 56:105-109, 1986.
6. Frank MM, Lawley TJ: Immune complexes and allergic disease. In Middleton E, Reed CE, Ellis EF, et al (eds): Allergy: Principles and Practice, 5th ed., St. Louis, Mosby, 1998.

7. Lawley TJ, Bielory L, Gascon P, et al: Prospective clinical and immunologic analysis of patients with serum sickness. N Engl J Med 311:1407-1413, 1984.
8. Lisak RP: Arthritis associated with circulating immune complexes following administration of intravenous immunoglobulin therapy in a patient with chronic inflammatory demyelinating polyneuropathy. J Neurol Sci 135:85-88, 1996.
9. Proctor BD, Murray PG, Joondeph BC: Bilateral anterior uveitis: A feature of streptokinase-induced serum sickness. N Engl J Med 330:576-577, 1994.
10. Roujeau JC, Stern RS: Severe adverse cutaneous reactions to drugs. N Engl J Med 331:1272-1285, 1994.
11. Stricker BH, Tijssen JG: Serum sickness-like reactions to cefaclor. J Clin Epidemiol 45:1177-1184, 1992.
12. Vial T, Pont J, Pham E, et al: Cefaclor-associated serum sickness-like disease: Eight cases and review of the literature. Ann Pharmacother 26:910-914, 1992.

13. FOOD ALLERGY AND INTOLERANCE

Suzanne S. Teuber, M.D.

1. How are reactions to foods categorized?

Adverse reactions are first split into toxic reactions to foods vs. nontoxic reactions. A toxic reaction to food affects all individuals who ingest the toxin in an amount sufficient to produce symptoms. Nontoxic food reactions are dependent upon host factors and can be divided into reactions that are immune-mediated (*food allergy* or *hypersensitivity*) or non–immune-mediated (*food intolerance*). Food intolerance can be due to pharmacologically active components, enzymatic deficiency, or unknown mechanisms.

Adverse Reactions to Foods[7]

Toxic
Bacterial enterotoxins
Fungal toxins
Solanine
Ciguatera poisoning
Saxitoxin
Scombroid fish poisoning

Nontoxic
Food Allergy: Immune Mediated
  IgE mediated
    Anaphylaxis (systemic reaction), mild to severe
    Food-dependent, exercise-induced anaphylaxis
    Oral allergy syndrome
    Food-induced asthma
    Contact urticaria
  Mixed IgE/non-IgE-mediated
    Atopic dermatitis
    Eosinophilic gastroenteritis
  Non-IgE-mediated
    Protein-induced enteropathy
    Celiac disease
    Protein-induced enterocolitis
    Protein-induced proctocolitis
    Dermatitis herpetiformis
    Heiner's syndrome
Food Intolerance: Nonimmune
  Enzyme deficiency
    Lactase deficiency
    Phenylketonuria
    Pancreatic insufficiency
  Pharmacologic sensitivity
    Caffeine
    Histamine

```
        Other vasoactive amines
        Capsaicin
        Alcohol
        Methylxanthines
    Psychologic
        Anorexia nervosa
        Bulimia
        Idiosyncratic food aversion
    Idiosyncratic
```

2. What is the frequency of food allergy vs. food intolerance?

- 5–8% of children have a food allergy. About 2.5% of infants develop cow's milk allergy.
- 1–2% of adults have a food allergy confirmed by oral challenges. Perhaps many more exhibit a mild food allergy termed oral allergy syndrome, but this is underreported.
- About 1% of households in a telephone survey reported a peanut or tree nut allergy.
- 25% of households report alteration of the diet due to either an unconfirmed "food allergy" or intolerance.
- Lactase deficiency is estimated to affect 25% of the United States population and up to 75% of the world's population.

3. Describe the clinical manifestations of IgE-mediated food allergy.

A full spectrum of clinical signs and symptoms are possible. Reactions often start immediately on contact with the food in the mouth, or within the first 1–2 minutes, in those with severe allergy. Reactions usually begin within 30 minutes, and rarely in up to 2 hours.

Clinical Manifestations of IgE-Mediated Food Allergy

SYSTEM	POSSIBLE SYMPTOMS	POSSIBLE SIGNS
Skin	Itching, generalized Itching of palms/soles	Flushing Urticaria
Ocular	Itching Tearing Swelling	Conjunctival injection Periorbital swelling
Upper respiratory	Itching of nose, palate, throat Sensation of swelling Difficulty speaking	Rhinorrhea Nasal obstruction Stridor
Lower respiratory	Shortness of breath Wheezing	Wheezing Obstruction by spirometry
Gastrointestinal	Nausea Abdominal cramps Diarrhea	Vomiting Hyperperistalsis Diarrhea
Genital tract	Vaginal itching Scrotal itching Uterine cramping	

(Table continued on next page.)

Clinical Manifestations of IgE-Mediated Food Allergy (cont.)

SYSTEM	POSSIBLE SYMPTOMS	POSSIBLE SIGNS
Cardiovascular	Light-headedness Difficulty walking Fainting	Hypotension Arrhythmia Tachycardia
Psychiatric	Fear Sense of doom	

4. How is food allergy diagnosed?

• **History**. This should focus on age of onset, symptoms, time between ingestion and reaction, reproducibility (does the reactions occur every time the food is eaten?), presence of atopic dermatitis, asthma, allergic rhinitis, or other atopy. The history also should focus on conditions that may be in the differential diagnosis of food allergy or intolerance, such as gastrointestinal conditions (hiatal hernia, pyloric stenosis, gall stones).

• **Physical examination**. Particular attention should be paid to finding signs of atopic disorders and the nutritional status.

• **Laboratory evaluation**

   If an IgE-mediated disorder is likely:

   • Prick skin tests (in severe anaphylaxis, consider the in vitro test). A negative skin test with a good quality extract is highly specific (95%) and suggests that the patient does not have an IgE-mediated food allergy.
   • Specific IgE in vitro (RAST, ELISA)

   If a non–IgE-mediated food allergy or intolerance is likely:

   • Antigliadin antibodies in suspected celiac disease
   • Breath hydrogen test for possible lactase deficiency
   • Referral for endoscopy, biopsy

• **Dietary elimination**. Usually, this only involves an elimination of one or two foods that are suspected by history and laboratory evaluation. However, in certain cases, a severe food restriction and substitution with an elemental diet for 2–6 weeks may be indicated to determine whether a chronic condition improves. For instance, a patient with severe atopic dermatitis or a patient with allergic eosinophilic gastroenteritis who is positive by RAST (radioallergosorbent test) to multiple commonly eaten foods may benefit from such a severe restriction. If improvement occurs, blinded food challenges can be performed to see which foods may be implicated. In gastrointestinal disorders, such as celiac disease, endoscopy and biopsies are coordinated with the elimination diet.

• **Oral challenges**. These are performed with incremental doses of the food, starting with an amount half of that reported to be the minimum to provoke symptoms. If 10 g of dried food or around 60 g of a wet food are ingested without reaction, it is very unlikely that the patient is sensitive to the food. Except in rare cases of immediate systemic IgE-mediated reactions to a pure, isolated food (e.g., walnuts from the shell, peanuts in the shell), supported by a positive skin test or in vitro-specific IgE assay, challenges are important to the

diagnosis but are underperformed. Many patients and physicians will stop the evaluation after the history or after the skin test or RAST. However, the history is falsely positive in 60% of cases; the skin test or RAST false-positive rate is 50%!

Consequences of *not* performing challenges—hypothetical case examples:

- A child with atopic dermatitis and positive RAST to milk, wheat, eggs, soy, corn, rice, and multiple pollens is placed on an extremely restrictive diet that impairs development. However, oral challenges show that the child clinically reacts with a morbilliform rash only after milk.
- An adult with chronic urticaria gives a history of worsening hives after wheat, any tomato product and corn products, including corn syrup and sweeteners. A RAST was positive for IgE to corn, wheat, tomatoes, and several other plant foods as well as extremely elevated IgE to grass pollens. Even after strict, bothersome elimination of these foods, he still has urticaria but says "it is not as frequent" and he follows this diet for 5 years. He then sees an allergist who suspects that it is quite likely that the food RASTs are falsely positive due to minor cross-reacting proteins between grass pollens and wheat, corn, and tomato. Double-blind, placebo-controlled challenges are subsequently performed and show no relationship between the suspected foods and the hives. Successful medical treatment is initiated.
- A teen has anaphylaxis after eating a Thai restaurant meal. He has never liked peanuts growing up. Skin testing is mildly positive to peanut. He and his family are advised how to avoid peanut and given epinephrine for self-injection. His mother subsequently prepares a dish at home with a dash of sesame seed oil. He goes into anaphylaxis and dies before anyone can find the epinephrine. He was actually sensitized to sesame seed. Postmortem RAST showed class 5 levels of IgE to sesame.

Types of oral challenges

- Open challenge: no blinding. Used in infants or children or after a negative double- or single-blind challenge in an adult.
- Single-blind: The food is hidden in another food that the patient tolerates or is hidden in opaque capsules. The physician is aware of whether it is a placebo or actual food challenge.
- Double-blind: A third party randomizes the placebo and actual food challenges.

The timing (immediate or delayed reactions expected), doses, and setting (hospital, clinic, home) depend on the type of reaction being considered.

- Challenges for some food intolerance reactions may consist of a series of four double-blind challenges using 10 g of wheat flour mixed in a milkshake (twice) vs. a tolerated potato flour (twice). This could be used for a patient who believes that wheat causes a sensation of "brain fog" and fatigue 4 hours after ingestion that lasts 24 hours. The patient would come to clinic to ingest the milkshake and then go home and record symptoms.

```
                    ┌─────────────────────────────────┐
                    │  History and Physical Examination │
                    └─────────────────────────────────┘
```

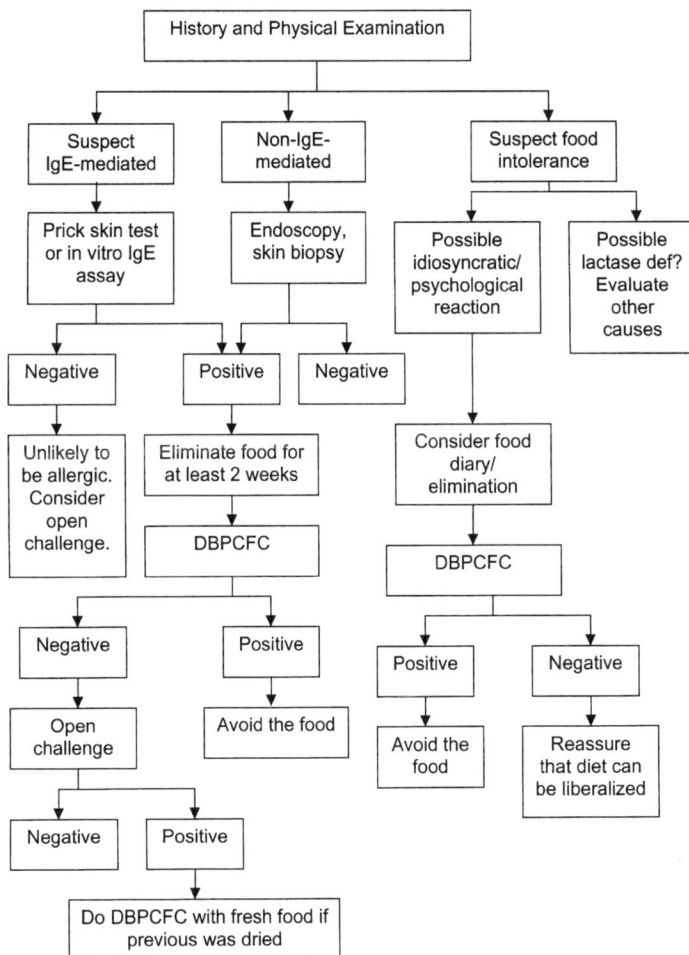

Algorithm for diagnosis of food allergy or intolerance. DBPCFC = double-blind, placebo-controlled food challenge. (Adapted from Sampson HA: Food allergy. Part 2: Immunopathogenesis and clinical disorders. J Allergy Clin Immunol 103:717–728, 1999.)

5. Can a person have an allergic reaction by just being near the food?

Yes. Fatal cases of anaphylaxis have been described in which shrimp or crab was boiled and the airborne proteins (which have been documented and quantitated in cooking steam) elicited severe anaphylactic reactions. Such reactions are possible to any food that is being cooked or handled in such a way that respirable particles containing allergenic proteins are present.

6. Is it true that people have had reactions to peanuts on airplanes?

Yes, it is true. People have had reactions to apparently airborne peanut dust on commercial airliners. The Food Allergy Network sponsored a survey that reported data on 31 people who had reported reactions to peanuts while in-flight. Fourteen of

these reactions were by inhalation. Two subjects were given epinephrine during the flight.

7. What is the most life-threatening kind of food allergy syndrome?

- IgE-mediated systemic reactions. A systemic reactions means that an allergic reaction is developing away from the immediate site of contact with the food. Someone who gets some itching in the mouth and throat when eating cantaloupe melon is said to have the oral allergy syndrome, which is felt to be a local reaction to the food. Someone who breaks out in generalized hives is having a systemic reaction. When a systemic reaction is severe, the term *anaphylaxis* is commonly used, but it is also correct to use the term when speaking about any systemic reaction. Modifiers of mild, moderate, or severe are often used in front of systemic reaction or anaphylaxis. There are no widely agreed upon definitions of different grades of anaphylaxis.
- The following manifestations can result in *death within minutes:*
    Laryngoedema
    Oral angioedema blocking the airway
    Bronchospasm
    Hypotension/cardiovascular collapse

8. List the risk factors for death from anaphylaxis.

- Failure to administer epinephrine early in the reaction
    Many patients do not have self-injectable epinephrine
    - Failure of physicians to prescribe epinephrine
    - Failure of patients to carry epinephrine
    - Failure of patients to keep the prescription up-to-date
    Many states do not allow all levels of emergency medical technicians to administer epinephrine in the field
- Underlying asthma
- A history of previous severe reactions
- Failure to activate the emergency medical system (EMS) after recognizing a reaction due to denial of the potential severity
- Failure to recognize biphasic anaphylaxis, which occurs when a systemic reaction initially seems to respond completely to therapy, only to recur within an hour or two
- Patient on beta-blockers and perhaps ACE inhibitors may have more severe anaphylaxis
- Approximately 150 people are believed to die each year in the US due to fatal food allergic reactions

9. Describe food-dependent, exercise-induced anaphylaxis.

- This is a systemic IgE-mediated reaction that only occurs when two criteria have been met: (1) ingestion of the implicated food; and (2) vigorous exercise within several hours of eating the food. When the food is eaten without exercise or the patient exercises vigorously without previously eating the food, no clinical reaction occurs. The unique juxtaposition of eating the allergenic food with the physiologic and metabolic changes incurred by exercise results in

mast cell activation. This has been studied in a double-blind fashion using treadmill tests.

- The disorder usually has an onset in young adulthood in atopic individuals.
- The foods implicated have included celery, wheat, fruit, peanut, fish, and crustaceans.

10. What is the oral allergy syndrome?

Itching, irritation, and mild swelling, or urticaria in or around the mouth as part of an immediate reaction to a fresh fruit or vegetable is called the oral allergy syndrome. By definition, this syndrome is not life threatening. There is concern however, that some cases of systemic food allergy may start with mild oral symptoms and evolve over continued exposures.

Characteristically, the involved food is only an allergen source when fresh, not cooked, as the proteins involved are usually heat labile. For example, someone may tolerate celery in soup, but not fresh. Additionally, this type of food allergy is purported to be strongly related to specific pollen allergy; studies have shown cross-reactive proteins present in the fruit or vegetable and common pollens. In vitro-specific IgE assays are often negative, as are skin prick tests with commercial fruit or vegetable extracts. If the fresh fruit or vegetable is macerated and pricked with the skin prick test needle, and then used to prick the patient's skin, an immediate wheal-and-flare reaction can often be demonstrated. This is called a "prick plus prick" skin test. There is a case report of a patient's oral allergy syndrome abating after a course of immunotherapy for coexistent pollen allergy.

11. What are some of the reported pollen/food cross-reactivities in the oral allergy syndrome?

Oral Allergy Syndrome Relationships

POLLEN	FOOD
Ragweed	Melons Bananas Cucumber
Birch	Apples Stone fruits (e.g., apricot, cherry, plum) Hazelnuts Carrot
Mugwort	Celery Carrot Some spices
Grass	Potato Tomato Peach

12. Should someone with peanut allergy avoid all legumes?

No. It is unusual, even in the setting of severe anaphylactic sensitivity, to be allergic to other legumes. About 5% of the time, a patient may react clinically (often much less severely) to one or two other specific legumes. However, it is extremely

common to show positive skin tests or RASTs to other legumes, even though these foods are tolerated clinically.

Cross-Reactivity Relationships in IgE-Mediated Food Allergy

FOOD	CROSS-REACTIVITIES
Peanut	Very rarely, soy, pea, or other bean
Cow's milk	Goat's milk, mare's milk, sheep's milk
Chicken egg	Other bird eggs Rarely, chicken meat
Shrimp	Other crustaceans (lobster, crab, crayfish) Rarely, mollusks (scallops, clam, oysters)
Fish	Other species, can be variable
Tree nuts	Other tree nuts, quite variable

13. Can a child with egg allergy get the MMR vaccine?

Yes. Most lots of MMR (measles, mumps, and rubella vaccine) have no detectable egg protein. Even with detectable egg protein, children have tolerated the MMR when given in a two-shot regimen: one-tenth of the dose is given, followed by the rest of the dose if there is no reaction within 30 minutes. Following this protocol, there have been no significant systemic reactions to the vaccine.

14. Is it all right for an adult with egg allergy to get the flu vaccine?

Most adults who report that they have egg allergy actually have no IgE discernible against egg when tested. Egg allergy is usually outgrown in childhood, or patients may be describing an idiosyncratic intolerance reaction (e.g., bloating with eating a lot of egg). Generally, a careful history reveals that the patient ingests egg routinely in small amounts in baked goods; these patients can be assured that the vaccine will be well tolerated.

15. How common is food-induced asthma?

It is uncommon for food allergy to present with the isolated symptom of bronchospasm. Most reactions to foods that include bronchospasm as a symptom include other symptoms as well (e.g., lip swelling, oral itching, rhinorrhea, periorbital edema). However, it has been shown that a small subset of patients with moderate-severe asthma may have food allergy contributing to their disease. Among asthmatics in general, surveys have found that 20–60% of patients believed that certain foods were a trigger. In one study, however, double-blind food challenges only showed positive results (drop in FEV1) in about 2.5% of those who believed they had food-induced asthma in a population that included both adults and children. The prevalence of positive food challenges increased to 6–8% of unselected pediatric asthmatics. Hence, the prevalence of food-induced asthma is lower than perceived by patients, but if diagnosed, the possibility for clinical improvement eliminating exposure to the specific food in a chronic asthma patient is real. A double-blind study of patients with food-induced asthma showed that in a subset of patients, the food allergy could be contributing to the immunopathology of asthma, as shown by increased bronchial hyperresponsivess.

16. Name and describe the food-induced immune-mediated gastrointestinal disorders.

1. **Eosinophilic gastroenteritis**
   - Age of onset: Infancy to young adult.
   - Outgrown?: Up to 50% of pediatric cases are related to food allergy and show IgE to common foods like cow's milk or soy; these cases tend to resolve over 2–3 years. Only a fraction of adult cases respond to an elimination diet and are therefore food-related.
   - Clinical characteristics: Abdominal pain, nausea, vomiting, failure to thrive, diarrhea, iron-deficiency anemia (sometimes), heme-positive stools, and peripheral eosinophilia.
   - Endoscopic findings: Antral gastritis with eosinophilic inflammation common and small bowel involvement are common. Some patients have prominent esophagitis or colitis.
   - Treatment: Assay for IgE to foods, try an elimination diet (may need elemental diet). If responsive, eliminate the offending foods. Otherwise, may need corticosteroids. No apparent long-term risk of malignancy.

2. **Food protein-induced enterocolitis**
   - Age of onset: 1 day to 9 months.
   - Outgrown?: Yes.
   - Clinical characteristics: Bloody diarrhea, emesis, failure to thrive, dehydration, fecal PMNs, leukocytosis, ill-appearing infant, may appear septic. Rapid improvement within a few days of restriction of the offending protein; usually cow's milk or soy. Diagnosis can be confirmed by hospitalization for a protein challenge at least 2 weeks after the infant is stable on a hydrolyzed formula. The infant is fed 0.6 g/kg body weight of hydrolyzed formula. Symptoms develop in less than 12 hours: leukocytosis; heme-positive and PMN-positive diarrhea; sometimes emesis; rarely shock.
   - Endoscopic findings: Diffuse colitis, crypt abscesses, chronic inflammation, sometimes with erosive gastritis, esophagitis, prominent eosinophilia and mild to moderate villous atrophy.
   - Treatment: Avoidance of the offending protein until about 18 months of age.

3. **Food protein-induced proctocolitis**
   - Age of onset: 4 days to 4 months.
   - Outgrown?: Yes.
   - Clinical characteristics: Well-appearing infant with blood-streaked or bloody stools, fecal PMNs, sometimes peripheral eosinophilia. Can occur in breast-fed infants.
   - Endoscopic findings: Eosinophilic rectal inflammation, sometimes colitis.
   - Treatment: Symptoms clear within several days of dietary manipulation. In breast-fed infants, maternal avoidance of cow's milk is indicated first, then egg and soy. In formula-fed infants, a switch to a highly hydrolyzed hypoallergenic formula is indicated. Infants will tolerate the offending protein by 9–12 months of age. No known long-term sequelae.

4. **Food protein-induced transient enteropathy** (excludes gluten enteropathy)
   - Age of onset: 2–18 months.
   - Outgrown?: Yes.

- Clinical characteristics: Anorexia, emesis, diarrhea, chronic sequelae of malabsorption.
- Endoscopic findings: Flattening of the small intestinal villi. Offending proteins: cow's milk, soy, rarely egg, chicken, fish.
- Treatment: Avoidance of the offending protein, usually by switching formulas to a highly hydrolyzed hypoallergenic formula. Infants usually outgrow this disorder by 9–12 months of age. If the onset was later, the reintroduction of the protein should be later. No known long-term sequelae.

5. **Gluten enteropathy/celiac disease**
   - Age of onset: 6 months to adult.
   - Outgrown?: No; it is a permanent condition.
   - Clinical characteristics, classically: Malabsorption syndrome, iron deficiency anemia, folate deficiency, steatorrhea, diarrhea, metabolic bone disease, weight loss, growth delay. Early diagnosis: Anemia, diarrhea, and weight loss or during evaluation for an associated disease; celiac disease may then be diagnosed in absence of gastrointestinal symptoms. IgA antigliadin antibodies and IgA antiendomysial antibodies are supportive of the diagnosis.
   - Associated diseases: Dermatitis herpetiformis, abdominal lymphoma, type I diabetes, IgA deficiency, recurrent aphthous ulcers, hyposplenism, hypo- and hyperthyroidism, myasthenia, sarcoidosis, and rare cerebellar atrophy.
   - Endoscopic findings: Small bowel villus flattening, crypt hyperplasia, intense lymphocytic infiltrates in the lamina propria, and many surface intraepithelial lymphocytes. In screening, a peroral capsule biopsy of the jejunum can be performed. To confirm the diagnosis, the biopsy should improve on a gluten-free diet. In some cases, it is necessary to again biopsy after a 3- to 6-month gluten challenge (daily gluten ingestion).
   - Treatment: Strict dietary avoidance of gluten. Gluten is a collection of poorly water-soluble seed storage proteins (often separated further as gliadins and glutelins) present in the closely related cereals wheat, oats, barley, and rye. Rice and corn are OK. The disease appears to be a multifactorial cell-mediated immune response triggered by the presence of these seed proteins.

17. **Define dermatitis herpetiformis.**
    - An intensely pruritic, bullous skin disease with small blisters in groups, usually on elbows, shoulders, knees, or buttocks highly associated with gluten enteropathy.
    - Biopsy shows IgA and C3 deposited in a granular fashion in the tips of the dermal papillae.
    - Almost all patients have an abnormal small bowel biopsy that is often asymptomatic.
    - Gluten avoidance normalizes the small bowel biopsy and often slowly improves the skin lesions (which may take a year).
    - Dapsone is often effective.

18. **What is Heiner's syndrome?**
    Also called Wilson-Heiner-Lahey syndrome, Heiner's syndrome comprises the constellation of cow's milk protein-induced occult rectal blood loss with anemia and

hypoproteinemia with pulmonary infiltrates in infants or toddlers being transitioned to cow's milk. The syndrome has only been reported in association with cow's milk, not cow's milk formulas. Biopsy of the lung shows IgG, IgA, and C3 deposition with iron-laden macrophages. Pulmonary symptoms and signs may recur during childhood with subsequent cow's milk exposure.

19. **What is the relationship between food allergy and atopic dermatitis?**
   - Approximately 33% of children with chronic moderate-severe atopic dermatitis have food allergy confirmed by double-blind, placebo-controlled food challenges. When the implicated foods are eliminated from the diet, the skin disease usually improves.
   - The food allergy is usually *not* apparent to the child or the family until the disease has been brought under control by aggressive local therapy and double-blind, placebo-controlled food challenges are performed. A positive challenge often presents as a morbilliform rash in the areas usually affected by atopic dermatitis rather than an urticarial response, along with nausea or abdominal pain in about half, and respiratory tract symptoms in slightly less than half.
   - Children are usually sensitive to only one or up to three foods confirmed by challenge even though skin tests or RASTs may show many positive foods.
   - Egg, cow's milk, peanut, soy, and wheat account for approximately 80% of positive double-blind challenges in the published series.

20. **Describe the main foods involved in IgE-mediated food allergies in children and adults.**
   The prevalence of a particular food allergy depends on cultural and geographic considerations. For example, in Japan, buckwheat and rice allergy are important among children. In Scandinavian countries, fish allergy is more prevalent. In Spain, fruit allergy may be the most common food allergy seen.
   In children in the US, studies using double-blind, placebo-controlled food challenges have shown that cow's milk, soy, egg, wheat, peanut, and fish are the most common food allergen sources. In adults, peanuts, tree nuts, crustaceans, and fish are the most common food allergen sources.

21. **Are the main allergens in foods fats, carbohydrates, or proteins?**
   Proteins. Many are glycoproteins, usually heat-stable. For example:
   - The main allergen in shrimp is a muscle protein called tropomyosin.
   - The main allergen in cow's milk is beta-lactoglobulin.
   - The main allergen in fish are proteins called parvalbumins, which control the calcium flux and are only found in fish and amphibians.
   - Both egg white and egg yolk contain allergens, although egg white appears to be more allergenic.
   - The main allergens in peanuts, soy, and tree nuts are seed storage proteins called albumins, vicilins, and legumins.

22. **Are IgE-mediated food allergies outgrown?**
   Only rare cases of peanut, tree nut, crustacean, or fish allergy are outgrown. These allergies tend to persist.

Approximately 85% of milk-, soy-, and egg-allergic children will tolerate the implicated food by age 3 years. If the reaction was anaphylactic and the level of IgE antibody is high, the development of tolerance is less likely. (Recall that most of the reactions to cow's milk are non-IgE-mediated gastrointestinal reactions.)

If a child has a low level of IgE to a food, there is a greater chance of developing tolerance to the food when rechallenged later as compared to those with high IgE. Incremental food challenges are very useful and allow liberalization of the diet after 1–3 years of avoidance. A child may still have a positive skin test or RAST and yet tolerate the food.

Food allergies that are acquired as a teen or as an adult do not seem to resolve.

23. Link sex with food allergy in four moves or less.
Sex → condoms → latex → cross-reactive foods.

24. Explain why some foods are cross-reactive with natural rubber latex.
Natural rubber latex is made from the sap of the *Hevea brasiliensis* tree, which is up to 30% by volume *cis*-1,4-polyisoprene. The *cis*-1,4-polyisoprene is the naturally occurring plant hydrocarbon that is vulcanized into natural rubber. The hydrocarbon exists in the sap as part of liquid rubber particles, surrounded by lipids, phospholipids, and proteins. The associated proteins are not excluded from the rubber-making process, and can be present in significant quantities in the natural rubber latex end product, for example, examination gloves. The addition of cornstarch powder to the gloves provides an excellent "carrier" for the proteins to adsorb to and become airborne or disseminated on mucosal or peritoneal surfaces. If gloves are specially treated to be powder-free or low in protein, it means that the additional steps of chlorination and leaching out of the proteins have occurred. Ordinary, powdered latex examination gloves can be a source of multiple protein allergens from the *Hevea brasiliensis* tree. Patients with "latex allergy" are allergic to these plant proteins. It is expected that some of these would cross-react with plant proteins from other sources.

25. Identify the foods that are most commonly reported to be cross-reactive with natural rubber latex.
- Banana, avocado, kiwi, and chestnut are the most common.
- Potato, tomato, apple, apricot, celery, cherry, fig, melon, papaya, peach, and nectarine have all been reported.
- About 20% of patients with clinically evident latex allergy also have a fruit allergy.

26. Why are food allergens hard to avoid?
In the US, labeling laws for processed or prepackaged foods are strict. All food ingredients must be declared. However, some of the lesser food ingredients are allowed to be listed ambiguously, such as "hydrolyzed vegetable protein," "natural flavoring," or "spices." Highly food-allergic patients may know to be wary of processed and packaged foods with ambiguous ingredients, but even if the label is clear, the food may still harbor a hidden allergen. All bets are off when considering restaurant foods! Fatal anaphylaxis to peanuts has occurred in an unsuspecting patron who ate chili in a fast-food restaurant (peanuts were the "secret ingredient")

and in a college student who ate eggrolls in which the ends were glued down with peanut butter. Contamination of utensils, cookware, or grills (shrimp/fish) can occur. Additionally, some restaurants use gourmet, expeller-pressed peanut or tree nut oils in salad dressings that contain relevant allergens. Highly processed peanut oil is tolerated in peanut-allergic individuals.

Reactions to Hidden Allergens

SOURCE OF ALLERGEN	REASON FOR NO DECLARATION ON LABEL	REASON CONSUMER MISSED THE ALLERGEN
Trace ingredient	Not required by law to explicitly state source: spice, natural flavoring, etc.	
Ingredient	Recent recipe change, labels not properly changed Error in labels—same labels used for two or more processing plants even though recipes differ at the different sites	Listed on label, but not expected by patient (e.g., milk in canned tuna) Listed on label, but an unfamiliar term was used (e.g., *vitellin*, *ovomucoid*, or *livetin* for egg)
Contaminant	Contaminated at wholesaler (e.g., tree nuts mixed) Rehashing or reworking (e.g., a small amount of batter left over from a similar product is mixed with a large amount of fresh batter) Traces of food allergen left on shared equipment contaminate the first products of the next batch (e.g., ice cream with peanuts contaminating a plain ice cream)	

27. Are there any treatments for food allergy?

- Avoidance is currently the only definite approach to both IgE-mediated and non–IgE-mediated food allergy disorders.
- Pollen immunotherapy or vaccination has been reported to cure a case of oral allergy syndrome.
- Oral cromolyn sodium has not been effective as a prophylactic medication.
- A randomized, double-blind trial of aqueous peanut extract immunotherapy showed that skin test reactivity was reduced after a course, but the risks of anaphylaxis were unacceptably high, and one patient tragically died from an administration error.
- Infusion with monoclonal antihuman IgE may prove useful for patients with life-threatening food allergy who are at high risk for accidental ingestion (e.g., peanut allergy), but this has not yet been reported in the literature.
- Clinical trials are planned wherein the patient is first treated with monoclonal antihuman IgE to deplete available IgE responsible for anaphylactic reactions, and then immunotherapy will be given with peanut extract.
- Future peptide therapy with T cell epitopes of food allergens, without the IgE-binding epitopes, and therapy with recombinant proteins that contain point mutations in the IgE-binding sites, rendering the protein unable to bind IgE, are possible.

28. What should you do for a patient who comes to your office with a history of life-threatening IgE-mediated food allergy?

- Prescribe epinephrine for self-injection—enough for two injections.
- Prescribe or instruct the patient to buy antihistamine in a liquid, chewable tablet, or rapidly dissolving tablet to be carried as an adjunctive treatment to the epinephrine.
- Advise that the patient should call emergency medical services at the start of a reaction; no one should wait to see if it is "a bad one." The patient should carry a cell phone if possible.
- The patient needs to have an emergency plan at all times; family members and friends need to be familiar with using epinephrine and how to call for help. If the patient is a child, the school needs to be involved. The Food Allergy Network, below, has many printed and audiovisual resources that can help with ensuring the safety of a child in the school setting.
- Advise the patient to obtain a MedicAlert bracelet or tag.
- Give the patient information on how to read food labels, on other names for the food (e.g., casein, whey, whey hydrolysate are all cow's milk), on the risk of ambiguous labels ("natural flavoring"), and on the risks of cross-contamination in processed foods or in restaurants.
- Link the patient with good resources such as:

   The Food Allergy Network, 10400 Eaton Place, Suite 107, Fairfax, VA 22030-2208. Toll-free phone: 1-800-822-2762 (www.foodallergy.org).

   American Academy of Allergy, Asthma, and Immunology, 611 East Wells St., Milwaukee, WI 53202. Toll-free phone: 1-800-822-2762 (www.aaaai.org).

   American Dietetic Association, 216 West Jackson Blvd., Chicago, IL 60606-6995. Phone: 312-899-0040 (www.eatright.org).

29. What are some of the unproven methods in food allergy diagnosis and treatment?

It is good to be aware of the following practices and to keep your eye out for others that sound "too good to be true." Such methods are sometimes applied by alternative medicine practitioners to people with chronic illnesses or conditions for which the etiology is unknown or for which medical management has been unsatisfactory. In addition, some people believe that certain subjective symptoms that they experience, such as fatigue, are related to certain foods or unknown foods and thus seek this type of evaluation or treatment.

- **Provocation-neutralization**. This is used by some physicians to "diagnose" and "treat" non-IgE-mediated "food allergy." A double-blind trial has shown this to be ineffective. Food extracts of various dilutions are either injected intradermally or given sublingually, and subjective symptoms over the next 10–20 minutes are recorded. If a symptom has occurred (e.g., sleepiness), then a different dilution of the food extract is given (either higher or lower) until the symptom is gone. Whatever dose of food extract was given that correlated with resolution of the symptom is called the neutralizing dose. Patients are then instructed to take the neutralizing dose sublingually or by injection prophylactically before exposure, after exposure for "treatment" or on a regular basis.

- The **4-day rotation diet or rotary diversified diet**. This diet has been promoted in the belief that foods are better tolerated if food groups are rotated completely so that foods from one group are only eaten every 4–5 days. For example, milk would only be consumed every 4 days. There are no clinical trials to substantiate this difficult-to-follow diet. Such a diet has been promoted by some health care practitioners to be used for subjective reactions purportedly due to foods (fatigue, weakness, and arthralgias).
- **Applied kinesiology testing**. Muscle strength in one arm is measured while vials containing the various foods are held in the patient's opposite hand. A drop in strength indicates "allergy" to the food. A blinded study has shown that results were nonreproducible.
- **Electrodermal testing**. Skin conductance is measured by placing one electrode in the patient's hand and another to various acupuncture points in the legs. A glass vial containing a food allergen is placed on an aluminum plate in the circuit. If food "allergy" is present, a drop in electrical conductance is measured. There are no controlled studies.
- **Food immune-complex-assay testing**. Normal individuals have been shown to have circulating immune complexes to commonly ingested foods. The intestinal mucosa is not impermeable and small quantities of food proteins circulate in the blood, which may become part of an immune complex that leads to elimination of the foreign protein. It has not yet been shown that any clinical diseases result from this process; such assays should be considered experimental only.
- **"IgG RAST" or food-specific IgG assays**. It is normal to produce some IgG and especially IgA to the foods that we commonly eat. When subclasses of IgG were described, there was great interest in IgG4 as marker for food allergy, but it has now been shown that normal people produce IgG4 to foods without clinical symptoms. Extremely high levels of IgG to food proteins, which can be visualized by the naked eye in a precipitin assay, are possibly involved in the pathogenesis of food-induced pulmonary hemosiderosis seen with cow's milk ingestion and reported in case reports with egg and pork. However, there is no proof of IgG antibody involvement in other types of adverse reactions to foods.

30. Can food allergies be prevented?

It is not clear whether food allergies in high-risk families (i.e, atopy in both parents or history of severe atopic dermatitis or food allergy in a sibling) can be prevented, but studies do suggest that by following certain dietary exclusions, the onset of atopic disorders may be delayed and the severity may be decreased.

- Consider maternal avoidance of peanut, tree nuts, shrimp, and fish in the last trimester of pregnancy as investigational only. Consider maternal avoidance of cow's milk, peanut, tree nuts, shrimp, and fish during breast-feeding as another investigational measure.
- Strongly encourage breast-feeding for at least 1 year.
- If supplemented, or when weaning, use extensively hydrolyzed hypoallergenic formulas.
- Delay solid foods until 6 months of age.

- Delay cow's milk and egg until over 12 months of age.
- Delay peanut, tree nuts, crustaceans, and fish until over age 2 years, perhaps longer.

BIBLIOGRAPHY

1. Bruijnzeel-Koomen C, Ortolani C, Aas K, et al: Adverse reactions to food. Allergy 50:623–635, 1995.
2. Bock SA, Sampson HA, Atkins FM, et al: Double-blind placebo-controlled food challenge as an office procedure: A manual. J Allergy Clin Immunol 82:986, 1988.
3. Frieri M, Kettelhut B (eds): Food Hypersensitivity and Adverse Reactions: A Practical Guide for Diagnosis and Management. New York, Marcel Dekker, 1999.
4. Metcalfe DD, Sampson HA, Simon RA (eds): Food Allergy: Adverse Reactions to Foods and Food Additives, 2nd ed. Cambridge, MA, Blackwell Science, 1997.
5. Parker SL, Leznoff A, Sussman G, et al: Characteristics of patients with food-related complaints. J Allergy Clin Immunol 86:503–511, 1990.
6. Sampson HA: Food allergy. Part 1: Diagnosis and management. J Allergy Clin Immunol 103:981–989, 1999.
7. Sampson HA: Food allergy. Part 2: Immunopathogenesis and clinical disorders. J Allergy Clin Immunol 103:717–728, 1999.
8. Terr AI: Unconventional theories and unproven methods in allergy. In Middleton E, Reed CE, Ellis EF, et al (eds): Allergy Priniciples and Practice, 5th ed., St. Louis, Mosby, 1998, pp 1767–1793.

14. INSECT ALLERGY

Rahmat Afrasiabi, M.D.

1. What is the overall prevalence of sting reactions in adults and children?
3.3% of adults and 0.4% to 0.8% of children develop systemic reaction following stings.

2. Of those people who develop systemic reaction following insect stings, what percentage has skin or RAST (radioallergosorbent test) test evidence of sensitization?
26% of people who have been stung by hymenoptera have RAST or skin test evidence of sensitization. Venom sensitization is rather common following a sting, occurring in 30 to 40% of those who had recently been stung. However, this figure could change depending on the time interval between stinging and testing. Persons stung more than 3 years prior to testing had a 15 to 20% positive skin or RAST test, suggesting that sensitization is often transient.

3. Is the frequency of sting reactions different in atopic versus nonatopic individuals?
The frequency of sting reactions do not differ between atopic, nonatopic, or unselected populations; however, the frequency of venom sensitivity on skin testing is greater in individuals with skin test sensitivity to inhalent allergens.

4. Describe the factors that affect the frequency and the risk of insect sting allergy.
- The rate of exposure is clearly an important factor and that is the reason that children, males, and adults who work or play outdoors, and beekeepers and their families are at higher risk of insect sting allergy.
- Agricultural and fruit-belt regions of the country have larger populations of the honeybee, whereas Polistes wasp sensitivity is more frequent in the central Gulf Coast states such as Texas and Louisiana.
- Multiple stings.
- Repeated stings in close proximity only weeks apart.

5. Is the pattern of venom skin test and RAST different?
The RAST test is negative in approximately 20% of skin test-positive individuals. However, approximately 10% of RAST-positive individuals have negative skin tests.

6. How many people die from insect sting allergy each year in the United States?
An estimated 40 to 50 people die each year from insect sting allergy. However, this figure may not reflect the real number of deaths because many unrecognized and unsuspected cases may have the label of myocardial infarction or cerebrovascular accident as the cause of death.

7. What is the fate of individuals with a history of insect sting allergy on subsequent stings?

The fate is somewhat unpredictable and there is considerable variability. Only 30 to 60% of sting-allergic patients have systemic reactions when deliberately challenged, even though the nonreactors may react to subsequent stings.

The frequency of recurrent systemic sting reactions in children is considerably lower. The children whose only systemic reaction has been cutaneous have only a 10% incidence of subsequent systemic reaction and the incidence of more severe reaction including respiratory or circulatory symptoms is 0.4%.

8. Describe the natural history of a large local reaction.

The recurrence rate appears to be high. To have a history of a large local reaction does not predict progression to systemic reaction. The eventual risk of anaphylaxis in these people is 5 to 10%. The factors favoring systemic reaction include multiple stings and repeat stings in proximity of few weeks.

9. What is the true incidence of immediate hypersensitivity to *Triatoma*?

The true incidence of immediate allergic reaction to *Triatoma* is unknown; however, a questionnaire survey by the California State Health Department found a 5% incidence of allergic reactions to *Triatoma* in Mariposa County.

10. State the common names of *Triatoma*.

Kissing bug or the cone-nosed bug.

11. What are the most commonly encountered species of *Triatoma* in the United States?

There are 10 *Triatoma* species in the United States. However, only 6 species are likely to be encountered in the continental United States:

1. *T. lectularius*
2. *T. gerstaeckeri*
3. *T. protracta*
4. *T. sanguisuga*
5. *T. rubida*
6. *T. recurva*

12. What is the primary host of *Triatoma protracta*?

The wood rat (genus *Neotoma*).

13. List some of the features of *Triatoma protracta* that have clinical and practical significance.

- *T. protracta* live in the nest of its primary host, the wood rat.
- Each summer, the adult bugs discur. It is during this time that the bites are common.
- *T. protracta* generally flies when the air temperature is above 20°C (65°F), but usually not more than 1 mile. The flights are primarily nocturnal.
- The insects are attracted by light to houses.
- Most bites occur when the host is asleep.

- In a nonallergic person, a triatoma bite is painless.
- The sensitive person usually wakes up with symptoms of impending anaphylaxis.

14. What is the source of _Triatoma_ antigens?
Salivary gland secretions.

15. Where in the United States are fire ants ubiquitous?
Southeastern United States and along the Gulf Coast.

16. What is a characteristic feature of a fire ant sting?
Sterile pustule.

17. Describe mosquitoes and allergic reactions to their bites.
There are 13 genera and 150 species of mosquitoes (Culicidae) found in the United States and Canada.

Most of the reports describe local reactions. In few published case reports, extensive local skin reactions, fever, and delayed systemic symptoms were described. Two of the three patients studied had positive skin tests and elevated IgE to whole-body extract. Using immunoblotting techniques, genus-specific and species-specific IgE antibodies to Aedes and Culex mosquitoes have been shown in sera of mosquito-sensitive persons.

18. Describe common systemic symptoms following hymenoptera stings.
- Systemic reactions, which occur up to 4 hours following sting, are defined as immediate reactions.
- Systemic reaction symptoms are generalized and manifest at sites remote from sting site. These symptoms may include generalized pruritus, urticaria, and laryngeal edema with feeling of tightness in the throat or closing feeling of throat and upper respiratory airway, bronchospasm with wheezing, and shortness of breath. Other symptoms include abdominal cramping, nausea and/or vomiting, and vascular collapse.

19. Which of the hymenoptera species leaves its stinger at the site of the sting?
Honeybee; however, in 4 to 8% of cases, vespid stingers and venom sacs also evulse.

20. What are the clinical presentations of delayed reactions following Hymenoptera stings?
- Delayed reactions usually occur more than 4 hours following sting
- Progressive swelling and erythema at the sting site
- Serum sicknesslike reactions
- Guillain-Barré syndrome
- Glomerulonephritis
- Influenza-like symptoms including fever, myalgia, and shaking chills 8 to 24 hours following honeybee sting have been reported

21. Describe the biochemical nature of allergens in honeybee, vespids, and fire ants.
Venom allergens are all proteins and most of them are enzymes. The most important allergens of honeybee are:

- APIM I, which is phospholipase A2.
- APIM II, which is hyaluronidase.
ᴧ • APIM III, which is melittin.
- APIM IV, which is acid phophatase.
The biochemical nature and the allergens of vespids are:
- DOLM I, which is phospholipase A.
- DOLM II, which is hyaluronidase.
- DOLM III, which is acid phosphatase.
✗ • DOLM IV, which is the common name of <u>antigen</u> 5.
The antigens of the fire ant include SOLI I, SOLI II, and SOLI III. SOLI II is phospholipase.

22. What tests are available to evaluate a patient with clinical history of systemic reaction to Hymenoptera?

Both skin test and RAST test are available for diagnosis. The lyophilized preparations of the five species within hymenoptera—honeybee, wasps, yellow jacket, yellow hornet, and white-faced hornet—are commercially available for use. Bumblebee venom has extensive cross-reactivity to honeybee venom. The persons who have history of systemic allergic reaction to bumblebee can be identified by honeybee skin test. The scratch test using venom concentration of 1 µg/mL is used for screening. If the initial scratch tests are negative, then venom concentration ranging between 1 ng/mL to 1 µg/mL is used in an intradermal skin test. The skin test should also include positive control using histamine and negative control using diluent.

23. Describe the sensitivity and specificity and clinical application of these tests.

- Skin test is more rapid and more sensitive than the RAST test. The RAST test is negative in approximately 20% of skin test-positive patients. However, in 10% of the subjects, the RAST test could be positive with a negative skin test. Therefore, the recommendation is to do both tests in a patient who has a strong history of systemic reaction and has negative skin test.
- Between 8% and 25% of people with sting sensitivity will have a negative skin test at venom concentrations below 1 µg/mL.

24. How early can these tests be done following a systemic reaction? Is there a waiting period following an anaphylactic reaction?

Skin test and RAST tests could be done at 2 weeks or more following anaphylaxis. Because of the consumption of specific IgE during anaphylaxis episodes, these tests may not be reliable early following anaphylaxis. If the tests are negative at 2 weeks following an episode of anaphylaxis, they can be repeated 4 weeks later.

25. Describe imported fire ant allergy diagnosis and treatment.

- There are two major imported fire ants: the black imported, or *Solenopsis richteri*, which is a native of Argentina and Uruguay, and the red imported fire ant, or *Solenopsis invecta*, originally a native of Argentina, Paraguay, and Brazil. Historically, they appear to have entered the United States through Mobile, Alabama.

- Fire ants are common in the southern states of the United States. Recent reports show that their habitat is expanding westward. They were recently spotted in Arizona, California, and New Mexico.
- There are three types of local reactions:
  a. Wheal-and-flare reactions
  b. Sterile pustule
  c. Large local reaction
  The pustules occur within 24-hours following sting and are pathognomonic for fire ant stings. No known treatment can effectively prevent pustules or accelerate their resolution.
- The symptoms of systemic reactions range from generalized urticaria, angioedema, pruritus, and erythema to life-threatening reactions of bronchospasm, laryngeal edema, or hypotension.
- The exact incidence of anaphylaxis to fire ants is not known. Surveys have reported that from 0.6% to 16% of individuals who are stung have anaphylactic reactions.
- The anaphylaxis may occur hours following sting. To date, more than 80 fatal anaphylaxes have been attributed to fire ant-induced anaphylaxis.
- Systemic reactions usually occur in individuals who have been sensitized through prior stings; however, there are individuals without a prior history of fire ant stings who develop anaphylaxis following their first exposure. It appears that these individuals have been sensitized by their prior exposure to *Vespula* (yellow jacket) venom. Both clinical and laboratory evidence supports cross-reactivity between *Vespula* and *Solenopsis* venom.
- Toxic reactions including seizures, mononeuritis, serum sickness, nephrotic syndrome, and worsening of preexisting cardiopulmonary conditions have been reported.
- 95% of fire ant venom is composed of water-insoluble alkaloids that have cytotoxic, hemolytic, antibacterial, and insecticidal properties, and are primarily 2,6 disubstituted piperidines. These alkaloids are the source of sterile pustules but do not induce IgE responses. The water-soluble proteins of *Solenopsis invecta* venom contain four major allergic proteins, Soli 1 to 4. Soli-1 has phospholipase A and B and has some immunologic cross-reactivity activity with vespid venoms.
- Two thirds of the venom proteins are comprised of Soli-2, which does not have any immunologic cross-reactivity with other hymenoptera venoms. Soli-3 is a member of the antigen-5 families of venom proteins without consistent cross-reactivity with vespid antigen-5.
- The commercially available IFA venoms are all whole-body venoms, which, unlike hymenoptera whole-body venom, contain significant and stable amounts of venom allergens. Skin test, ELISA (enzyme-linked immunosorbent assay), and RAST can be used to confirm a history of systemic reaction to imported fire ant. Several studies found venom RAST superior to whole-body RAST. The venom ELISA has similar sensitivity.
- Immunotherapy with whole-body extract of imported fire ant has been done in the last 30 years by injecting dilution of whole-body venom on a weekly basis with gradual increase in dose until reaching an empiric maintenance dose of

0.5 mL of 1:10 dilution of the 1:10 weight/volume stock whole-body venom solution is reached. Maintenance doses are usually given every 4 to 6 weeks.

26. Describe the avoidance techniques for individuals with history of sting sensitivity to Hymenoptera.
- Avoid wearing bright and light-colored clothes that could attract bees.
- Avoid wearing scents and perfumes.
- Wear gloves and long pants while working in gardens.
- Avoid drinking out of uncovered opened soda cans left outside.
- Wear shoes, long pants, or slacks when walking in grass fields.
- Use insecticides specially designed to kill Hymenoptera.

27. What advice do you give to your patients with history of anaphylaxis to triatoma to minimize his/her exposure to kissing bugs?
- Trap wood rats in immediate vicinity (100 yards) if in rural setting, and certainly in dwelling, if wood rat nest is found.
- Check attic, basements, and crawl spaces for wood rat nests.
- If nest is found, trap the rat, destroy the nest, and treat area with malathion 2% emulsifiable concentrate.
- Block wood rat access to structures with ¼-inch hardware cloth; check periodically.
- Weather-strip all doors and windows that are open.
- Be sure pet doors close with no openings greater than ¹⁄₁₆-inch.
- Do not bring outdoor furniture into the house, as you may bring in *Triatoma* with it.
- Use gravity flap covers on outside of exhaust ports for fans and air conditioning.
- Keep outdoor lighting to a minimum.
- Curtains should be drawn in lighted rooms at night.
- Do not use ultraviolet insect traps.
- Inspect dark quiet area (along baseboard, behind curtains, in the furniture, in closets) weekly during triatoma season (mid-spring to mid-fall).
- Scrutinize sleeping area. Bedding should be inspected each evening before retiring. A bed net (available from outdoor/sporting goods stores) is the best exclusionary device while sleeping and should be tucked in at all times.
- Except in known cases of infestation, insecticides are of little value. Safe levels of residual insecticides will not immediately prevent *Triatoma* from gaining access and biting.
- Do not attempt to destroy the local wood rat population, as doing so is ineffective. Consider seasonal (spring and fall) dusting of local wood rats with carbaryl 2% dust to control insect.

28. What are the methods that you can use to control imported fire ants?
- Basic methods are broadcast applications, individual mound treatments, or both.
- Chemical barriers and spot treatments may be helpful.
- Broadcast applications using a bait containing a slow-acting toxicant (hydramethylnon) dissolved in an attractant food source such as soybean oil. Corn grits that have absorbed the toxicant-containing oil are an easily broadcast carrier.

- Because the toxicant used is a slow-acting chemical, there is enough time for the worker ants to feed the queen and other ants before the worker ants die.
- This method results in the Queen either dying or no longer producing eggs, leading to the eventual demise of the colony.

29. List the three most important steps in the treatment of anaphylaxis following an insect sting.
1. Epinephrine.
2. Epinephrine.
3. Epinephrine.

30. How much epinephrine should be used in adults and children?
- 0.3 mL of 1:1000 for adults.
- 0.3 mL of 1:2000 for children weighing less than 30 kg.

31. Explain the epinephrine-containing kits that are available to treat anaphylaxis.

1. Ana-kit contains a syringe preloaded with two 0.5 mL doses of 1:1000 epinephrine, along with chewable antihistamine tablets, a tourniquet, and alcohol swab. A problems with this kit is that patients frequently take the tablets first and wait until the symptoms worsen before using the syringes.

2. EpiPen, EpiPen Jr, Epi-EZ-Pen, and Epi-EZ-Pen Jr contain 0.3mL of 1:000, 0.3mL of 1:2000, 0.3mL of 1:1000, and 0.3mL of 1:2000 epinephrine, respectively. These forms of epinephrine-containing devices are easier to use and are more practical. However, only one dose is available. All patients should be instructed how to use the EpiPen and the Epi-EZ-Pen, which has a practice pen available with it. Patients should also be instructed not to make a mistake and use the practice pen in the treatment of anaphylaxis. The pharmacist should also further train the patients. There have been fatalities reported as a result of patients not knowing how to use the EpiPen. So, it is critical to spend some time with the patient to ensure that the patient fully understands how and when the EpiPen should be used, and that any delay in the treatment of anaphylaxis could be disastrous. Patients should carry the epinephrine kit at all times. The kits should be stored at room temperature and protected from exposure to sunlight. The other available kits include min-I-Jet, Anahelp, and Fasject.

32. Describe step-by-step management of anaphylaxis following insect sting.

1. Aqueous epinephrine 1:1000 (1 mg/mL) administered subcutaneously or intramuscularly in a dose of 0.01 mg/kg of body weight up to a maximum of 0.3 mL. If hypotension exists, lower the dose (1–5 μg/kg) using 1:10,000 (0.1 mg/mL) preparation can be used intravenously by infusion.

2. Parenteral H1-antihistamine, usually diphenhydramine, is commonly administered. Remember that the use of antihistamines as the only treatment of urticaria and cutaneous angioedema, which appears to have become a common practice in many emergency rooms, should be discouraged. Epinephrine should be used for these milder forms of anaphylaxis, and it is very effective in reversing itching and urticaria.

3. The combination of H1- and H2-antihistamines may be more effective in the treatment and prevention of histamine-induced falls in diastolic blood pressure.

4. Glucocorticoids should be used systemically. Their use could help up-regulate the beta-receptors; they might also interfere with arachidonic acid metabolism and the synthesis of leukotrienes and prostaglandins. Their use may prevent late-phase reactions. Patients should be informed about the potential risks of parenteral use of steroids, including avascular necrosis of the head of femur, which could potentially lead to hip replacement.

5. Intravenous glucagon at the dose of 50 μg/kg as intravenous bolus should be administered for the treatment of anaphylaxis in the patients who are on beta-blockers, as these patients do not usually respond to the usual doses of epinephrine. Persistent hypotension may respond to intravenous glucagon, which has the unique property of activating adenyl cyclase independent of beta-receptors, leading to increase in intracellular cyclic-AMP. Because of its vasodilator property could sometimes lead to hypotension.

6. Patients whose only manifestations are urticaria and cutaneous angioedema can be discharged after clearance of these symptoms. These patients should be prescribed an epinephrine kit and instructed on how to use it in case of recurrence of their symptoms. Because of the biphasic nature of some of the anaphylactic reactions, it is prudent that patients be given an injection of epinephrine in suspension (Sus-Phrine, 1:200) 0.005 mL/kg (maximum dose 0.3 mL) at the time of discharge.

Patients who present with significant bronchospasm or hypotension, or who do not live close to a medical care facility, should be admitted to the hospital or kept for observation for 8 to 12 hours before their discharge.

All the patients should be given written instruction on insect avoidance, a prescription for epinephrine with several refills, and instruction on how to use it, as well as a referral to the pharmacist for further training. Referral to an allergist for follow-up evaluation should be arranged.

33. Is immunotherapy indicated for children who have a history of urticaria as the only manifestation of systemic reaction to hymenoptera stings?

No. To answer this question and similar questions, a natural history study was designed at Johns Hopkins University. Two hundred forty-two children ages 3 to 16 years whose only reactions were mild generalized reactions (cutaneous angioedema and or urticaria) were randomly assigned to two groups. One group (68 children) received venom immunotherapy. The second group (174 children) received no treatment; only 1 (1.2%) of 84 stings in the children receiving venom immunotherapy caused a mild systemic reaction. Eighteen (9.2%) of 196 stings in untreated children produced systemic reactions. None of these reactions were more severe than their original sting reactions. The conclusion of this study was that immunotherapy was of little medical benefit, so there is no reason to treat these children with venom immunotherapy.

34. Is there any indication for evaluation and immunotherapy for a large local reaction following Hymenoptera sting?

The majority of individuals presenting with large local reactions following sting as the only manifestation have demonstrable venom-specific IgE antibodies. A very small group of these individuals, however, will develop anaphylaxis after future stings, therefore skin or RAST tests, as well as immunotherapy, are not indicated for these individuals.

35. How effective is the immunotherapy for Hymenoptera?
  • The rate of protection varies depending on the maintenance dose and whether the immunotherapy is for vespid or honeybee.
  • At the usual maintenance dose of 100 µg, 98% of the adults and children on vespid immunotherapy have clinical protection.
  • The clinical protection for honeybee is reported to be at 80%.
  • The clinical protection is reduced at the lower maintenance dose. At a maintenance dose of 50 µg, the clinical protection for adults following sting challenge will drop to 79% from the 98% at 100 µg maintenance dose.

36. When can immunotherapy for Hymenoptera safely be discontinued?
Most studies suggest that the venom immunotherapy can be discontinued after 3 to 5 years of treatment, irrespective of the status of venom skin and RAST tests. However, immunotherapy should be continued for a total of 5 years for individuals who had anaphylactic shock before immunotherapy, or for those individuals who have experienced systemic reaction during the course of treatment. A 5-year period is also indicated for individuals who are sensitive to honeybee stings. The decision to continue or discontinue immunotherapy should be individualized.

37. How safe is the immunotherapy for Hymenoptera?
Systemic reaction does occur during venom immunotherapy. Up to 12% of individuals on venom immunotherapy have allergic reactions during the treatment during build up and during the maintenance. The systemic reactions are more common with honeybee and wasp immunotherapy.

38. What are the safety precautions that should be implemented during venom immunotherapy?
  • Patients should be advised to stay in the office for 30 minutes following injection.
  • Patients should sit in the visible part of the office under supervision.
  • Patients should avoid using the bathroom after they receive their injections, because if they develop serious reaction and faint, they may not be accessible for treatment.
  • Patients should carry their epinephrine kit even when they come for immunotherapy.

39. What are the indications for venom immunotherapy?
  • Adults who have experienced a systemic reaction including urticaria, cutaneous angioedema, respiratory symptoms, and cardiovascular collapse with positive skin or RAST test.
  • Children with respiratory symptoms and cardiovascular collapse.

40. Should the decision to administer venom immunotherapy be individualized?
Yes. The decision should be individualized and should consider many factors, including medical, financial, and logistics.

41. Is immunotherapy available for *Triatoma*?
  • Successful immunotherapy for *Triatoma protracta*-induced anaphylaxis has been reported for 5 patients who were treated with a 1000-unit maintenance dosage developed by Dr. Andrew Saxon and his colleagues at UCLA.

- The standardized antigen was developed by RAST-inhibition assay, which was defined as the amount of antigen that inhibited 50% of the maximum binding of 10 μl of the reference serum and equaled to 0.4 units.
- The antigens were extracted from salivary gland of *Triatoma* colonies.
- The 5 patients showed excellent protection at 28 to 33 weeks of therapy during bite challenges. All patients had a local reaction similar to positive skin test reaction during bite challenges.
- Skin test reactivity was not lost while the patient showed excellent protection without systemic reaction after bite challenges.

BIBLIOGRAPHY

1. Golden DBK: Epidemiology of allergy to insect venoms and stings. Allergy Proceed 10:103–107, 1989.
2. Kemp SF, Deshazo RD, Moffitt JE, et al: Expanding habitat of imported fire ant (*Solenopsis invecta*): A public health concern. J Allergy Clin Immunol 105:683–691, 2000.
3. Middleton EJR (ed): Allergy: Principles and Practice, 5th ed. St. Louis, MO, CV Mosby, 1998, pp 1063–1072.
4. Reisman RE: Studies of the natural history of insect sting allergy. Allergy Proceed 10:97–101, 1989.
5. Rohr AS, Marshall NA, Saxon A: Successful immunotherapy for *Triatoma protracta*-induced anaphylaxis. J Allergy Immunol 73:369–375, 1984.

15. DRUG HYPERSENSITIVITY

Bruce T. *Ryhal*, M.D.

1. What characteristics define a drug hypersensitivity reaction?

Drug hypersensitivity is a subset of the broad category of adverse drug reactions. Most adverse drug reactions are not hypersensitivity responses; instead, they represent a side effect, an overdose, a drug-drug interaction, or other effect related to the dose or pharmacology of the drug. According to a recent consensus statement, hypersensitivity reactions involve immunity and differ from drug intolerance or idiosyncratic reactions, which are mediated by nonimmune processes of physiology or metabolism. Several important clinical characteristics help to define a hypersensitivity/immunologic drug reaction:

- The symptoms and signs should correspond to possible mechanisms of immune damage.
- The reaction generally should not occur early on first exposure to a medication, because specific immunologic memory for a drug usually does not exist prior to the drug's first administration.
- The reaction should recur on reexposure to the drug, and the response triggered after the second exposure will typically be more rapid in onset.
- The drug involved should have a chemical structure capable of eliciting an immune response.
- Because immunity is specific, the reaction should not be a universal, dose-dependent pharmacologic effect of the drug.

Defining a drug reaction as a possible hypersensitivity response guides plans for further diagnosis and treatment of an affected patient.

2. Is there a distinction between drug allergy and drug hypersensitivity?

Drug allergy has such a variety of meanings depending on context that some have suggested abandoning medical use of the term. In allergy and immunology specialty textbooks, allergy usually means IgE-mediated, or immediate-type, hypersensitivity. In many general medical texts and journals, drug allergy is used interchangeably with the term drug hypersensitivity. In institutional medical charts, drug allergy is commonly used to mean almost any adverse reaction to a medication. In lay usage, the word allergy can denote many types of untoward reaction; remember this when taking a medical history. The more precise specialty definitions (IgE-mediated or immediate-type hypersensitivity) apply in this chapter. These distinctions are not merely academic; they have consequences for clinical evaluation and management.

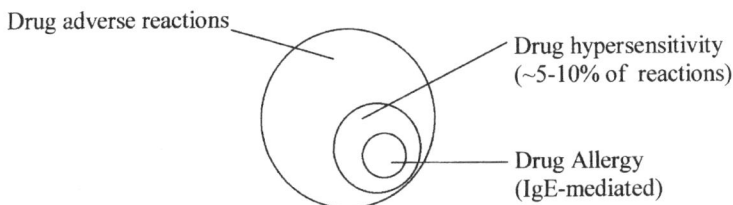

Drug adverse reactions

Drug hypersensitivity (~5-10% of reactions)

Drug Allergy (IgE-mediated)

3. How does an anaphylactoid reaction differ from anaphylaxis?

Anaphylactic reactions involve specific IgE-mediated mast cell and/or basophil degranulation and mediator release. Clinical findings can include urticaria, angioedema, bronchospasm, and hypotension. Anaphylactoid reactions may clinically simulate anaphylaxis and involve mast cells, but they do not involve specific IgE and therefore are not true drug hypersensitivity reactions. Anaphylactoid events may occur after first exposure to a drug.

4. What is the difference between desensitization and a graded challenge?

To be desensitized, a patient must show evidence, usually by a positive skin test, of prior sensitization. Desensitization therefore applies most accurately to the reduction of IgE-mediated hypersensitivity. Graded challenge is the term used to describe the practice of administering incremental doses of a drug to a patient with some other suspected type of adverse drug reaction. Increasingly, though, the term desensitization is used to denote a form of graded challenge (as in aspirin desensitization) involving physiologic processes that may not include IgE.

5. What are the known mechanisms of immune damage that have been associated with drug hypersensitivity?

The Gell and Coombs classification of human hypersensitivity provides models for understanding immunologic drug reactions. A Type I reaction is IgE-mediated and constitutes an immediate hypersensitivity response. Type II hypersensitivity involves antibody-mediated cytotoxicity. Immune complex reactions are termed Type III. Cell-mediated immunity causes Type IV hypersensitivity. For the majority of suspected hypersensitivity reactions, the exact mechanism of involvement of the immune system is not fully known, and some drug reactions may involve multiple pathways.

6. Describe the pathogenesis of Type I hypersensitivity reactions and some examples of it.

Type I hypersensitivity reactions are true drug allergies. They are elicited by the binding of some form of the drug to specific IgE attached to Fcε receptors on mast cells. Degranulation and activation of the mast cell occurs with release of histamine and other preformed and newly synthesized mediators of inflammation. Clinical findings include urticaria, angioedema, bronchospasm, and anaphylaxis.

The proposed mechanism for this type of reaction involves a period of exposure to the drug in a manner likely to favor a Th2 response and IgE production. The initial step in this sensitization process begins with entry of the drug into an appropriate antigen-presenting cell (APC). High-molecular-weight weight protein drugs may be directly processed, whereas low-molecular-weight protein drugs may require haptenization to proteins and peptides to be recognized as antigenic (or allergenic). In the APC endosome compartment, the processed drug-peptide fragments are bound to newly synthesized MHC Class II molecules and transported to the cell surface. The MHC-antigen complexes at the cell surface are presented with costimulatory molecules on the APC to CD4+ T cells which produce cytokines, such as IL-4, that stimulate IgE production by B cells.

Drugs such as penicillin that can bind to human proteins and create allergenic haptens are the most common cause of Type I hypersensitivity. Other drugs that

produce this type of reaction are proteins, generally of a high molecular weight, such as:

- Antithymocyte globulin
- Chymopapain
- Heterologous antiserum
- Insulin
- Protamine
- Recombinant GM-CSF
- Streptokinase
- Tetanus toxoid

7. Describe the mechanism of a Type II hypersensitivity reaction.

Type II hypersensitivity involves toxicity due to antibody directed against antigens on or near the cell surface. Specific antibodies are necessary to initiate this form of cytotoxic reaction, but in contrast to Type I reactions, the antibodies are typically of the IgG or IgM class. An example of this type of reaction is Coombs-positive hemolytic anemia in which penicillin exposure results in the production of antibodies directed against penicillin-coated erythrocytes, causing lysis of the cells. Other examples are:

- Granulocytopenia due to phenothiazines and sulfonamides
- Immune-induced thrombocytopenia due to sulfonamides, quinidine, or heparin
- Methicillin-induced nephritis
- Methyldopa-induced immunohemolytic anemia

The clinical manifestations of Type II reactions depend largely upon which target cell is involved.

8. What are the clinical and pathologic features of a Type III hypersensitivity reaction? Give some examples of a Type III hypersensitivity reaction.

Type III hypersensitivity involves damage resulting from immune complex deposition in tissue and blood vessels. Antibodies are usually of the IgG or IgM class and arise with ongoing exposure to the drug or to a similar drug. Antigen-antibody complexes are created that may activate complement. Medications that elicit this type of reaction can be proteins with a long half-life in the body, such as those found in heterologous antiserum. The clinical manifestations often resemble serum sickness (skin rash, fever, lymphadenopathy, and arthralgia) and occur 1 to 3 weeks after drug administration. Penicillin and cefaclor have been associated with a serum sicknesslike illness, although the mechanism of this syndrome appears to be more complex, and in the case of cefaclor, seems not to involve significant antigen-antibody reactions.

9. Describe the proposed pathogenesis of a Type IV hypersensitivity reaction.

In Type IV hypersensitivity, or delayed hypersensitivity, cell-mediated cytotoxicity is responsible for the various clinical symptoms. Both CD4+ and CD8+ T cells mediate Type IV responses. The proposed mechanism involves binding of drug haptens to intracellular or extracellular proteins for presentation by MHC molecules to drug-specific T cells. Subsequent T cell cytokine release, together with the production of other mediators of cytotoxicity, creates the inflammatory response that is

seen in conditions such as delayed-type hypersensitivity skin disease. Examples include contact dermatitis induced by:
- Ethylenediamine
- Neomycin
- Topical anesthetics
- Topical antihistamines
- Topical corticosteroids

10. What mechanisms of drug hypersensitivity may exist outside the Gell and Coombs classification?

Multiple mechanisms have been proposed to explain the many drug reactions that have suspected immunologic characteristics but that do not fit simply into any of the Type I through Type IV classifications.

It is suspected that many of the morbilliform (maculopapular) rashes, which are commonly seen after several days of drug administration, are caused by specific T cell responses. A proposed mechanism, occurring in cells that express major histocompatibility complex (MHC) Class I (nucleated cells), involves the binding of drugs to intracellular proteins, which are then degraded in the intracellular proteasome complex. The drug-peptide conjugates are then taken to the endoplasmic reticulum for binding to MHC Class I molecules and transport to the cell surface. Specific CD8+ T cells that recognize the antigen-peptides bound to MHC Class I molecules may then mediate inflammation and cytotoxicity. Infiltration of the skin with specific CD4+ T cells also might occur by delayed-type hypersensitivity mechanisms. Cutaneous lymphocyte-associated antigen (CLA) on circulating T lymphocytes may act as the homing receptor for drug-specific T cells to target areas of skin.

The innate immune system, which has lesser specificity, may augment some drug reactions and may not need prior exposure to the drug or its metabolites in order to be activated. The innate system has pattern recognition receptors that protect the body against a broad range of foreign substances with certain characteristic structures. Innate immunity activated by a concomitant infectious process, such as a viral illness, has been proposed to modulate the immunologic response to drugs.

Syndromes that mimic autoimmunity, such the procainamide-induced lupus-like syndrome, represent another pathway of damage. An autoimmune form of hepatitis is associated with anticytochrome P450 autoantibodies induced by drugs such as halothane.

Some nonpeptide drugs, such as penicillin and sulfamethoxazole, can be presented to T cells through association with MHC independent of covalent processing, but the precise clinical significance of this finding is unclear.

11. Describe the most important methods available for arriving at a clinical diagnosis of a suspected hypersensitivity drug reaction.

The medical history and physical exam are the most important tools for arriving at a diagnosis of drug hypersensitivity. Confusion often results when multiple drugs have been administered and a reaction has occurred. A complete list of all medications taken by the patient and the time and dates of administration must be recorded. Information should be collected regarding the patient's prior reactions and any previous exposure to the suspected medications. Knowledge of the pharmacology and side

effects of the drugs, as well as the general risk of hypersensitivity for each drug taken, is important. An assessment of the patient's individual risk for drug hypersensitivity should be made. Alternative causes, such as infection, should be excluded. The physical exam can help define the type of reaction, which can then be correlated with the time course of administration of the various drugs to suggest a plausible cause and mechanism. Very limited diagnostic testing is available for most drug reactions.

12. Who is at risk for drug hypersensitivity?

Several categories of patients may be at greater risk for drug hypersensitivity. The elderly are more susceptible to adverse drug reactions, and females are more likely to acquire autoimmune disease. Patients who have had previous immune reactions to one or more drugs may be at greater risk, especially if they have reacted to a chemically similar medication. Higher risk patients may show genetic variation in drug metabolic enzymes. Patients with concomitant viral infections are more likely to develop hypersensitivity. A common example is the morbilliform rash that is often seen in patients with mononucleosis who are given amoxicillin. Patients with AIDS also have more drug-induced morbilliform cutaneous reactions, typically occurring 1 to 2 weeks into treatment with the drug, and especially with sulfonamides. Atopy by itself does not appear to be a risk factor for reactions to nonprotein drugs.

The method of delivery of a drug also affects the risk for reaction. Topical administration is the most likely to result in sensitization; oral ingestion is the least likely to cause an immune reaction, and parenteral delivery is intermediate in risk of sensitization.

13. Name the dermatologic syndromes that can result from drug hypersensitivity.

Drug reactions are most commonly heralded by skin changes, partly because they are the most noticeable, and because the skin is an active metabolic and immunologic organ. Clinical syndromes include:

- Cutaneous vasculitis
- Eczema
- Erythema multiforme/Stevens-Johnson syndrome/toxic epidermal necrolysis
- Erythema nodosum
- Erythroderma (exfoliative dermatitis)
- Fixed drug eruptions
- Lichenoid eruptions
- Morbilliform rashes
- Photoallergic reactions
- Urticaria/angioedema

14. What are the causes and characteristics of drug-induced urticaria?

Drug-induced urticaria is due to release of mast cell mediators and occurs most often because of a Type I hypersensitivity reaction, although Type III and pseudoallergic reactions may also result in this syndrome. Lesions are typically erythematous wheals that are pruritic and blanch on pressure. The lesions are evanescent and, if marked, will usually vanish and/or relocate within 24 hours. Angioedema, or soft tissue swelling, may occur with an urticarial reaction and, when present, is often most visible on the face and perioral region. Severe, systemic mast cell mediator release

results in anaphylaxis, so urticarial reactions are of significant concern. Examples of medications likely to induce urticaria include many of the drugs that cause Type I hypersensitivity. Aspirin and related drugs can cause an urticarial rash through leukotriene mechanisms not involving specific immunity.

15. Describe the clinical features of drug-induced morbilliform reactions.

Drug-induced morbilliform reactions are among the most common of all drug reactions. The morbilliform rashes typically begin on the trunk as small, maculopapular, blanching areas of erythema, and may spread to involve the limbs. The palms and soles are often spared. Pruritus is variable. The lesions can become confluent. The rash usually develops within 1 to 3 weeks of initiating a drug, and medications that have been used for a long time (months or years) in the patient are rarely suspect. Some of these reactions may resolve despite continued use of the drug, but this course of action is not riskless, because some more-serious reactions may have a morbilliform initial appearance. Most cases resolve with symptomatic treatment and discontinuation of the drug.

16. How are erythema multiforme, Stevens-Johnson syndrome, and toxic epidermal necrolysis (TEN) related to drug hypersensitivity?

This group of diseases shares some clinical and pathologic features. Ten to 20% of cases of erythema multiforme are attributed to drug reactions. Erythema multiforme may begin early after drug administration and manifests as erythematous target lesions with central bullae. The individual lesions are nonblanching, have varying shapes, and persist in a specific location for a week or more instead of relocating, as do urticarial lesions, within 24 hours. Erythema multiforme major involves multiple mucosal surfaces in addition to the skin and presents with more systemic symptoms. Patients with the Stevens-Johnson syndrome have purpuric macules and blisters with prominent trunk and face involvement.

Toxic epidermal necrolysis presents with fever, diffuse erythema, and edema evolving into widespread bullae formation with skin detachment. It is thought that drugs cause most cases of TEN. A proposed immune mechanism accounting for TEN is keratinocyte apoptosis mediated by Fas (CD95) and Fas ligand (FasL). An increase in activated CLA+ T cells has also been reported.

Selected medications associated with these types of drug reactions include:
• Allopurinol
• Anticonvulsants
• Barbiturates
• NSAIDs
• Penicillins
• Sulfonamides

17. How does drug-induced erythroderma differ from TEN?

Drug-induced erythroderma may be confused with TEN but it is a less-serious disease. Diffuse erythema with scaling and exfoliation occurs in the erythroderma syndrome although full thickness epidermal detachment is not found. Many drugs, including vancomycin, sulfonamides, and penicillins, may cause exfoliative dermatitis. Erythroderma has been referred to as the red-man syndrome, although the

term red-man is also used to describe the immediate and transient histamine flush caused in some patients by vancomycin infusion.

18. What are fixed drug eruptions?

Fixed drug eruptions are typically well circumscribed, erythematous papules and plaques that recur at the same site each time a drug is administered. The lesions are commonly found around the oral, anal, and genital areas and often occur less than 8 hours after readministration of a drug. They may be pruritic or cause a burning dysesthesia. The characteristic recurrence at a specific site suggests immunologic memory, perhaps related to skin T cells. Drugs that may cause this reaction include:

- Acetaminophen
- Barbiturates
- NSAIDs
- Oral contraceptives
- Phenolphthalein
- Sulfonamides

19. Describe the characteristics of drug-allergy-associated eczema.

The clinical symptom of eczema occurs most commonly with topical administration of a drug, although systemic administration may cause some cases. Eczema consists of disrupted skin with varying degrees of erythema, vesiculation, scaling, and thickening. Many drugs may cause contact dermatitis with eczema after topical administration, presumably through Type IV hypersensitivity mechanisms. Medications that may cause eczema through systemic administration include penicillin, bleomycin, and gold.

20. Are lichenoid eruptions associated with drug hypersensitivity?

Lichenoid drug eruptions are rashes that clinically resemble lichen planus. The drug-induced lesions are well circumscribed, violaceous or red papules with occasional scaling. They may appear after several months of drug administration. Drugs that have been associated with this type of eruption include:

- Antimalarials
- β-Blockers
- Captopril
- Dapsone
- Furosemide
- Gold
- Methyldopa
- Penicillamine
- Sildenafil

21. Is drug hypersensitivity involved in photoallergic responses?

Light-induced rashes may be of several types. Photoirritant or phototoxic dermatitis is nonimmune in etiology and usually occurs rapidly after administration of the drug together with sun exposure. Examples of phototoxic drugs include tetracyclines, phenothiazines, and NSAIDs. A photoallergic response, which occurs after a

period of sensitization, is often delayed in onset and resembles a contact dermatitis. Examples of photoallergic reactions include the pruritic, inflammatory skin reactions seen on light-exposed areas after administration of medications such as:

- Fluoroquinolones
- Griseofulvin
- Sulfonamides
- Thiazides

22. What are some systemic syndromes associated with drug hypersensitivity?

Anaphylaxis may be seen after drug exposure and is a systemic syndrome consisting of urticaria, bronchoconstriction, and hypotension. True anaphylaxis is due to a Type I hypersensitivity reaction, and usually occurs with minutes (rarely hours) of exposure to a drug.

Drug-induced lupus-like syndromes may occur after use of hydralazine or procainamide. Clinical symptoms resolve promptly when these medications are discontinued.

Various forms of vasculitis can occur due to drug hypersensitivity and may be systemic or limited to the skin. Drug-induced urticarial vasculitis is similar to urticaria in appearance but has skin lesions that are more persistent. Drugs can cause hypersensitivity vasculitis, which affects postcapillary venules and causes non-blanching, purpuric papules ("palpable purpura") that are most numerous on the lower extremities. Henoch-Schönlein purpura may also be triggered by medications. Drugs associated with vasculitis include:

- Allopurinol
- Granulocyte colony-stimulating factor
- Penicillin
- Propylthiouracil
- Sulfonamides
- Thiazides

23. Do drugs cause hypersensitivity reactions that predominantly affect a single organ system?

Single-organ systems other than the skin may be the focus of a drug hypersensitivity reaction. Selected examples are listed below:

TARGET ORGAN	CLINICAL FINDINGS	DRUGS
Lungs	Pneumonia with eosinophilia	Penicillin Nitrofurantoin NSAIDs Sulfonamides
	Alveolar or interstitial infiltrates	Methotrexate Melphalan
Kidney	Interstitial nephritis	Methicillin Sulfonamides
	Membranous glomerulonephritis	Allopurinol Gold
Liver	Hepatitis	Halothane Sulfonamides
	Hepatitis with cholestatic jaundice	Phenothiazines

24. What types of diagnostic testing are available to evaluate drug reactions?

Only limited testing is available for most drug-hypersensitivity conditions. Some studies may be helpful to confirm a clinical diagnosis. Commonly used tests include:

- Drug challenge
- Autoantibodies including Coombs test and antiplatelet antibodies
- Epicutaneous, intradermal, and patch skin testing
- In vitro antibody testing with RAST and/or ELISA
- Serum β-tryptase
- Skin biopsy
- Tests for immune complexes or complement activation including C3, C4, cryoglobulins, and C1q-binding assays

Tests with limited or research availability include:

- Cytotoxic testing
- In vitro lymphocyte transformation
- Isolation of specific T cell clones
- Leukocyte histamine release assays

25. Describe the uses and limitations of testing for drug hypersensitivity.

Testing can be utilized in some instances to confirm or to exclude a specific immune mechanism. A Type I reaction with anaphylaxis can be confirmed by an elevated serum β-tryptase, although this test will not identify the causative agent. For a limited number of drugs, the risk of a Type I reaction can be determined by epicutaneous and intradermal skin testing. Skin testing has clear predictive value for Type I immune reactions due to penicillin, insulin, chymopapain, tetanus toxoid, protamine, and streptokinase. Although occasionally used to test other drugs such as cephalosporins, the negative predictive value for these substances is not accurately known. The negative predictive value is critical because it represents the likelihood that a negative test will correlate with safe administration of the drug. Skin testing is inaccurate for most drugs that are not high-molecular-weight protein drugs. In vivo metabolites and hapten-protein conjugates may cause an adverse reaction in circumstances in which the native drug does not. Skin testing may also give false positive results, because many drugs act as irritants, even at dilute concentrations. Radioallergosorbent (RAST) and enzyme-linked immunosorbent (ELISA) tests are also available; they quantitatively assay IgE antibody to some drugs. These tests may be less sensitive than skin tests, but can be used in patients who cannot stop antihistamines or who have dermographism.

Type II hypersensitivity reactions can be evaluated in the laboratory with tests for autoantibodies such as Coombs and antiplatelet antibodies, though these tests will not confirm the involvement of a specific drug. Type III reactions may show abnormalities on measurement of C3, C4, cryoglobulins, and C1q-binding assays.

Type IV hypersensitivity, when due to contact dermatitis, can be tested with specific patch testing. Lymphocyte proliferation testing and isolation of specific T cell clones are research tools for evaluating Type IV reactions.

Although testing can demonstrate lack of sensitization at a particular point in time, the risk of later sensitization cannot be entirely excluded.

26. What investigative options exist if specific testing for a drug is not available?

If specific testing is not available, the clinician can discontinue all or selected drugs and observe the results. After the clinical symptoms have resolved, a graded drug challenge is an optional procedure.

27. How is a drug challenge used to test and treat patients?

An incremental or graded drug challenge can help determine whether a patient will have an adverse reaction to a specific drug. A graded drug challenge is based on the assumption that small doses of a medication are less likely to have major toxic effects than full doses. Incremental drug challenge is not true desensitization because no immune sensitization is demonstrated before the challenge. In fact, if sensitization is proven, such as with a positive skin test, a desensitization protocol should be used instead. Usually, desensitization protocols involve more drug dilutions and are more cautious than graded challenges. A graded challenge should not be attempted where the drug is suspected to have caused mucocutaneous bullous skin disease, TEN, or vasculitis, because these disorders are associated with considerable morbidity and mortality. Protocols for graded challenge are available for many drugs including sulfonamides, aspirin, NSAIDs, acyclovir, zidovudine, pentamidine, and penicillamine. Depending on the severity of the possible reaction, required monitoring for a challenge may vary from an ICU setting to a carefully observed office environment. The patient's historical reaction to the medication and the likelihood of known reactions to the drug can help estimate risk.

28. What is the role of penicillin testing in the evaluation of a patient with a history of a penicillin reaction? How is it performed?

Penicillin skin testing is the model for much of drug hypersensitivity testing. As with all immediate hypersensitivity skin testing, penicillin skin tests are predictive of IgE-mediated reactions only. Serum sickness-type reactions, hemolytic anemia, and nonurticarial rashes are not excluded by a negative test. To achieve maximum predictive value, testing must be performed with both major and minor determinant materials. Major determinant mix is available commercially as PrePen, which is benzylpenicilloyl-polylysine, and will detect approximately 80% of penicillin-sensitized patients. The remainder of sensitized patients will have significant IgE-mediated reactions only to minor determinant mix, which is not available commercially. Benzylpenicillin (penicillin G) is used as the sole minor determinant test in many centers. Approximately 93 to 97% of patients who are skin test-negative to PrePen and penicillin G will tolerate penicillin administration. If minor determinant mix is synthesized and used according to published protocols, nearly 99% of skin test-negative patients can be administered penicillin safely. Active components of synthesized minor determinant mix include benzylpenicilloate and benzylpenilloate. For all testing reagents, intradermal testing follows a prick test.

29. How can testing evaluate possible hypersensitivity reactions to muscle relaxants, local anesthetics, and agents used in general anesthesia?

Both hypersensitivity and pseudoallergic reactions can occur during local and general anesthesia. Often it is difficult to determine the cause because multiple drugs are administered during these procedures. Protocols are available for testing anesthetic

agents and muscle relaxants (neuromuscular agents). The protocols for anesthetic agents represent a combination of skin testing and graded challenge, because specific IgE has not been demonstrated for most of these drugs. Although specific IgE has been found for some muscle relaxants, skin tests for these medications tend to have a low predictive value. Good negative predictive values for skin testing of local anesthetics allow patients with negative results to safely receive these agents.

30. What types of treatment are available for drug hypersensitivity?
In nearly all cases, the suspected drug should be discontinued. Some rare cases that constitute only minor reactions, such as morbilliform rashes, can be treated through if no substitute medication is available. However, a morbilliform eruption may be the initial manifestation of a potentially fatal reaction such as TEN. Specific treatment is directed at the presenting symptoms, such as urticaria or anaphylaxis. Desensitization for some medications can allow continued use of the drug. TEN requires special attention, and most patients are managed the same as those with major burns. Systemic corticosteroids are harmful in advanced TEN. At least one uncontrolled report suggests that infusion of intravenous immune serum globulin (IVIG) may be effective for TEN.

31. What types of drugs can be substituted for a medication that has caused a hypersensitivity reaction?
The therapeutic indication for a drug often persists despite the need for withdrawal of the medication. Cross-reactivity between structurally similar drugs can be anticipated, therefore structurally unrelated drugs are the preferred substitute. Oral forms of substitute drugs are usually safer and less likely to cause sensitization.

32. Can other beta lactams or cephalosporins be used in the penicillin-allergic individual?
Closely related beta lactams, such as amoxicillin or ampicillin, should not be used in the penicillin-allergic patient. Carbapenems (such as imipenem) are cross-reactive with penicillin. Monobactams (such as aztreonam) generally do not cross-react. Use of cephalosporins in penicillin skin test-positive patients poses an estimated 2% risk of reaction, and the safest course is to use a desensitization protocol if a cephalosporin is necessary for such patients. Skin testing for cephalosporins has unclear predictive value. Patients who give a vague history of a nonanaphylactic reaction to penicillin, and who have never been penicillin skin tested, probably have a less than 1% risk of reacting to a cephalosporin. First- and second-generation cephalosporins are more likely than third-generation drugs to cause allergic reactions in penicillin-sensitive individuals.

33. When is drug desensitization appropriate?
When substitution is impossible and the drug is necessary, drug allergic patients may undergo a desensitization protocol. Extremely dilute solutions (such as a 10,000-fold dilution) of the drug are administered initially, with a gradual increase in concentration and amount. A successful protocol results in antigen-specific mast cell desensitization, enabling full concentrations of the drug to be given. Oral desensitization is the safest route. After desensitization, the drug must be continually

administered until the required course is completed. Return of clinical sensitivity can occur on cessation of the drug. Penicillin desensitization has been the most successful. Protocols termed desensitization have been published for sulfonamides and aspirin, but they are more accurately called graded challenges.

34. What is a pseudoallergic reaction?

A pseudoallergic reaction has the clinical manifestations of an immediate hypersensitivity reaction but without involvement of IgE. Some medications, such as opiates, radiocontrast media (RCM), and vancomycin, can cause direct histamine release. Other drugs, such as the angiotensin-converting enzyme inhibitors, act through kinin mechanisms and may cause angioedema and cough. Other pathways that produce pseudoallergic responses include complement activation (protamine), leukotriene synthesis (aspirin and NSAIDs), and irritant bronchospasm (sulfites).

35. Why is the anaphylactoid reaction to RCM in high-risk patients prevented by pretreatment rather than desensitization?

Because radiocontrast materials can cause mast cell mediator release without involvement of specific IgE, a densensitization protocol will not prevent RCM reactions and skin testing will not be helpful. Patients who require RCM and who have had a previous reaction to RCM should receive pretreatment with corticosteroids, antihistamines, and possibly adrenergic agents to decrease the risk of an adverse reaction. Use of nonionic contrast materials can also decrease the likelihood of mast cell activation in individuals at risk.

36. Describe the clinical and biochemical characteristics of salicylate reactions.

Salicylates cause pseudoallergic/anaphylactoid reactions in some individuals through inhibition of cyclooxygenase (COX), and through subsequent changes in prostaglandin and leukotriene production. Skin testing is not helpful in determining at-risk patients because no specific IgE is involved. Weak inhibitors of COX, such as acetaminophen and salsalate, are better tolerated in ASA-sensitive patients, although cross-sensitivity may occur, especially at high doses. The COX-2 inhibitors have not been widely investigated at this writing. The manufacturer's labeling on COX-2 inhibitors includes a warning for cross-sensitivity with ASA. Preliminary studies indicate that the risk for cross-reactivity between ASA and COX-2 inhibitors is much less than with older NSAIDs; this would be predicted on theoretical grounds. A graded challenge, which is often called desensitization, can render ASA-sensitive patients tolerant.

37. How is drug hypersensitivity related to drug metabolism?

Risk of hypersensitivity may depend upon alterations in an individual patient's drug metabolism. An example is the anticonvulsant hypersensitivity syndrome, which is characterized by fever, maculopapular rash, and lymphadenopathy. There may also be eosinophilia and diffuse inflammation of the liver and kidney. This syndrome may follow, within weeks to months, the administration of aromatic anticonvulsants such as phenytoin, carbamazepine, and phenobarbital. Susceptibility to this type of hypersensitivity disorder may be due to the presence of a defined alteration

in drug metabolism. Increased risk of immunologic damage has been proposed to increase with metabolic variation in the biotransformation of other drugs as well.

DRUG	CLINICAL SYNDROME	METABOLIC ALTERATION	REACTIVE METABOLITE
Anticonvulsants	Anticonvulsant hypersensitivity syndrome	Hereditary deficiency of epoxide hydrolase	Arene oxides
Sulfamethoxazole	Skin rash	Slow N-acetylation or decreased glutathione	Sulfamethoxazole hydroxylamine
Cefaclor	Serum-sicknesslike reaction	Hereditary variation in cefaclor metabolism	Cefaclor metabolites
Procainamide	Drug-induced lupus	Slow acetylators	Hydroxylamino-procainamide

The link between toxicity and immunity may be the contribution of reactive metabolites to the formation of an immunogenic product. This product may trigger the specific immune system ("drug-hapten model"), or it may activate the innate immune system ("danger model"), which could proceed to modulate a more complex adaptive immune response. Pharmacogenetic screening for metabolic variants may someday decrease the incidence of adverse immunologic drug reactions.

38. After receiving a medication, can a patient have a hypersensitivity reaction that is not due to the active drug or its metabolites?

Excipients, preservatives, and contaminants can cause a hypersensitivity response. For example, pharmaceutical components such as gelatin, egg proteins, and benzylalkonium chloride have been associated with drug allergy.

39. Does the health care professional have a responsibility to report drug hypersensitivity?

As a category of adverse drug reaction, serious drug hypersensitivity reactions may be reported through MedWatch (1-800-FDA-1088), the FDA medical products reporting system. Except for adverse events associated with vaccines, reporting is voluntary at the federal level for health professionals. However, reports are encouraged because underreporting of reactions is a major concern. Some states and local agencies may have additional reporting requirements.

BIBLIOGRAPHY

1. Adkinson NF: Drug allergy. In Middleton E, Reed CE, Ellis EF, et al (eds): Allergy: Principles and Practice, 5th ed. St. Louis, Mosby, 1998, pp 1212–1224.
2. Beltrani VS: Cutaneous manifestations of adverse drug reactions. Immunol Allergy Clin N Am 18:867–895, 1998.
3. Bernstein IL, Gruchalla RS, Lee RE et al (eds): Disease management of drug hypersensitivity: A practice parameter. Ann Allergy Asthma Immunol 83:665–700, 1998.
4. Borish L, Tilles SA: Immune mechanisms of drug allergy. Immunol Allergy Clin N Am 18:717–729, 1999.
5. Dykewicz MS: Drug allergy. In Slavin RG, Reisman RE (eds): Expert Guide to Allergy and Immunology, Philadelphia, American College of Physicians, 1999, pp 127–160.
6. Kalish RS, Askenase PW: Molecular mechanism of CD8+ T-cell-mediated delayed hypersensitivity: Implications for allergies, asthma and autoimmunity. J Allergy Clin Immunol 103:192–199, 1999.
7. Leyva L, Torres MJ, Posadas S, et al: Anticonvulsant-induced toxic epidermal necrolysis: Monitoring the immunologic response. J Allergy Clin Immunol 105:157–165, 2000.

8. Macy E, Richter PK, Falkoff R, et al: Skin testing with penicilloate and penilloate prepared by an improved method: Amoxicillin oral challenge in patients with negative skin test response to penicillin reagents. J Allergy Clin Immunol 100:586–591, 1997.

9. Moscicki RA, Sockin SM, Corsello BF, et al: Anaphylaxis during induction of general anesthesia: Subsequent evaluation and management. J Allergy Clin Immunol 86:325–332, 1990.

10. Nicklas RA, Bernstein IL, Li JT, et al (eds): The diagnosis and management of anaphylaxis. J Allergy Clin Immunol 101:S465–S528, 1998.

11. Roujeau JC, Stern RC: Severe adverse cutaneous reactions to drugs. N Engl J Med 331:1272–1285, 1994.

12. Saxon A, Beall GN, Rohr AS, et al: Immediate hypersensitivity reactions to beta-lactam antibiotics. Ann Intern Med 107:204–215, 1987.

13. Stern RS, Wintroub BU: Cutaneous reactions to drugs. In Freedberg IM, Eisen AZ, Wolff K, et al (eds): Fitzpatrick's Dermatology in General Medicine, 5th ed. New York, McGraw-Hill, 1999, pp 1633–1642.

14. Szczeklik A, Stevenson DD: Aspirin-induced asthma: Advances in pathogenesis and management. J Allergy Clin Immunol 104:5–13, 1999.

15. Viard I, Wehrli P, Bullani R, et al: Inhibition of toxic epidermal necrolysis by blockade of CD95 with human intravenous immunoglobulin. Science 282:490–493, 1998.

16. Vittorio CC, Muglia JJ: Anticonvulsant hypersensitivity syndrome. Arch Intern Med 155:2285-2290, 1995.

17. Uetrecht JP: New concepts in immunology relevant to idiosyncratic drug reactions: the "danger hypothesis" and innate immune system. Chem Res Toxicol 12:387-395, 1999.

16. HYPERSENSITIVITY PNEUMONITIS/ ALLERGIC BRONCHOPULMONARY ASPERGILLOSIS

Robert D. Watson, Ph.D., M.D.

HYPERSENSITIVITY PNEUMONITIS (HP)

1. What is hypersensitivity pneumonitis also known as?
It is also known as extrinsic allergic alveolitis. There are many types of HP, known by many different names, depending on the antigen or dust involved. The classic form of HP is called Farmer's Lung. See table.

2. What are the causative agents of HP?
Fine biologic dusts or small chemicals that can be inhaled into the smallest airways, are responsible for initiating the immune response that is responsible for HP. These biologic, organic dusts contain materials that are antigenic, and the small chemicals can be haptens when combined with proteins. See table.

3. Who gets HP?
HP usually develops after prolonged and/or intermittent exposure to antigens at high or low levels. Atopy is not a risk factor. Although uncommon, HP can occur in young children. It is interesting to note that smokers are less susceptible to HP. ↑ ✗

Hypersensitivity Pneumonitis Antigens

BACTERIA	
Including mainly thermophilic actinomycetes, and other aquatic bacterial species.	
DISEASE	SOURCE
Farmer's lung	Moldy hay, grain, compost
Bagassosis, composter's lung	Moldy sugar cane; moldy residential compost
Ventilation pneumonitis	Humidifier/air conditioner
Mushroom worker's lung	Mushroom compost
Machine worker's lung	Metalworking fluid aerosols
Humidifier lung	Cool mist humidifiers

FUNGI	
Including *Aspergillus*; *Alternaria*; *Penicillium*; *Pullularia*; *Trichosporon*; *Cryptostroma*; and *Rhodotorula* species.	
DISEASE	SOURCE
Woodworker's lung	Moldy wood dust
Suberosis	Moldy cork dust
Cheese worker's lung	Cheese mold
Sequoiosis	Moldy wood dust
Summer-type HP	Japanese house dust
Maple bark stripper's disease	Wet maple bark
Malt worker's lung	Moldy barley dust

(Table continued on next page.)

199

Hypersensitivity Pneumonitis Antigens (cont.)

ANIMAL PROTEINS	
Including avian, bovine, porcine, rat, and mollusk shell proteins.	
DISEASE	SOURCE
Bird breeder's disease	Pigeon, duck, turkey, parakeet
Laboratory worker's lung	Rat urine
Oyster shell lung	Shell dust
INSECT PROTEINS	
Including Sitophilus *granarius* and silkworm larvae.	
DISEASE	SOURCE
Wheat weevil disease	Infested wheat flour
Sericulturist's lung disease	Cocoon fluff
AMEBAE	
DISEASE	SOURCE
Ventilation pneumonitis	Contaminated ventilation system
CHEMICALS	
Including toluene diisocyanate (TDI), diphenylmethane diisocyanate (MDI), phthalic anhydride, and trimetallic anhydride.	
DISEASE	SOURCE
Paint refinisher's disease	Urethane, paint catalyst
Bathtub refinisher's disease	Urethane, paint catalyst; resin; adhesive; foam
Epoxy resin worker's lung	Epoxy resin
Plastic worker's lung	Plastics industry

Other sources of HP antigen include medicines such as amiodarone, gold, procarbazine, minocycline, chlorambucil, sulfasalazine, and beta-adrenergic blockers, and soybean hulls in veterinary feed.

4. Is HP a new disease?

Ramazzini, the father of occupational medicine, first described HP in 1713, and farmer's lung was described in England in 1932.

5. What is HP's prevalence?

Fink and Zacharisen recently reviewed this question. In the past, the prevalence of farmer's lung in an agricultural community ranged from 2.3 to 8.6%. Fortunately, the prevalence has been reduced with changes in farming methods. In individuals with high exposure to contaminated air conditioning systems, the prevalence ranges from 15 to 60%, and in pigeon breeders, it ranges from 6 to 21%.

6. How does HP present?

There are two main presentations for HP: acute and chronic. A subacute presentation is sometimes described and can be helpful. The presentations and prognoses are very different.

7. What are the differences between these presentations?

Understanding the differences between the two presentations is key to understanding HP. The **acute** presentation is much more dramatic, with fever up to 40°C, chills, fatigue, headache, and myalgia, as well as respiratory signs and symptoms. Leukocytosis is common. Clinically these patients appear to have acute pneumonia until it is recognized that the symptoms resolve within 24 hours of removal from the

antigen exposure (usually in the workplace), and recur within 4 to 6 hours of reexposure. **Antigen levels are typically high**.

The **chronic** form is much more **insidious** and difficult to diagnose. Patients complain of progressive dyspnea, cough, and of systemic symptoms including nonspecific malaise, with anorexia, weight loss, fatigue, and weakness. They are often afebrile. Typically, the **antigen exposure is prolonged and at a lower level**, such as having a bird or two in the home. These patients are felt to have had subclinical disease for years before the damage becomes apparent. The chronic form can also be the culmination of repeated acute episodes.

The **subacute** form is between the acute and chronic forms, with progressively worsening fatigue, dyspnea, and cough over a period of days to weeks. The systemic findings of the acute form are not always present.

8. What questions should be asked regarding the patient's occupation and hobbies if HP is being considered?

The patient should be asked about:
- Pet and other animal exposures, particularly birds
- Flood- or water-damaged environments
- The presence of humidifiers, dehumidifiers, evaporative coolers, or vaporizers
- Occupational or hobby exposure to organic dusts or chemicals, particularly hay and silo exposures
- The use of feather clothing or bedding
- The presence of visible mold in home or work environments
- Temporal patterns such as improvement after vacations, possibly weekends, away from work or hobbies
- Worsening symptoms upon reintroduction to a particular environment

9. What are the main physical findings?

In **acute** HP, the patients appear ill. They have dry cough, dyspnea, and chest tightness. Bilateral crackles can be heard, suggesting a clinical diagnosis of acute pneumonia.

Patients with **chronic** HP present with progressive exertional dyspnea, but minimal physical findings are found until they have late, severe disease. They may have cyanosis, dyspnea, and crackles.

10. What are the main x-ray findings?

The chest x-ray may be normal or show nodular infiltrates in the acute form, and show diffuse fibrosis in the chronic form. During an acute attack, the chest x-ray may have soft, patchy densities in both lung fields. These parenchymal densities often coalesce. Between episodes, the chest x-ray may be normal in acute HP.

In subacute and chronic HP, the CT scan is more useful than conventional chest x-ray. The CT scan can also be useful in distinguishing chronic HP from idiopathic pulmonary fibrosis and sarcoidosis. In chronic HP, the CT scan findings include ground glass opacities, centrilobular nodules, and a bronchocentric pattern of emphysema. In end-stage disease, the chest x-ray may show diffuse fibrosis, including parenchymal contracture or honeycombing.

Sarcoid CT - granulomas & lymphadenopathy

IPF - peripheral int. densities

11. What are the spirometry findings?

In acute HP, the typical pulmonary function abnormality is decreased volume or restriction. In some patients, there is dual phase, with a drop in flow rates like an early asthmatic response, followed by a late response. Unlike the late asthmatic response, in the late HP response, a decreased volume is found rather than decreased flow rate. In chronic HP, a mixed pattern can be found, with obstruction and/or restriction.

12. How else can you distinguish HP from asthma?

Arterial blood gasses can further differentiate asthma from HP, because carbon monoxide diffusing capacity (DLCO) is decreased in HP. Because both asthma and HP can express an early and a late response after exposure, performing spirometry pre- and postexposure may be of limited usefulness in distinguishing asthma from HP. Hypoxemia is worsened by exercise in HP. Hypoxemia and hypercapnia, even at rest, may be found in late disease.

13. What are the main diseases to consider in the differential diagnosis?

The differential diagnosis also depends on the clinical presentation. Initially, the acute form with systemic symptoms, presents like acute pneumonia. Later, when a temporal pattern is noticed, other illnesses such as building-related illness, organic dust toxic syndrome (ODTS), and occupational asthma need to be considered. These illnesses are much more common than HP. ODTS illnesses are pulmonary disorders without fever or abnormal chest x-ray findings, and are caused by heavy exposures to organic dusts and toxins.

In chronic HP, other disorders with restrictive lung disease and fibrosis need to be considered, such as sarcoid, eosinophilic granuloma, idiopathic pulmonary fibrosis, and bronchiolitis obliterans with organizing pneumonia (BOOP) (or cryptogenic organizing pneumonia (COP) in Europe). Most patients with BOOP, which is an interstitial pulmonary illness that often presents with systemic symptoms, also respond to systemic corticosteroids. Open-lung biopsy is necessary to differentiate these disorders.

14. What is the role of an industrial hygienist in HP?

Their role is to analyze the suspected environment for the presence of HP antigens or other triggers, and to recommend environmental changes or other avoidance measures, so as to minimize production of, or exposure to these antigens.

15. Describe the pathophysiology.

HP includes a spectrum of lymphocytic and granulomatous interstitial and alveolar filling disorders. Inflammatory cells include mainly lymphocytes, macrophages, plasma cells, and some neutrophils. Macrophages with foamy cytoplasm, surrounded by mononuclear cells may be specific for HP. Later, interstitial fibrosis with honeycombing, as in idiopathic pulmonary fibrosis, is found. Hilar adenopathy and systemic organ involvement are not part of HP, which helps to differentiate it from sarcoid.

16. What immunologic parameters are involved?

Although cell-mediated and humoral immunity are involved, the immunology is not understood. IgE is not felt to be important. IgG is probably involved in all patients,

although some patients have specific elevations in IgA or IgM. It is not known whether complement has a significant role, although IgG, which is pivotal in HP, fixes complement. Complement levels do not decrease in HP as in immune complex-mediated diseases, and immune complexes have not been found in bronchoalveolar lavage fluid (BAL). It is also not known which regulatory or cell-mediated functions promote HP in the presence of specific antibody. CD8+ T lymphocytes are elevated and probably have an important regulatory role involving alveolar macrophages. These macrophages appear to be directly involved in the pathogenesis of HP.

Clearly, both host and antigen factors are necessary:

• Many persons with exposure develop specific antibody, without any identifiable illness.
• Antigen must be of a small enough size to penetrate the smallest airways, and must be present at higher levels intermittently, or at lower levels chronically, to be capable of causing disease.

17. What tests should be considered for the evaluation?

Pulmonary function testing, including spirometry, blood gasses, lung volumes, diffusion capacity, and possibly exercise challenge should be done in patients suspected of having HP. Peripheral blood leukocytosis is common, usually without eosinophilia. The search for antigens is based on the exposure history. Depending on the environment, different antigens are suspected and the search may involve an industrial hygienist. Several laboratories offer a "hypersensitivity panel" to screen for precipitins (usually IgG) directed against the most common HP antigens. The tests are done by using Ouchterlony gel diffusion or ELISA techniques. Skin tests have not been consistently useful and are without significant advantage over serologic methods for identification of antigen-specific IgG. The skin test demonstrates an Arthus reaction, which detects antigen, IgG antibody, and complement, and which occurs in 4 to 6 hours.

18. Are invasive tests needed for the diagnosis of HP?

Although other tests are usually adequate for a diagnosis, open lung biopsy may be needed to diagnose the cause of pulmonary fibrosis. Needle biopsies are generally inadequate, because large biopsy samples are needed. Immunofluorescent studies may detect antigen, even in late-stage HP. Bronchoalveolar lavage is not diagnostic because findings in symptomatic and nonsymptomatic patients overlap.

19. Are the serologic tests diagnostic?

A positive IgG antibody is not diagnostic of HP, nor does a negative test exclude HP:
• Inadequate testing materials can be responsible for a negative test.
• A positive test confirms exposure to antigen, but not the presence of disease. Positive results are also found in 50% of exposed individuals, without disease. A positive test is important to support the clinical suspicions, indicating sufficient exposure to generate an immune response.

20. How is the diagnosis made?

In early HP, information regarding the clinical history, physical examination, spirometry, radiologic findings, and laboratory results, including blood-gas

analysis and serology, are used to make the putative diagnosis. Spirometry before and after workplace or hobby exposure can help to confirm the trigger, and possibly the diagnosis.

21. What are the most important diagnostic criteria?

The most important part of making a diagnosis of HP is a high index of suspicion. There is no pathognomonic test. The elimination of symptoms and prevention of recurrences confirm the diagnosis after complete removal from the suspected antigen. As such, identification of the causative antigen is a critical part of the diagnosis. Occasionally, materials from the suspected environment can be tested for antigens. Inhalation challenge is not usually required. If, however, an association with environmental exposure cannot be confirmed, a lung biopsy may be needed. This is more likely in chronic HP.

22. How is HP treated?

Avoidance of the identified antigen is an essential part of the treatment of HP. This can involve the use of air filters, dust masks, removal of the antigen from the environment, or removal of the patient from the environment. Identification of the antigen may also help prevent the development of HP in coworkers.

23. What medicines are used to treat HP?

Patients with acute HP usually respond dramatically to systemic corticosteroids, starting at prednisone doses of 60 to 80 mg per day. However, this **must not be used as a substitute for avoidance measures because corticosteroids do not prevent the disease's progression to irreversible pulmonary fibrosis**. The dose and duration of treatment depend on the individual clinical and laboratory response. Typically, larger doses are continued for 2 to 3 weeks, and then slowly tapered over a period of 4 to 6 months. Bronchodilators may be tried in the early part of an acute episode, but are generally not helpful because they do not treat the underlying pulmonary pathology.

24. Do all HP patients respond to treatment?

In early HP, patients with acute disease respond well to avoidance measures. However, once sensitized, small doses of antigen can trigger flares. Chronic HP may not respond to corticosteroids or even avoidance measures. Some patients require prolonged low-dose prednisone, but the response is variable. Patients with chronic findings, such as fibrosis and honeycombing, have irreversible damage that will not respond to any treatments, whereas the active inflammatory processes may improve. In some patients the disease can progress even after rigorous avoidance measures are instituted, and all patients should be monitored for several years. Desensitization is not indicated because the disease is not IgE mediated.

25. How is treatment monitored?

Clinical and laboratory parameters are followed, including spirometric, radiologic, and blood-gas studies. Serology is not useful for monitoring treatment because antibody levels persist for many years.

26. If prednisone works, why don't inhaled corticosteroids work?

Inhaled corticosteroids have not been shown to be efficacious, but higher doses, as are possible with the newer products have not yet been adequately studied.

27. What is the prognosis?

With early diagnosis, and institution of antigen-avoidance measures, the prognosis is excellent. In HP patients, removal of antigen usually reverses the damage. In chronic HP, the damage is irreversible and may progress even with antigen avoidance. Often, these patients do not respond well to corticosteroids.

28. Are there predictors of a poor prognosis?

> 6 months prednisone
- Clubbing

A poor response after 6 months of prednisone suggests a poor prognosis, as does the presence of clubbing.

Most deaths, although uncommon in HP, occur in the chronic presentation; they can, however, also occur in the acute presentation.

ALLERGIC BRONCHOPULMONARY ASPERGILLOSIS (ABPA)

29. What clinical presentation suggests ABPA?

Chronic, refractory asthma or cystic fibrosis, particularly in steroid-dependent patients suggests ABPA.

30. What are the causative agents of ABPA?

There are more than 150 species of *Aspergillus* molds. The *fumigatus* species is the agent involved in greater than 80% of ABPA, although other species, such as *niger*, *flavus*, and *terreus*, can also be involved. The spores are 2.0 to 3.5 microns in diameter, allowing deposition into the smaller airways. Healthy lungs, however, can clear these spores.

31. Where do you find *Aspergillus* molds?

Aspergillus molds are ubiquitous, and, like other molds, are commonly found in moist environments of organic materials. They can be found in agricultural environments such as hay, soil, and compost; indoors in damp areas; and in bird excrement. *Aspergillus* is thermotolerant, growing at temperatures ranging from 15°C to 53°C, and optimally at 37°C.

32. What other diseases are associated with *Aspergillus*?

Aspergillus-allergic asthma, allergic *Aspergillus* sinusitis, chronic necrotizing pneumonia, hypersensitivity pneumonitis, invasive aspergillosis, and aspergilloma. The patient's genetics and immune responses determine whether these diseases will occur upon exposure.

33. What is the prevalence of ABPA?

Up to 10% of cystic fibrosis patients may have ABPA. In one study from India, 15% of children fulfilled the criteria for ABPA. Occupation and geographical regions are important because of the distribution of the *Aspergillus* molds. Six percent

of *Aspergillus*-positive skin test patients with asthma have ABPA. Sometimes, retrospectively, the onset of ABPA in childhood is suspected.

34. Is ABPA a new disease?
Hinson first described ABPA in 1932.

35. Describe the stages of illness.
ABPA has been classified into five stages:
- Acute. These patients typically present with asthma, but they have extremely elevated IgE, eosinophilia, pulmonary infiltrates, and *Aspergillus*-specific IgG and IgE. They respond to prednisone.
- Remission. The asthma is under control and the chest x-ray is normal. IgE levels are still elevated, but closer to normal. *Aspergillus*-specific IgG and IgE may be normal. Remission may last for many years.
- Exacerbation. This is a repeat of the acute phase, and is recognized when the serum IgE increases, usually by more than double. Systemic symptoms such as dyspnea, fever, myalgia, and sputum production are not uncommon. This phase also responds to prednisone and is treated like the acute phase.
- Steroid dependent. The disease flares when tapering of the corticosteroid dose is attempted. IgE levels can be extremely high (over 30,000 ng/mL) and may remain above 5,000 ng/mL without disease activity, but can also be normal. Chest x-ray findings usually, but not consistently, show bronchiectasis.
- End-stage fibrosis. These patients have irreversible lung damage that may progress to respiratory failure. Serologic findings are variable. Spirometry shows irreversible obstruction and restriction. With treatment, most patients do not progress to this stage.

36. What are the main physical findings of ABPA?
In earlier stages, patients typically present with an asthmalike picture of wheeze, shortness of breath, chest tightness, and brown mucus plugs, which are sometimes blood-streaked. The asthma is not necessarily severe; however, patients do not respond to less-aggressive asthma treatments and require systemic corticosteroids.

37. How do the end-stage fibrosis patients present clinically?
They present with shortness of breath, cyanosis, cor pulmonale, rales, and sometimes clubbing.

38. What are the main x-ray findings?
In the earlier stages of ABPA, intermittent pulmonary infiltrates are found on the chest x-ray. This can help differentiate between an asthma attack and a flare of ABPA. The chest x-ray can also show consolidation, which is much more remarkable than would be expected from the clinical presentation.

In later stages, irreversible radiologic findings include central bronchiectasis and pulmonary fibrosis. Central bronchiectasis is suggestive of ABPA, but may require a CT scan for detection. CT scan has generally superseded bronchography, which was widely used in the past. Mucoid impaction is common.

39. At what stage of ABPA is the diagnosis usually made?

Diagnosis is usually made at the corticosteroid-dependent stage. Earlier diagnosis requires a very high index of suspicion.

40. Why is early diagnosis of ABPA important?

Early diagnosis is important before the development of irreversible late-stage disease, which is usually preventable with treatment.

41. Describe the pathophysiology.

Little is known about the pathophysiology of ABPA. Clearly, however, ABPA is not an infection with *Aspergillus per se*, but immunologic responses to the mold that colonizes the airway. These include CD4+ Th2 and CD3+ T lymphocyte, and B lymphocyte activation.

In ABPA, the *Aspergillus*-specific IgE and total IgE are much higher than in asthma. Specific IgE and IgG are both elevated, and presumed to be relevant. Of particular interest is why most atopic patients with *Aspergillus* exposure develop specific IgE, but don't get ABPA. A possible mechanism in the development of ABPA is a modification of the cellular immune response and/or immune regulators by *Aspergillus* toxins or binding proteins. A shift towards Th2 production could cause increased immunoglobulin production.

42. What tests should be considered for the evaluation?

If suspected clinically, the diagnosis is confirmed serologically and radiologically. Initial tests could include allergy skin testing for *Aspergillus*, total IgE, and a chest x-ray. If these tests support the diagnosis of ABPA, further testing, such as those listed in the diagnostic criteria, should be done. They include *Aspergillus*-specific IgG and IgE serologies, CBC with eosinophil count, and possibly sputum analysis with culture and staining.

43. Can *Aspergillus* be isolated from the sputum?

Yes, although after corticosteroid treatment, *Aspergillus* may be absent in up to 40% of patients. *Aspergillus* isolation from sputum is not diagnostic, although repeatedly positive cultures warrants further evaluation of ABPA.

44. What is the differential diagnosis?

The main diagnosis to consider in a child with asthma symptoms and recurrent pneumonia is cystic fibrosis. Other diagnoses include parasitic infections such as visceral larval migrans, Churg-Strauss vasculitis, and eosinophilic pneumonia. Chronic obstructive pulmonary disease (COPD) needs to be considered in a patient with obstructive lung disease, particularly because some COPD patients can respond to corticosteroids. In the younger patient, alpha$_1$-antiproteinase (alpha$_1$-antitrypsin) deficiency should also be considered. These illnesses, however, do not have the chest x-ray findings typical of ABPA, nor the IgE spikes.

45. What are the diagnostic criteria for ABPA?

In the US, the diagnostic criteria are:
• Asthma

- Immediate cutaneous reactivity to *A. fumigatus* (or mixed *Aspergillus* species)
- Precipitating IgG antibodies to *A. fumigatus*
- Elevated total IgE (> 1000 ng/ml)
- Elevated IgE antibodies to *A. fumigatus*. The level should be double that found in patients with *Aspergillus*-related atopic disease, such as allergic rhinitis or asthma.
- Central bronchiectasis
- Infiltrates on chest x-ray, which may be absent between flares of ABPA.
- Eosinophilia coincident with chest x-ray infiltrates; this finding may not be present while on corticosteroids.

46. How is the diagnosis established?

There is no worldwide consensus on the diagnosis of ABPA, but the above are the commonly used criteria in the US. It has been suggested that the first five criteria, plus one other, are necessary to confirm to diagnosis.

47. How is ABPA treated?

The mainstay of ABPA treatment remains oral corticosteroids. A usual treatment regimen is prednisone, 0.5 mg/kg per day for 2 to 3 weeks, which is then changed to alternate-day doses for 2 to 3 months. After the serum IgE has diminished by two thirds, the prednisone is tapered, and possibly discontinued.

48. How is the treatment monitored?

Total serum IgE is measured frequently, often monthly initially, and less often as the disease stabilizes. This is useful to aid in both tapering the prednisone dose and in identifying ABPA flares. Serial spirometry and the chest x-ray are also useful.

49. How do you distinguish between an asthma attack and a flare of ABPA?

An asthma attack associated with a marked increase in IgE (at least double) and pulmonary infiltrates on chest x-ray suggest an ABPA flare. With these findings, the patient will need aggressive treatment with systemic corticosteroids. This differentiation can be particularly difficult in cystic fibrosis.

50. Are there other treatments besides systemic corticosteroids?

Leon and Craig reviewed the medical literature regarding the use of antifungals in the treatment of ABPA. Oral corticosteroids are still the recommended treatment, but more studies are needed regarding the use of antifungals. Antifungals may be tried as an adjunctive treatment in patients who require high-dose steroids. Inhaled corticosteroids have not been shown to consistently prevent ABPA recurrences, although the newer, high-dose, inhaled corticosteroids need further investigation. Inhaled corticosteroids are used for treatment of the asthma associated with ABPA. *Aspergillus* immunotherapy is not recommended. Exposure to high levels of *Aspergillus* should be avoided, although complete avoidance is practically impossible. It is important to attempt avoidance measures, however, even if only to prevent disease in family members. Avoidance of asthma triggers, whether mold or otherwise, is necessary for the patient's asthma treatment.

51. What is the prognosis?

With the exception of end-stage ABPA, the prognosis is favorable if the disease is monitored and treated aggressively. Progression of the disease can usually be prevented with the early use of systemic corticosteroids, although the disease can flare, even after years of remission.

BIBLIOGRAPHY

1. Chetty A, Menon RK, Malviya AN: Allergic bronchopulmonary aspergillosis. India J Pediatr 49:203–205, 1982.
2. Cockrill BA, Hales CA: Allergic bronchopulmonary aspergillosis. Annu Rev Med 50:303–316, 1999.
3. Daroowalla F, Raghu G: Hypersensitivity pneumonitis. Compr Ther 23:244–248, 1997.
4. Fink JN, Zacharisen MC: Hypersensitivity pneumonitis. In Middleton E, et al (eds): Allergy, Principles & Practice, 5th ed., New York, Mosby, 1998, pp 994–1004.
5. Greenberger PA: Allergic bronchopulmonary aspergillosis. In Middleton E, et al (eds): Allergy, Principles & Practice, 5th ed. New York, Mosby, 1998, pp 981–993.
6. Hinson KFW, Moon AJ, Plummer NS: Bronchopulmonary aspergillosis: A review and report of eight new cases. Thorax 7:317–333, 1952.
7. Knutsen AP, Mueller KR, Hutcheson PS, Slavin RG: Serum anti-*Aspergillus fumigatus* antibodies by immunoblot and ELISA in cystic fibrosis with allergic bronchopulmonary aspergillosis. J Allergy Clin Immunol 93:926–931, 1994.
8. Krasnick J, Meuwissen HJ, Nakao MA, et al: Hypersensitivity pneumonitis: Problems in diagnosis. J Allergy Clin Immunol 97:1027–1030, 1996.
9. Leon EE, Craig TJ: Antifungals in the treatment of allergic bronchopulmonary aspergillosis. Ann Allergy Asthma Immunol 82(6):511–516, 1999.
10. Patterson R, Roberts M: Classification and staging of allergic bronchopulmonary aspergillosis. In Patterson R, Greenberger P, Roberts M (eds): Allergic Bronchopulmonary Aspergillosis. Providence, RI, Oceanside Publications, 1995, pp 5–10.
11. Sansores R, Salas J, Chapela R, et al: Clubbing in hypersensitivity pneumonitis, its prevalence and possible prognostic role. Arch Intern Med 150:1849–1851, 1990.
12. Seltzer JM: Building-related illness. J Allergy Clin Immunol 94:351–362, 1994.
13. Viswanath PK, Banerjee B, Greenberger PA, Fink JN: Allergic bronchopulmonary aspergillosis: Challenges in diagnosis. Medscape Resp Care 3(6), 1999.
14. Yoshizawa Y, Miyake S, Sumi Y, et al: A follow-up study of pulmonary function tests, bronchoalveolar lavage cells, and humoral and cellular immunity in bird fancier's lung. J Allergy Clin Immunol 96:122–129, 1995.
15. Zacharisen MC: Hypersensitivity pneumonitis: Knowing what to look for. J Resp Dis 20:523–533, 1999.

Immune wrup

Bacterial Cell

- Bacterial inf / Viral
  Strep, Staph, H flu entero

a) Recurrent Sinopulm. infections >6-8 inf / yr x10 yr

b) Recurrent Pneumonia

c) CNS infections (meningitis viral / bact)

- Failure to thrive
  recurrent infection
  but can also be
  because of

- d) GI - GE giardiasis ≤ 2 episodes/y x10 yr

- CBC ē diff + platelets
- Ig — total
  — IgG, A, M.
  G >600, A 50-125
  M > 75-150 mg
  <200 mg% needs IVIG
  no immune protection

Antibody titres
Dip
Tetanus } protein
H flu - conjugate

* normal IgA - precludes B cell defects

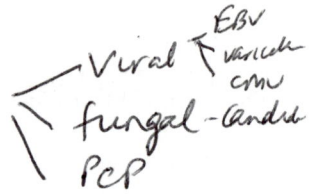

T cell

— Viral ← EBV, varicella, CMV
— fungal - candida
— PCP

Chronic infection ē resp./intestinal virus

CBC ē diff
Total T cell - CD_3
CD_4 / CD_8 1.5-3.?
>2 yrs Anergy
CXR - thymic shadow

Neutrophils

- gram -ve - Pseudo
- gram +ve Staph
- Asp., Candida, Nocardia

- mild recurrent Skin inf
- systemic shock

Comp

Early comp
C_1, C_4, C_2 - gram +ve
C_5-9 - neisseria
C_3 - gm + + Neisseria
Δ CH_{50}, C_3, C_4

17. PRIMARY IMMUNODEFICIENCIES

Richard S. DeMera, M.D.

1. What are the four major components of the immune system?
- Antibody-mediated (B-cell) immunity
- Cell-mediated (T-cell) immunity
- Phagocytosis
- Complement system

Their role is to protect the body from the constant assault by bacterial, viral, fungal, protozoal, and nonreplicating agents, which, if left unchecked, can produce infection and disease.

2. What organisms are most common in patients with T-cell defects?
Viral and fungal organisms. These are aggressive opportunistic pathogens that the patients are unable to clear. The most common viral pathogens are cytomegalovirus, Epstein-Barr virus, severe varicella, and chronic infections with respiratory and intestinal viruses. The most common fungal pathogens are *Candida* and *Pneumocystis carinii*. T-cells are essential for controlling viral and fungal pathogens, but they also provide helper function to B-cells for effective antibody responses. When a macrophage or dendritic cell takes up a pathogen, it degrades its antigen and presents it on the cell surface of T-cells. This causes T-cells to induce the maturation of B-cells through the release of cytokines. Therefore, T-cell defects can present as a combined T-cell–B-cell defect, and bacterial sepsis is not unusual in these patients.

3. What are the most common organisms seen in patients with B-cell defects?
These patients commonly present with recurrent sinopulmonary infections and septicemias with encapsulated bacteria. The most common bacteria found are streptococci, staphylococci, and *Haemophilus* organisms. They are also susceptible to invasive disease with enteroviruses, which can lead to chronic viral meningitis. Also, severe and chronic gastrointestinal disease from giardiasis is not uncommon.

4. What are the most common organisms seen in patients with phagocytic or granulocytic defects?
These patients susceptibility to infection may range from mild recurrent skin infections to severe fatal systemic infections. Staphylococcal disease is very common because this organism is normally eliminated by phagocytosis and superoxide-mediated killing in granulocytes. They can also present with gram-negative infections especially *Pseudomonas*. These patients usually have little difficulty with viral infections. Some fungal and protozoal infections, such as *Aspergillus*, *Candida*, and *Nocardia*, can be overwhelming in some of the more severe disorders.

5. What are the most common organisms seen in complement defects?
The complement system involves more than 30 proteins encoded throughout the genome. Complement deficiencies can present with increased susceptibility to

infections, angioedema, or rheumatologic disorders. Patients with deficiencies in the early components (C1, C4, C2,) present with recurrent bacterial infections, most commonly gram-positive infections. Invasive neisserial infections are commonly seen in patients with defects in the terminal lytic components (C5–C9) and alternative pathway components. A deficiency of the pivotal factor (C3) is rare, but when it occurs, the patient may present with gram-positive and neisserial infections.

6. What clues can help identify a child with an impaired immunity?

It is important to note first that normal children average six to eight respiratory infections per year for the first 10 years of life. They can also have up to six episodes of otitis media and two of gastroenteritis per year for the first 2–3 years. Healthy children will generally handle these infections well. On the other hand, children with an impaired immune system do not handle infections well. They have more severe infections that persist for uncommonly long periods with frequent recurrences. Normal therapy is not as effective in these children. They frequently show a failure to thrive and often are fall below average in weight, height, and developmental skills. Some of these children will appear to be normal and respond well to therapy, but they will have much more frequent episodes, and a high index of suspicion is needed to make the diagnosis. Infants will have protection from transplacentally acquired IgG for the first 3–6 months of life. After this passive protection subsides, their underlying impaired immunity will manifest itself. Chronic skin rashes are common in the first year of life in immunodeficient infants. They also have a higher incidence of other congenital disorders such as developmental anomalies of the face, skeleton, heart, and intestines and disorders of pigmentation of hair.

7. Which initial tests must a physician consider when evaluating a patient with a suspected immunodeficiency?

In all immunodeficiencies, a complete blood count with platelets and differential should be done. If an antibody deficiency is suspected, quantitative immunoglobulins should be ordered, and, if normal, IgG subclasses should be considered. Antibody titers of diphtheria, tetanus, and *Haemophilus influenzae* should also be drawn. If the titers are low, booster shots should be given and responses checked in 2–3 weeks. If a T-cell deficiency is suspected, a chest x-ray is indicated to try to identify a thymic shadow. T-cell surface markers such as CD3 (mature T-cells), CD4 (mature T-helper cells), CD8 (mature cytotoxic T-cells), CD11 (leukocytes), and CD56 (natural killer cells) should also be obtained. Evaluation of delayed hypersensitivity can be determined with a skin test to *Candida albicans* antigen. Anergy is a clue to a T-cell deficiency but cannot be determined in those younger than 2 years of age. When a phagocytic or neutrophilic defect is suspected, a neutrophil count and a flow cytometric respiratory burst assay using fluorescent dye can help make the diagnosis. A CH-50 assay is a good initial screening test for complement defects.

8. Which four primary immunodeficiencies commonly present during adulthood?

• Common variable immunodeficiency
• Selective IgA deficiency

• IgG subclass deficiency
• Complement deficiency

These diseases can have immune defects that develop in adult life, such as common variable immunodeficiency, or the defect may be present from birth. When present from birth, the defect is usually mild and therefore symptoms are not experienced until adulthood.

9. Which four childhood primary immunodeficiencies can present during adulthood?
• Adenosine deaminase deficiency
• Wiskott-Aldrich syndrome
• X-linked agammaglobulinemia
• Chronic granulomatous disease

These diseases traditionally present during childhood but some patients may have a delayed onset of symptoms due to a milder clinical phenotype of the genetic defect.

10. What are the clinical features of X-linked agammaglobulinemia (XLA)?

XLA is an antibody deficiency that affects only males, although females can be carriers. Manifestations usually present by 5–6 months of age, at which time the passively transferred maternal IgG reaches its lowest levels. Because they have no B-cells (low or zero concentrations of all immunoglobulin subtypes), these patients usually develop high-grade bacterial infections from such organisms as *Streptococcus pneumoniae*, *Haemophilus influenzae*, and staphylococci. These can present as sepsis, meningitis, sinusitis, pneumonia, septic arthritis, cellulitis, abscess, recurrent otitis media, bronchitis, and dermatitis. These tend to not respond completely to prompt appropriate antibiotic therapy, and some patients may continue to have symptoms and illness without periods of well-being. Despite repeated infections, their tonsils and lymph nodes are small or absent, but the spleen is of normal size. Circulating T-cells are increased and function normally; therefore, they respond well to viral infections. The diagnosis is based on the absence or markedly reduced levels of all five immunoglobulin classes (IgG, IgA, IgM, IgE, IgD). Some patients with agammaglobulinemia may not present until early childhood. They can present with other complaints such as abnormal dental decay, chronic conjunctivitis, and malabsorption. Malabsorption, when severe, can cause failure to thrive with retardation of height and weight. *Giardia lamblia* is the most common cause of the malabsorption.

11. What is the treatment for XLA?

Treatment consist of life-long intravenous gammaglobulin replacement and prophylactic antibiotic therapy or acute treatment when necessary. The optimal dose and frequency of intravenous immunoglobulin (IVIG) must be determined for each patient. The usual dose consist of 350–500 mg/kg of body weight administered each month. This usually will keep the patient free of chronic infection except they are still vulnerable to chronic enteroviral infection of the central nervous system.

12. What is the genetic defect in XLA?

A tyrosine kinase protein, known as **Bruton tyrosine kinase** (Btk), is missing in this disease. This enzyme was named in honor of its discoverer, Dr. Ogden

Bruton, who is recognized as making the first clinical description and precise diagnosis of an immunodeficiency disorder. Tyrosine kinases are found in high levels in all B lineage cells. They are involved in the regulation of B-cell proliferation and differentiation. It is thought that the genetic defect may be located on the mid-portion of the long arm of chromosome X (Xq21.3-22).

13. What is the cause of X-linked immunodeficiency with hyper IgM?

This is an antibody (B-cell) disorder that is similar to XLA. Seventy-percent of the patients with this disorder have the X-linked form. The mode of inheritance of the remaining 30% is not as clear cut. In this disease there are very low concentrations of IgG (< 150 mg/dL), no IgA, or IgE, but unlike XLA IgM is elevated as well as IgD. Patients with X-linked immunodeficiency cannot synthesize the CD 40 ligand. This ligand is expressed on activated T-cells. CD 40 is a B-cell surface marker that is expressed throughout B-cell differentiation. The interaction of the CD40 ligand with CD40 on B-lymphocytes is required for effective isotype switching. When it is not present, B-cells cannot switch from IgM production to IgA, IgE, or IgG. The defect has been placed at the distal end of the long arm of the X chromosome at Xq26.

14. What is a unique feature commonly observed in patients with X-linked immunodeficiency with hyper-IgM?

A characteristic feature often observed in these patients is lymphoid hypertrophy. In the second decade of life, there may be uncontrolled proliferation of plasma cells from the IgM cells. The proliferation of these cells can be fatal with an extensive invasion of the gastrointestinal tract, gallbladder, and liver. Patients with this disease also have an increased risk of abdominal cancers.

15. What is the triad in Wiskott-Aldrich syndrome?

Wiskott-Aldrich syndrome (WAS) is a combined T-cell-B–cell disorder. It is an X-linked recessive disease characterized by the triad of eczema, thrombocytopenia, and recurrent pyogenic infections. The triad only occurs together 27% of the time. Twenty percent have thrombocytopenia only, whereas 5% have only immunodeficiency. Eczema usually appears by one year of age and is usually moderate to severe. Thrombocytopenia is present at birth and is characterized by normal-appearing megakaryocytes, but the platelets are small and defective with shortened survival times. Platelet counts may be in the range of 5000–100,000/µl. The infections are typically caused by encapsulated bacteria such as *Streptococcus pneumoniae* and *Haemophilus influenzae*, which cause recurrent bouts of otitis media, pneumonia, meningitis, and sepsis. There is also an increased susceptibility to viruses and opportunistic infections.

16. What is the defect in WAS?

The molecular defect is due to a mutation of the gene encoding the WAS protein. This protein, whose complete function is unknown, is thought have an important role in organization of the cytoskeleton through polymerization with actin. T-cells tend to be the most affected. Without the WAS protein there will be a loss of T-cell surface microvilli, decreased platelet size, and defective T-cell and platelet

function. Affected male patients tend to have normal levels of IgG, low levels of IgM, and elevated levels of IgE and IgA. They have an impaired humoral response to make specific antibodies to polysaccharide antigens and have a poor response to protein antigens. Over time the number of T-cells progressively decreases while the number of B-cells progressively expands.

$$IgG \rightarrow$$
$$m \downarrow$$
$$E/A \uparrow$$

17. How is WAS treated?

Bone marrow transplantation (BMT) can be curative. If BMT is not an option, IVIG can be effective with the prompt and aggressive use of antibiotics. Splenectomy, when combined with antibiotic prophylaxis, can increase survival by increasing the platelet number and thereby controlling bleeding complications.

18. What is the diagnosis in an infant with an interrupted type B aortic arch, truncus arteriosus, and hypocalcemia and no thymus?

DiGeorge syndrome (thymic hypoplasia).

19. What is DiGeorge syndrome?

DiGeorge syndrome is a T-cell deficiency (usually only partial) due to a deletion in chromosome 22q11. This causes abnormal migration of the 3rd and 4th branchial pouches during embryogenesis leading to hypoplasia or aplasia of the thymus and parathyroids, truncal cardiovascular malformations, and abnormal facies. This syndrome is one of the few immunodeficiency disorders associated with symptoms immediately following birth.

Neonatal tetany, one of these symptoms, is frequently seen during the first 24 hours of life. It is caused by the hypocalcemia associated with hypoparathyroidism from the lack of the parathyroids. Symptoms from congenital heart disease, due to the cardiac malformations, are also seen soon after birth. The abnormal facies consist of low-set ears, fish-shaped mouth, notched ear pinnae, micrognathia, hypertelorism, and an antimongoloid slant of the eyes.

The immunodeficiency is highly variable, depending on the degree of thymic hypoplasia. T-cell immunity is usually absent at birth, as indicated by lymphocytopenia and depressed numbers of circulating T-cells. Recurrent or chronic infection, depending on the degree of thymic hypoplasia, can occur with various viral, bacterial, fungal, or protozoal organisms. More than 90% of the patients will have only a mild immune defect that can often be transient. Most patients with DiGeorge syndrome have normal B-cell immunity, but some have low immunoglobulin levels and will fail to make specific antibodies following immunization.

20. How is DiGeorge syndrome treated?

The management of hypocalcemia should be the first concern. It is rarely controlled with supplementation alone. Calcium needs to be given in conjunction with vitamin D or parathyroid hormone. Congenital heart disease often can cause congestive heart failure and may require immediate surgical correction. Prophylaxis can prevent infections depending on the CD4 counts. Bone marrow transplantation is the treatment of choice for severe types if an HLA-identical donor is available. If a donor cannot be found, the fetal thymus transplantation, which was the treatment of choice before BMT, could be performed.

21. What is severe combined immunodeficiency (SCID)?

SCID is a rare and fatal syndrome characterized by severe deficiencies of both B- and T-cell function. There are several forms that all result in the same clinical picture. Usually, affected infants present by 3 months of age with persistent thrush or severe nonresolving diaper rash. They sometimes present shortly after birth with a hyperpigmented morbilliform rash, due to the transplacental passage of maternal lymphocytes, causing a graft-versus-host reaction. Growth and development can be normal in the first 3 months, but then weight and growth slow, and failure to thrive becomes dramatic. At this time they may develop intractable diarrhea or a persistent cough from interstitial pneumonia caused by *Pneumocystis carinii*. Death can occur rapidly from infections such as cytomegalovirus, herpes, adenovirus, and varicella. A diagnosis of SCID is therefore a medical emergency.

Infants with SCID have profound lymphopenia (< 1000 lymphocytes/mm^3) and therefore are not capable of cell-mediated immunity. They cannot respond to an allogenic stimulus or a specific antigen such as tetanus toxoid. The thymus fails to become a lymphoid organ, and its shadow cannot be seen on a chest film. Serum immunoglobulin concentrations are low except in the X-linked form where the number of B-cells can be normal or elevated, but they fail to mature and function normally.

X-/linkm   T⁻ B⁺ NK⁻

22. What is the main treatment for SCID?

SCID is a pediatric emergency. The treatment is BMT. If BMT is done in the first 3 months of life, the patient will have a $> 95\%$ chance for survival; if not done, the result is almost always fatal.

23. Name the most common form of SCID.

Of the many forms of SCID, the most common is X-linked SCID (42% of SCID in the US), which has been mapped to Xq13. The genetic defect has been identified as a mutation of the γ chain of the interleukin-2 (IL-2) receptor. This γ chain is also a component of the IL-4, IL-7, IL-9, and IL-15 receptors and several myeloid cytokine receptors.

ADA
T⁻ B⁺
NK⁻

24. Twenty percent of patients with SCID lack what enzyme, which functions in the purine salvage pathway?

Adenosine deaminase (ADA). ADA deficiency is autosomal recessive and accounts for approximately 15% of all SCID cases. It is caused by mutations within the gene encoding ADA on chromosome 20. ADA is involved in purine metabolism by catalyzing the conversion of adenosine and deoxyadenosine into inosine and deoxyinosine. The lack of ADA leads to build up of deoxyadenosine triphosphate (dATP), which results in inhibition of ribonucleotide reductase and subsequent depletion of deoxyribonucleoside triphosphates. This becomes toxic to many cells but most importantly T-cells. Eighty to ninety percent of patients with ADA deficiency have complete absence of T-cell and B-cell immunity, as in SCID. The remaining patients may have mild to moderate abnormalities in T-cell and B-cell function. Patients with ADA deficiency and SCID may have unique radiographic abnormalities such as flaring of the anterior ribs, abnormal contour and articulation of posterior ribs and transverse processes, thick growth-arrest lines, and an abnormal bony pelvis. Treatment for this disorder is the same as for SCID: BMT and subsequent

return of immunologic function. Patients also can be treated with bovine ADA conjugated to polyethylene glycol 2–3 times a week to reduce the levels of toxic metabolites.

25. What is the most common clinically significant primary immunodeficiency that presents in adulthood?

Common variable immunodeficiency (CVID). CVID is an antibody (B-cell) immunodeficiency disorder. The cause of this heterogeneous group of diseases is unknown. Because it is a heterogeneous group of undifferentiated diseases, there are many forms of inheritance (autosomal recessive, autosomal dominant, and X-linked). All are characterized by defective antibody formation and decreased levels of immunoglobulins. CVID occurs with a frequency of 1 in 75,000 people. It is equally distributed between men and women. It can occur between infancy and old age and peaks at 6–10 years of age and 26–30 years of age. More than two-thirds of these patients were adults when the diagnosis was made. The total immunoglobulin level is below 300 mg/dL, and the IgG level is usually below 250 mg/dL. IgM and IgA may be absent or present in normal amounts. Circulating B-cells in the peripheral blood may be decreased but are usually normal. Undetectable antibody titers following specific immunization can help diagnose patients who have borderline immunoglobulin levels. Cell-mediated immunity, especially later in the disease, may be suppressed.

26. Describe the clinical manifestations of CVID.

Patients commonly present initially with chronic sinusitis, but chronic otitis media, bronchitis, and pneumonia also are very common. The most common respiratory pathogen is an encapsulated bacteria such as pneumococcus or *Staphylococcus*, but mycoplasma and unencapsulated *Haemophilus influenzae* can also be a cause. Organisms such as *Giardia lamblia*, *Salmonella*, *Shigella*, and *Campylobacter jejuni* can lead to malabsorption. These can cause diarrhea in 50% of patients with CVID. Opportunistic infections such as *Pneumocystis carinii*, herpes zoster, and fungi can play a prominent role in CVID. Around 30% of patients with CVID will develop an autoimmune disease such as systemic lupus erythematosus, autoimmune thyroiditis, primary biliary cirrhosis, hemolytic anemia, and arthritis. These can precede, start concurrently with, or follow the onset of infections. CVID patients also have an increased risk for inflammatory bowel diseases such as Crohn's disease, celiac disease, and lymphoid hyperplasia. Leukemia, lymphoma (300 times more frequent in women with CVID than men), and gastric carcinoma (50 fold increase) occur with increased frequency.

27. How is CVID treated?

Monthly IVIG treatments (300–400 mg/kg) are given to maintain IgG trough levels greater than 500 mg/dL. Antibiotics are frequently needed in addition to the IVIG. The major complication of CVID is chronic lung disease, which can develop despite adequate immunoglobulin therapy.

28. What is the most common primary immunodeficiency?

Selective IgA deficiency is the most common primary immunodeficiency with an incidence as high as 1 in 350.

29. What are the four criteria that define selective IgA deficiency?
1. Serum IgA levels < 5.0 mg/dL
2. Normal serum IgG and IgM levels
3. Normal cell-mediated immunity
4. Normal antibody production

30. True or False: Most patients with selective IgA deficiency are clinically normal?
True. Most patients are clinically normal, but some present with recurrent infections, the most common being upper respiratory tract infections. These patients also can have a higher incidence of allergic, collagen vascular, and gastrointestinal disorders. The cause is unknown.

31. Can IVIG be used in treating symptomatic patients with selective IgA deficiency?
No. Actually IVIG is contraindicated in these patients because they can have anti-IgA antibodies, which can cause anaphylactic reactions. These antibodies also can be present in blood products and can cause transfusion reactions. Therefore, these patients should only be given washed packed red blood cells. A way to safely replace the deficient IgA has not yet been developed. Appropriate antibiotics should be used in symptomatic patients.

32. What autosomal-recessive disorder is characterized by oculocutaneous albinism and susceptibility to recurrent respiratory tract infections?
Chédiak-Higashi syndrome. Chédiak-Higashi syndrome is a phagocytic dysfunction disease. It is a rare multisystem autosomal-recessive disorder caused by mutations in a gene on chromosome 1.

33. What is the characteristic feature of Chédiak-Higashi syndrome?
The characteristic feature is giant lysosomal granules found in almost all cells in the body including neutrophils, renal tubular cells, gastric mucosal cells, melanocytes, and hepatocytes. Patients suffer from recurrent bacterial infections due to abnormal neutrophil chemotaxis, decreased natural killer cell activity, and abnormal intracellular killing of organisms. Patients also may have partial albinism, central nervous system abnormalities, and a high incidence of lymphoreticular cancers.

34. What disease is characterized by an abnormal immune response to infection with Epstein-Barr virus (EBV)?
X-linked lymphoproliferative disease (XLP) or Duncan's disease. This is a combined antibody (B-cell) and cellular (T-cell) disorder that is characterized by a hereditary susceptibility to EBV infection. Patients are usually immunologically normal prior to EBV infection. After infection, hypogammaglobulinemia, inverted helper/suppressor T-cell ratios, defective interferon gamma production, and decreased natural killer (NK) cell activity are seen. After EBV infection, cytotoxic T-cells recognize EBV-infected autologous B-cells. This can cause severe progressive mononucleosis with liver failure and death (73% of patients). The mortality rate is 75% by age 10 and almost 100% by age 40. BMT has been curative in some patients, especially if done by age 12.

35. Patients with CD8 lymphocytopenia who present with severe infections similar to SCID patients have what deficiency?

Zeta-chain associated protein 70 (ZAP-70) deficiency. This rare deficiency is inherited as an autosomal-recessive trait and is due to mutations in the gene for ZAP-70 which is on chromosome 2 at position q12. ZAP-70 is a tyrosine kinase important in T-cell reactivity signaling. The number of CD4 cells is normal or elevated, but they are not functional and there are essentially no CD8 cells. Immunoglobulin concentrations can be low, normal, or high. Patients present with severe, recurrent, often fatal infections similar to those in SCID patients.

36. Infants with histories of delayed separation of the umbilical cord, gingivitis, recurrent skin infections, recurrent otitis media, pneumonia, and septicemia have what deficiency?

Leukocyte adhesion deficiency-1 (LAD-1). LAD-1 is a phagocytic dysfunction disorder. Its onset is within the first weeks of life, usually presenting with delayed separation of the umbilical cord. Recurrent pyogenic infections with such organisms as *Staphylococcus aureus*, *Pseudomonas aeruginosa*, *Klebsiella*, *Proteus*, and enterococci are common. Recurrent skin infections, perianal abscesses, periodontal disease, pneumonia, and septicemia are seen as the patient grows older. There are two different clinical phenotypes: moderate and severe. The inheritance pattern is autosomal recessive for both. The severe phenotype tends to be fatal in the first years of life. Early aggressive treatment with antibiotics is the standard therapy. BMT has also been curative in children with the severe phenotype.

37. What three leukocyte adhesion heterodimers are deficient in LAD-1?

- Leukocyte function associated antigen-1 (LFA-1)—found on B-, T-, and NK cells
- Complement receptor type 3 (CR3)—found on neutrophils, monocytes, macrophages, eosinophils, and NK cells
- p150,95—a complement receptor

These molecules are deficient due to a mutation of the gene encoding CD18, the common β chain of the leukocyte adhesion proteins. Phagocytic cells are decreased to the degree that CD18 expression is absent, and they are incapable of migrating into areas of infection.

38. What is LAD-2?

In LAD-2, there is a defect in fructose metabolism that results in the absence of sialyl Lewis x, a neutrophil receptor for E-selectin. E-selectin is an adhesion molecule on activated endothelial cells of blood vessels. Without sialyl Lewis x, neutrophil rolling and chemotaxis are lacking. This results in recurrent bacterial infections, pronounced neutrophilia, and mental retardation.

39. What severe immunodeficiency is characterized by development soon after birth of generalized erythroderma and desquamation, failure to thrive, diarrhea, hepatosplenomegaly, hypereosinophilia, and greatly elevated serum IgE levels and eosinophilia?

Omenn's syndrome. It is a combined T-cell and B-cell immunodeficiency. There are no circulating B-cells except IgE. T-cells are increased in circulation as well as

in tissue, but they do not respond normally to mitogens or antigens. This syndrome is often fatal during the first 5 months of life unless BMT is done.

40. A child who must use a wheelchair by 10–12 years of age might have what immunodeficient disease?

Ataxia telangiectasia. This autosomal-recessive disorder is characterized by progressive cerebellar ataxia, which becomes evident soon after the child starts to walk but may not occur until the child is 4–6 years of age. These patients have variable cellular and humoral immunodeficiencies. They have frequent sinopulmonary infections, and chronic pneumonia and bronchiectasis are common causes of death. Telangiectasia usually presents by 2 years of age in the bulbar conjunctiva and subsequently on the bridge of the nose, on the ears, or in the antecubital fossa. Neurologic symptoms, such as dysconjugate gaze, choreoathetoid movements, mental retardation, and extrapyramidal and posterior column signs, develop as the patient becomes older. Secondary sexual characteristics rarely develop at puberty.

41. Which immunoglobulin levels are normal or depleted in ataxia telangiectasia?

Fifty to eighty percent of these patients will have IgA deficiency. IgE concentrations are usually low. IgM is usually present in normal numbers although it may be of the low–molecular-weight variety. IgG levels are usually normal, but IgG2 subclass deficiency is commonly present. CD4 levels are usually low. NK cell activity is normal.

42. What is the underlying defect in ataxia telangiectasia?

The defect is thought to be an abnormal DNA repair mechanism, with a possible deficiency in recombinase, but a unifying defect has not been found. A high frequency of chromosomal breaks have been found on chromosomes 7 and 14.

43. What percentage of patients with ataxia telangiectasia develops cancer?

Fifteen percent of these patients will develop cancer. They most commonly develop cancers of the lymphoreticular type, with T-cell malignancy being the most common.

44. What syndrome is characterized by recurrent staphylococcal abscesses of the skin, lungs, and viscera and dermatitis in children with coarse facial features?

Hyperimmunoglobulinemia E syndrome. These patients have eosinophilia and very high levels of IgE, whereas IgG, IgM, and IgA levels are normal. Other bacteria can cause infections as well as fungi, specifically *Candida* and *Aspergillus* species. There are variable defects of cellular and humoral response to previously encountered antigens, and defective neutrophil chemotaxis is found in one-third of patients. The immunologic defect at this time is unknown, but recent reports indicate that a mutation in the gene encoding the α chain of the IL-4 receptor may be implicated.

45. What is the treatment for hyper-IgE syndrome?

Continuous treatment with antistaphylococcal antibiotics usually results in a good prognosis. With no treatment, progressive lung disease develops and there is a much worse prognosis.

46. What is transient hypogammaglobulinemia of infancy?

This rare disorder generally appears in young children with lower than normal immunoglobulin concentrations who respond normally to protein antigens such as diphtheria and tetanus. Most of these patients remain immunologically competent throughout their lives, but a small subset will develop other immune abnormalities.

47. What primary immunodeficiency is commonly associated with IgG2 subclass deficiency?

IgA deficiency.

48. What are the clinical manifestations of purine nucleoside phosphorylase (PNP) deficiency?

This is an autosomal-recessive disease with a combined B-cell and T-cell disorder. Its presentation is similar to ADA deficiency. Deaths can occur from generalized vaccinia, varicella, lymphosarcoma, and graft-versus-host disease. Two-thirds of patients have neurologic abnormalities ranging from spasticity to mental retardation. One-third of patients develop autoimmune diseases including, most commonly, autoimmune hemolytic anemia. Unlike ADA deficiency, patients with PNP deficiency have normal bone x-rays. BMT is the treatment of choice.

49. What is the immunologic defect in PNP deficiency?

PNP is necessary for the normal catabolism of purines. It catalyzes the conversion of inosine, deoxyinosine, guanosine, and deoxyguanosine to hypoxanthine and guanine. In PNP, deoxyguanosine has been shown to result in the accumulation of deoxyguanosine triphosphate (dGTP). These elevated levels become toxic and impair the cells ability to proliferate. The toxic effects of elevated dGTP affects T-lymphocytes more than B-lymphocytes. The defects in the gene encoding PNP are located on chromosome 14.

50. What are the clinical manifestations of chronic granulomatous disease (CGD)?

This phagocytic dysfunction disease presents during infancy with infections to organisms that are catalase-positive (*Staphylococcus aureus*, *Salmonella*, and *Pseudomonas* species) but not to organisms that are catalase-negative (*Streptococcus pneumoniae* or *Haemophilus influenzae*). Other organisms such as *Staphylococcus epidermidis*, *Serratia marcescens*, *Escherichia coli*, *Candida*, and *Aspergillus* can also play a prominent role. Marked lymphadenopathy, hepatosplenomegaly, and draining lymph nodes are not infrequent.

Abscesses are also very common and require surgical drainage when present. Osteomyelitis is more commonly found in CGD than any other immunodeficiency. Sixty-five percent of patients with CGD have an X-linked mode of inheritance, and the rest have an autosomal-recessive mode of inheritance.

51. What is the immunologic defect in CGD?

The defect is the inability of the phagocyte to kill ingested organisms such as bacteria and fungi. This is due to the absence of one of the nicotinamide adenine dinucleotide phosphate oxidase subunits, which is involved in the oxidative burst

triggered by phagocytosis. Diagnosis is made by a nitroblue tetrazolium (NBT) or a chemoluminescence assay. Patients' leukocytes have absent NBT dye reduction and reduced chemoluminescence, whereas carriers may have normal or reduced values.

52. What is the treatment for CGD?

Aggressive antibiotic therapy has reduced the high mortality rate seen in young children with CGD. Fungal infections have now become a common cause of death in these patients. If these infections respond to initial treatment, chronic antifungal therapy appears to be effective in preventing relapses. Interferon gamma has been shown to decrease the number of serious infections in a recent study. BMT has not been as successful as it has been in other immunodeficiencies. The chronic indolent bacterial or fungal infections seen in CGD are difficult to control when chemotherapy is given to prevent graft rejection but when successful is curative.

53. What is chronic mucocutaneous candidiasis (CMC)?

CMC is due to a defect in T-cell immunity resulting in susceptibility to chronic candidal infection. The disorder may appear by 1 year of age or may be delayed until the second decade. Candida infection is found in multiple locations including the nails, skin, and mucous membranes. It is usually a superficial infection, and dissemination is rare. CMC patients also rarely develop infections with other fungal agents. Beside candida, patients can also have frequent bacterial and viral infections, bacterial being more common. Endocrine and autoimmune abnormalities are not uncommon.

Hypoparathyroidism with hypocalcemia and Addison's disease are the two most common endocrine disorders. The underlying immunologic defect is still unknown. Oral antifungals are the mainstay of therapy, but no treatment can prevent the endocrinopathies.

54. Cellular immunodeficiency with immunoglobulins is also known by what name?

Nezelof syndrome. This syndrome is characterized by failure to thrive, CMC, lung infections, urinary tract infections, diarrhea, and gram-negative sepsis. It is caused by incomplete T-cell dysfunction. Patients are lymphopenic with low levels of CD4 and CD8. Their immunoglobulins cannot make specific antibodies to antigens, but the number of immunoglobulins is normal or elevated.

55. How is Nezelof syndrome different from other forms of SCID?

In Nezelof syndrome, serum immunoglobulins and lymphoid tissue are present unlike most forms of SCID.

56. Nezelof syndrome presents very similarly to AIDS. How do you distinguish the two?

In Nezelof syndrome, the CD4 and CD8 levels are low, but their ratio is usually normal unlike AIDS. T-cell function is usually abnormal from birth in Nezelof syndrome but is normal in the early stages of HIV.

57. Patients with normal serum immunoglobulins, normal IgG subclass levels, and normal antibody response to protein antigens (i.e., diphtheria and tetanus) might have what immunodeficiency?

Polysaccharide antibody deficiency. This syndrome is usually seen in young children, but many will eventually develop an antibody response.

58. Patients who simultaneously develop recurrent infections, agranulocytosis, pancytopenia, hemolytic anemia, and eosinophilia or eosinopenia have what immunodeficiency?

Immunodeficiency with thymoma. These patients have panhypoglobulinemia with low or absent B-cells. T-cells, on the other hand, are normal in number and function. These patients also have higher incidence of myasthenia gravis, diabetes, amyloidosis, chronic hepatitis, and nonthymic cancer. Thymoma is usually discovered on routine x-ray, and occasionally it is detected prior to the development of immunodeficiency.

Removal of the thymoma does not result in improvement of immunodeficiency. IVIG can help to control recurrent infections and chronic diarrhea. The overall prognosis is poor. Death from infection, aplastic anemia, and thrombocytopenia is common.

59. What is the clinical significance of an IgG subclass deficiency?

It is still unclear at this time. There are four IgG subclasses numbered IgG1, IgG2, IgG3, and IgG4. There are biological differences between each subclass, but no subclass has such a unique biological activity that the others cannot assume its function. IgG2 subclass deficiency is the most significant of the four. It is associated with IgA deficiency and is seen in patients with repeated infections with encapsulated bacteria. However, many patients with IgG2 subclass deficiency are clinically normal. Therefore, it is important to evaluate patients with IgG2 deficiency on an individual basis.

60. A patient with eczema, chronic diarrhea, malabsorption, and recurrent sinopulmonary infections might be lacking what nutrient?

Zinc. Patients who cannot absorb zinc, an autosomal recessive trait, develop a clinical syndrome called acrodermatitis enteropathica and exhibit the above clinical features. They can be hypogammaglobulinemic and may also have T-cell defects. Treatment with zinc, IV or high-dose oral, resolves the symptoms.

61. Patients with the metabolic disease type I hereditary oroticaciduria have what clinical features?

Increased number of infections
Lymphopenia
Decreased numbers of T-cells
Impaired T-cell function
Growth failure
Megaloblastic anemia
Recurrent diarrhea

62. What cell deficiency has been found in Chédiak-Higashi syndrome, X-linked lymphoproliferative syndrome, LAD-1, and SCID?

NK cell deficiency. The function of NK cells is to lyse a number of target cells, including tumor cells and a broad range of virus-infected cells when activated by IL-2 or interferon gamma. NK cell deficiency is not an isolated immunodeficiency but is found in the above disorders. Patients can present with recurrent severe infections from varicella, herpes viruses, cytomegalovirus, and herpes simplex. Antivirals (acute and prophylactic) are the only treatment.

BIBLIOGRAPHY

1. Aruffo A, Hollenbaugh D, Wu LH, Ochs HD: The molecular basis of X-linked agammaglobulinemia, hyper-IgM syndrome, and severe combined immunodeficiency in humans. Curr Opin Hematol 1:12–18, 1994.
2. Buckley RH, Schiff RI, Schiff SE, et al: Human severe combined immunodeficiency (SCID): Genetic, phenotypic and functional diversity in 108 infants. J Pediatr 130:378–387, 1997.
3. Buckley RH: Primary immunodeficiency diseases. In Middleton E, et al (eds): Allergy Principles and Practice. St. Louis, Mosby, 1998, pp 713–734.
4. Cunningham-Rundles C, Bodian C: Common variable immunodeficiency: Clinical and immunological features of 248 patients. Clin Immunol 92:34–48, 1999.
5. Liblau RS, Bach JF: Selective IgA deficiency and autoimmunity. Int Arch Allergy Immunol 99:16–27, 1992.
6. Lipnick RN, Iliopoulos A, Salata K, et al: Leukocyte adhesion deficiency: Report of a case and review of the literature. Clin Exp Rheumatol 14:95–98, 1996.
7. Minegishi Y, Rohrer J, Conley ME: Recent progress in the diagnosis and treatment of patients with defects in early B-cell development. Curr Opin Pediatr 11:528–532, 1999.
8. Myers LA, Riester DE, Schiff RI, et al: Bone marrow transplantation for SCID in the neonatal period. J Allergy Clin Immunol 99S:101, 1997.
9. Nelson RP: Immunodeficiencies. In Slavin RG, et al (eds): Expert Guide to Allergy and Immunology. Philadelphia, American College of Physicians, 1999, pp 189–207.
10. Paller AS: Immunodeficiency syndromes. X-linked agammaglobulinemia, common variable immunodeficiency, Chediak-Higashi syndrome, Wiskott-Aldrich syndrome, and X-linked lymphoproliferative disorder. Dermatol Clin 13:65–71, 1995.
11. Rosen FS, Cooper MD, Wedgwood RJP: The primary immunodeficiencies. N Engl J Med 333:431–440, 1995.
12. Rosen FS, Janeway CA: The gamma globulins. Part III: The antibody deficiency syndromes. N Engl J Med 275:769–775, 1966.
13. Sicherer SH, Winkelstein JA: Primary immunodeficiency diseases in adults. JAMA 279:58–61, 1998.
14. Stites DP, Terr AI, Parslow TG (eds): Immunodeficiencies. Medical Immunology. Stamford, CT, Appleton & Lange 1997.
15. Ten RM: Primary immunodeficiencies. Mayo Clin Proc 73:865–872, 1998.
16. Thrasher AJ, Kinnon C: The Wiskott-Aldrich syndrome. Clin Exp Immunol 120:2–9, 2000.
17. Tsukada S, Saffran DC, Rawlings DJ, et al: Deficient expression of a B-cell cytoplasmic tyrosine kinase in human X-linked agammaglobulinemia. Cell 72:279–290, 1993.
18. World Health Organization Scientific Group: Primary immunodeficiency diseases. Clin Exp Immunol 109(suppl):1–28, 1997.

18. IMMUNOTHERAPY

Massoud Mahmoudi, D.O., Ph.D., and Stanley M. Naguwa, M.D.

1. What is immunotherapy?

Immunotherapy is the repeated administration of specific allergen(s) to patients with IgE-mediated conditions to provide protection against the allergic symptoms and inflammation.

2. Describe the immunologic changes that occur in immunotherapy.

Several immunologic changes occur in patients treated with immunotherapy, including a reduction in mediator release from mast cells and basophils. Total serum IgE does not change, but specific IgE antibody titer decreases over time. There is an increase in specific IgG titer, early-on IgG1, and later IgG4; CD8+ and T lymphocytes increase; serum interleukin-2R (IL-2R) and RceII/CD23 on B lymphocytes decrease. One hypothesis of the mechanism of immunotherapy indicates a shift from Th-2–type to Th-1–type response. Th-2 response produces IL-4 and IL-5 which promotes the allergic reaction, whereas Th1 produces IFN-γ and ameliorates the allergic reaction. The shift of Th-2 to Th-1 response is hypothesized to occur as a result of either selective down-regulation (anergy) of the Th-2 response or induction of immune deviation by IL-12. The Table summarizes the immunologic changes.

Immunologic Changes Associated with Allergen Immunotherapy

PARAMETER	TREATED SUBJECTS	UNTREATED SUBJECTS
Specific IgE Ab titer	Decreased over time	No change
Post-seasonal specific IgE rise	Decreased	No change
Specific IgG titer	Increased	No change
Auto-anti-idiotype (anti-IgE) antibody	Appears after 6–10 months	Undetectable
Total serum IgE	No change	No change
Ag-specific basophil histamine release	Decreased	No change
Ag-specific nasal mediator release	Decreased	No change
Skin test late-phase response	Decreased	No change
Bronchial early antigen response	Decreased	No change
Bronchial late-phase response	Variable	No change
Serum neutrophil/eosinophil chemotactic activity	Decreased	No change
Spontaneous mononuclear cell HRF production	Decreased	No change
Seasonal serum ECP level	Decreased	No change
Ag-specific CD4+ T-cell proliferation	Decreased	No change
Ag-specific CD8+ T-cell proliferation	Increased	No change
Ag-specific lymphocyte IL-2 production	Decreased	No Change

Treated and untreated subjects were compared with nonallergic controls.
Ab = antibody; Ag = antigen; HRF = histamine-releasing factor; ECP = eosinophil cationic protein.
Reprinted with permission from the American College of Physicians–American Society of Internal Medicine.

225

3. On what is the decision to start immunotherapy based?

Diseases in which there is documented benefit of allergy immunotherapy include allergic rhinitis, allergic conjunctivitis, allergic asthma, and hymenoptera venom hypersensitivity. Immunotherapy for allergic conjunctivitis is less effective than allergic rhinitis, and there is no controlled study to support the effect of immunotherapy on food allergy. The following is a list of recommendations when considering the start of immunotherapy:

- Inform the patient of limitations of immunotherapy benefit.
- Discuss alternative measures to immunotherapy; for example, avoidance and symptomatic relief, using medications.
- Discuss avoidance measures. If allergic symptoms are due to specific allergens, for example, cat and dust mites, avoidance per se would make a great impact in the prevention of symptoms. The extent of such exposures can be investigated with thorough history taking.
- Discuss the possible development of mild to life-threatening reactions as a result of immunotherapy.
- Inform the patient about the period of immunotherapy and that it may or may not benefit the symptoms.
- Give the patient enough time to make a decision about starting immunotherapy.
- Persistence of symptoms for two consecutive seasons and failure of medications or avoidance measures is a reasonable indication of starting immunotherapy.

4. List the precautions/contraindications of immunotherapy.

- Pregnancy: It is an accepted practice to continue immunotherapy during pregnancy, but the dose of immunotherapy should not be increased.
- Immunodeficiency/autoimmune diseases: There are relative contraindications due to possible interference with the immune system.
- Unstable asthma.
- Patient on beta-blocker medication: In case of anaphylaxis with immunotherapy, epinephrine may not be effective in reversing the condition. Therefore, it is recommended that the patient switch to an antihypertensive of a different class, if possible.
- Malignancy.
- Noncompliant patient.

	Start	Maintenance	Dose increase
Pregnancy	NR	P	NR
Beta blockers	NR		
Ace inhibitors	NR		
Unstable asthma	NR	NR	NR
Immunodeficiency	NR		
Autoimmune diseases	NR		
Malignancy	NR		
Noncompliant patients	NR		

[NR: not recommended, P: permitted]

5. Describe the time course of immunotherapy.

The duration of immunotherapy is usually 4 to 5 years. If there is no improvement in symptoms after a approximately 1 year, the immunotherapy should be stopped. If

there is an improvement of the symptoms, the immunotherapy should be continued for an additional 3 to 4 years. If symptoms recur after immunotherapy is discontinued after a 5-year course, the patient should be reevaluated for a second course of immunotherapy.

6. Explain what a maintenance dose is.

It is the dose of an allergen extract that controls the patient's symptoms and that is tolerated without systemic reaction. The maintenance dose varies among individuals, because the level of sensitivity to a specific allergen is different among patients. Doses of 5 to 20 µg are reported for domestic mites, cat dander, rag weed pollen, and hymenoptera venom. However, some patients are not able to tolerate these doses, thus, allergen doses should be tailored individually.

7. Are systemic reactions to immunotherapy predictable?

The systemic reactions in individuals receiving immunotherapy are never predictable. However, there are situations and circumstances that increase the chance of systemic reactions. Precautionary measures should include:

1. Assuring administration of a correct dose of allergen.
2. Use of a correct route of immunotherapy; i.e., subcutaneous injection as opposed to intramuscular or intravenous injection.
3. Administration of allergen extract to a stable patient. The immunotherapy should be postponed in patients with unstable asthma or acute illness.

Systemic reactions are more likely to occur with:

• Start-up doses of immunotherapy.
• Dosage increase.
• Use of a new vial of allergen extract (particularly with non-standardized allergens).
• Patients with past history of systemic reactions to immunotherapy.
• Beta-blocker medications. Patients on beta-blockers are less responsive to epinephrine treatment of a systemic reaction.

8. How common are systemic reactions and fatalities due to immunotherapy?

Systemic reactions, especially when there is no fatal outcome, are not usually reported. Therefore, the prevalence is unknown. In one report by the committee on allergen standardization of the American Academy of Allergy, Asthma, and Immunology, 46 fatalities due to postskin test/immunotherapy have been reported since 1945. Thirty of the fatalities reported had sufficient information for analysis for the period 1959–1984, of which 24 were postimmunotherapy and 6 were postskin testing. Of the 24 fatalities postimmunotherapy, 4 had experienced previous reactions, 11 had shown a high degree of sensitivity, and 4 had received a new preparation of extract. In a subsequent survey of fatalities associated with immunotherapy for the period 1985–1989, the same committee reported 17 additional fatalities. It was estimated that the fatality rate from immunotherapy in the United States is 1 per 2 million dose administrations.

9. What is the recommended observation period after administration of allergen extract in the office?

The American Academy of Allergy, Asthma, and Immunology position statement on treatment of systemic reactions caused by immunotherapy recommends an

observation period of 20 minutes (longer for high-risk patients) to prevent serious, or possibly fatal, reactions postimmunotherapy.

10. List and describe the steps in hymenoptera venom immunotherapy.

1. Determine bee sting history and identify the species, if possible.

2. Inquire about the type of reaction; i.e., small or large, local, or systemic. Ask in detail about the symptoms; i.e., urticaria, angioedema, shortness of breath, wheezing, feeling of suffocation.

3. Inquire whether the patient is on beta-blocker medication.

4. Ask about the history of any others stings, particularly when and what kind of reactions occurred.

5. Determine patient's occupation. Is it an outdoor or indoor occupation? If outdoor, is the patient in danger of being stung in the future?

6. Test for venom-specific IgE by skin testing and/or RAST.

7. The European Academy of Allergology and Clinical Immunology (EAACI), subcommittee on insect venom allergy reports the following as indications for venom immunotherapy. Patients with positive skin test or venom-specific serum IgE who have severe reactions, that is, respiratory and cardiovascular symptoms, should be started on venom immunotherapy. However, there is no indication for venom immunotherapy for the patient with a severe systemic reaction and negative testing. Immunotherapy for patients with mild to moderate reactions—that is, urticaria, angioedema (unless at high risk for repeated stings), large local or unusual reactions with positive or negative testing—is not indicated.

8. The immunotherapy subcommittee also recommends venom immunotherapy for beekeepers (presently working or not) with a history of recent anaphylaxis.

11. Can venom immunotherapy be used in infancy and children?

The EAACI subcommittee on insect venom allergy recommends venom immunotherapy for children (before age 5 years) with great exposure who have severe reactions, such as children of beekeepers. Children and young adults have less severe allergic reactions and fewer fatalities than elderly adults.

12. Should anything special be done for patients who are on beta-blocker medication and in need of immunotherapy?

Because of concern about beta-blockers and immunotherapy, the American Academy of Allergy, Asthma, and Immunology issued a position statement. Where possible, another class of medications, which is safe and effective, should be substituted for beta-blockers. The risk and benefit of immunotherapy initiation should be thoroughly discussed with individuals who are unable to substitute beta-blockers. The recommendations include labeling of the charts with a warning regarding the potential danger and risk of such combinations for patients on beta-blockers and allergen extract preparations.

13. Define allergen extract.

It is a preparation of a specific allergen(s) obtained from trees, grasses, weed pollens, mold spores, dust mites, cats, dogs, feathers, and the like, and purified with a designated unit dose. Not all allergen extracts are standardized at this time; consequently,

there is variation among companies in preparations of nonstandardized extracts. There are variations on the designated unit dose as well. A common unit used is weight per volume. It simply measures the gram(s) of allergen extract per known volume. For example: a gram of an extract in 100 ml of solution makes a 1% solution and is designated 1:100 W:V. Another unit system is the Noon pollen unit, which is designated as 0.001 mg of pollen extract. Other systems of unit doses are used, such as the protein nitrogen unit or the total nitrogen unit. The standardized preparations have a unit dose of BAU (biologic allergenic unit), or allergen units (AU).

14. What is the goal in making an allergen extract preparation?
An ideal allergen extract preparation is one that conserves immunogenicity, has longevity, and is absorbed slowly. The alum precipitation method retards absorption. Pyridine or aqueous-extracted alum-precipitated extracts have been used. The advantage of the aqueous preparation over pyridine preparation is that it incurs a less-systemic reaction. The disadvantage of alum-precipitated extracts is its limited availability. Other allergen-extract preparations include formaldehyde or glutaraldehyde-treated extracts, both with reduced allergenicity.

15. List the office equipment needed for administration of immunotherapy.
The following equipment is recommended by the American Academy of Allergy, Asthma and Immunology:
• Stethoscope and sphygmomanometer
• Tourniquets, syringes, hypodermic needles, and large bore (14-gauge) needles
• Aqueous epinephrine HCl 1:1000
• Equipment for administration of oxygen
• Equipment for administration of intravenous fluids
• Oral airways
• Diphenhydramine or similar antihistamine for injection
• Aminophyllin for intravenous administration
• Corticosteroids for intravenous injections
• Vasopressor
H2 antihistamine for intravenous injection may be desirable.

16. What is the route of allergen immunotherapy? Are there any alternatives?
Allergen immunotherapy is administered subcutaneously, but other routes, such as oral/sublingual, nasal, and intrabronchial have been suggested. Although administration of an allergen extract by an oral/sublingual route has the potential to be more convenient, its drawbacks include possible gastrointestinal side effects, high doses needed, and prolonged time to become effective. The European Academy of Allergology and Clinical Immunology (EAACI) Immunotherapy subcommittee's position paper raised the issues of cost and safety of oral immunotherapy. The report noted a significant difference in the cost of oral immunotherapy over sublingual administration. The other issue was lack of safety data. The necessity of more controlled trials to address risk and limitations, and to understand the mechanism of oral immunotherapy was also noted by the subcommittee. The subcommittee was unable to recommend sublingual immunotherapy due to lack of sufficient beneficial data. In a recent position paper, the World Health Organization reviewed recent studies on

oral immunotherapy and did not recommend it due to lack of clinical efficacy of the therapy.

Intranasal preparations of allergen extracts, although not approved by the Food and Drug Administration, are reportedly effective in reducing symptoms of seasonal and perennial allergic rhinitis. In one study, local nasal immunotherapy, consisting of a birch pollen allergen in powder form or a placebo, was administered to two 15-patient groups. The 22-week-long study consisted of 14 weeks of build-up phase and 8 weeks of maintenance therapy. During the pollen season, a significant reduction in medication score was noted; after treatment, a significant increase in the specific nasal threshold dose was noted as well. In a double-blind, placebo-controlled study, the efficacy and safety of parietaria pollen nasal immunotherapy in allergic rhinitis patients were investigated. Patients were divided into two random groups of 13, a treatment group and the placebo group. Nasal immunotherapy, in the form of a macronized powder of parietaria pollen, was administered. The mean weekly nasal symptom scores and the specific nasal threshold to the pollen extract and drug consumption were significantly different in the treated group as compared to the placebo group.

17. Describe the dose schedules of immunotherapy. Distinguish conventional from rapid immunotherapy.

The goal of immunotherapy is to reach a tolerable dose of an allergen extract that is able to minimize and control symptoms of allergic rhinitis/asthma and to protect against severe systemic reactions, as in the case of venom hymenoptera hypersensitivity. There are several protocols that have been used to reach this goal, namely rush, daily, cluster, and conventional schedules. The aim of all protocols is to quickly reach a maintenance dose, with the conventional schedule slower than the others. The following is an example of one of the conventional dose schedule: allergen extract is diluted from 1:10 to have final dilutions of 1:10, 1:100, 1:1000, 1:10,000, and 1:100,000. The usual starting point is 0.05 ml of a 1:10,000 dilution vial. At times, with hypersensitive patients, the starting vial is a 1:100,000 dilution. The injections are weekly/biweekly and the dose is increased incrementally: 0.1, 0.15, 0.20, 0.30. 0.40, and 0.50 cc. If the injections are tolerated. The procedure is repeated with the next higher concentration until a maintenance dose is reached. The desired maintenance dose is 0.50 ml of 1:100 dilution equivalent to 2,500 protein nitrogen units (PNUs) or 5 to 20 µg of allergen. Those patients who cannot tolerate this dose should be on a lower maintenance dose. The maintenance dose may be given weekly for 1 month and then every other week for 1 month. Thereafter, the interval between doses can be increased to 3 to 4 weeks.

18. What are reasonable goals of immunotherapy?

An allergist needs to discuss the benefits and possible harm of immunotherapy and outcome expectations with the patient. Immunotherapy is beneficial in specific diseases, such as allergic rhinitis, allergic conjunctivitis, allergic asthma, and hymenoptera hypersensitivity. Whether immunotherapy will help the particular patient, and if it will help, to what extent it will do so, is unpredictable. A complete disappearance of symptoms on a maintenance dose of immunotherapy is ideal; the reality, however, is that a patient might continue having symptoms, although with less severity

and frequency as compared to the preimmunotherapy period. Patients need to know that the level of benefit varies among individuals. The chance of having no benefit from immunotherapy should be discussed with the patient, as well. For a patient who benefits from immunotherapy, a reasonable goal is to use the medications less often and in lower doses. The severity of symptoms should also decrease and reach a tolerable level.

19. Name the factors that can cause failure of immunotherapy and describe how they can be addressed.

1. Compliance of the patient. The issue of compliance has a great impact on the outcome of immunotherapy. The patient should be informed of a long-term commitment to complete the course of immunotherapy, that is, the time needed to spend coming to the office for weekly/biweekly injections initially, and at longer intervals after reaching the maintenance dose.

2. Change of allergen sensitivity. When a patient does not respond to immunotherapy, it may be due to the development of allergies to a new allergen. This can be true when a patient on immunotherapy moves to a different geographic region where the patient is exposed to new and different allergens. With this suspicion, a patient should be tested to allergens common to the new area and after confirmation of new allergen sensitivity, the new allergen(s) can then be added to the immunotherapy regimen.

3. Patient intolerance. Repeated systemic reactions and inability to advance the dose of an allergen extract to an effective dose is a troublesome situation. If the dose given is not effective, the immunotherapy should be stopped.

4. Unreliability of initial allergy testing. Inaccurate test results can be due to mislabeling the allergen bottle(s) used for testing, or mixing a wrong allergen to which the patient is not allergic. This occurs rarely, but is possible. Using an expired extract or using incorrectly prepared dilutions are also possibilities of ineffective immunotherapy.

5. Insufficient allergen for clinical efficacy.

It is known that low-dose immunotherapy is considered ineffective. Therefore, administration of allergen extract should follow a conventional immunotherapy regimen.

BIBLIOGRAPHY

1. American Academy of Allergy and Immunology: Position statement. Guidelines to minimize the risk from systemic reactions caused by immunotherapy with allergenic extracts. J Allergy Clin Immunol 93:811–812, 1994.
2. Anderson JA, Kaliner M, Kaplan AP, et al: American Academy of Allergy and Immunology. Position statement. The waiting period after allergen skin testing and immunotherapy. J Allergy Clin Immunol 85:526–527, 1990.
3. Andri L, Senna G, Andri G, et al: Local nasal immunotherapy for birch allergic rhinitis with extract in powder form. Clin Exp Allergy 25:1092–1099, 1995.
4. Bielory L: Allergic and immunologic disorders of the eye. In Middleton, E Jr, Reed CE, Ellis EF, et al (eds): Allergy Principles and Practice, vol 2, 5th ed. St. Louis, Mosby, 1998, pp 1148–1161.
5. Bousquet J, Lockey RF, Malling HJ: Allergen immunotherapy: Therapeutic vaccines for allergic diseases. WHO position paper. Allergy 53:1–42, 1998.
6. Bousquet JB, Lockey RF, Mailling HJ, et al: Allergen immunotherapy: Therapeutic vaccines for allergic diseases. World Health Organization paper, an executive summary. Ann Allergy Asthma Immunol 81:401–405, 1998.
7. D'Amato G, Lobefalo G, Liccardi G, et al: A double-blind, placebo-controlled trial of local nasal immunotherapy in allergic rhinitis to parietaria pollen. Clin Exp Allergy 25:141–148, 1995.

8. Durham SR, Till SJ: Immunologic changes associated with allergen immunotherapy. J Allergy Clin Immunol 102:157–164, 1998.
9. Horwitz RJ, Bush RK: Allergens and other factors important in atopic disease. In Patterson R, Grammer LC, Greenberger PA, et al (eds): Allergic Diseases: Diagnosis and Management, 5th ed, Philadelphia, Lippincott-Williams and Wilkins, 1997, pp 75–129.
10. Kaplan AP, Anderson JA, Valentine MD, et al (American Academy of Allergy and Immunology): Position statement. Beta-adrenergic blockers, immunotherapy, and skin testing. J Allergy Clin Immunol 84:129–130, 1989.
11. Ledford DK: Immunotherapy for allergic diseases. In Condemi JJ, Dykewicz MS (eds): Allergy and Immunology, Medical Knowledge Self-Assessment Program, 2nd ed, Philadelphia, American College of Physicians, 1997, pp 143–152.
12. Lockey RF, Benedict LM, Turkeltaub PC, et al: Fatalities from immunotherapy (IT) and skin testing (ST). J Allergy Clin Immunol 79:660–677, 1987.
13. Malling HJ, Weeke B: Position paper: Immunotherapy. Allergy 48(Suppl):7–35, 1993.
14. Muller U, Mosbech H: Position paper: Immunotherapy with hymenoptera venoms. Allergy 48:36–46, 1993.
15. Nelson HS: Immunotherapy for inhalant allergens. In Middleton, E Jr, Reed CE, Ellis EF, et al (eds): Allergy Principles and Practice, vol. 2, 5th ed, St. Louis, CV Mosby, 1998, pp 1050–1062.
16. Nicklas RA, Bernstein IL, Blessing-Moore J, et al (eds): Practice parameters for allergen immunotherapy. J Allergy Clin Immunol 98:1001–1011, 1996.
17. Reid MJ, Lockey RF, Turkeltaub PC, et al: Survey of fatalities from skin testing and immunotherapy 1985-1989. J Allergy Clin Immunol 92:6–15, 1993.
18. Sale SR, Patterson R. Immunotherapy. In: Korenblat PE, Wedner HJ (eds): Allergy Theory and Practice, 2nd ed, Philadelphia, WB Saunders, 1992, pp 279–294.

19. COMPLEMENTARY MEDICINE

Katherine E. Gundling, M.D.

1. What is the relationship of zinc to asthma severity?

Patients with low dietary zinc intake may suffer from increased bronchial hyperreactivity. Other clinical clues of zinc deficiency include diarrhea and acrodermatitis. Asthmatics should maintain a healthy diet that includes food with natural zinc content. Whether supplemental zinc improves clinical outcome in asthmatics is uncertain and under investigation.

2. Which botanical agents have a history of traditional use for asthma?

- *Coffee* has been used traditionally as an antiasthmatic in Europe. Caffeine is a bronchodilator and the humidity from steam serves to hydrate mucous membranes.
- *Black and green tea* contain lesser amounts of caffeine; additionally, the term *theophylline* actually originates from tea leaf.
- *Ma huang* has been used in China for generations as a stimulant and treatment for asthma. The active ingredient, ephedrine, is closely related biochemically to pseudoephedrine, phenylpropanolamine and amphetamine. It can be obtained over the counter as a dietary supplement in the United States, although it has been associated with numerous amphetaminelike adverse effects.
- *Ginkgo biloba* has been used in several cultures to reduce symptoms of asthma. Extracts have been shown to inhibit platelet-activating factor, which provides a theoretical basis for the observation of improvement of asthma-related cough. Clinical evidence is lacking, however.
- *Datura stramonium* leaves were smoked as tobacco in India and became a popular remedy for asthma exacerbation in the United States and Europe in the nineteenth and twentieth centuries. This botanical agent contains a bronchodilator.

3. Describe the effects of caffeine on pulmonary function studies.

Whether or not patients use caffeine for its bronchodilating effects, they should be advised to hold their caffe lattes in the 4 hours prior to pulmonary function studies. A Cochrane Collaboration review found sufficient data to conclude that caffeine from just three cups of coffee is enough to interfere with measurements of pulmonary function and reversibility due to bronchodilators.

4. Does acupuncture reduce bronchospasm?

Evidence does not yet support the use of acupuncture for bronchospasm. A Cochrane Collaboration systematic review analyzed 59 clinical studies, 7 of which met methodologic criteria for review. Two suggested benefit compared to dummy acupuncture and five revealed no significant difference between treatment and sham acupuncture. However, only one study individualized treatment and another contained only four patients with reversible disease. None of the trials was directly comparable to the others. Based on existing data, acupuncture should not be used in place of pharmaceutic agents for treatment of reactive airway disease. The use of

acupuncture as part of an entire program of traditional Chinese medicine is even less well studied.

5. Which complementary therapy is most frequently recommended to asthmatic patients by health care professionals?

Change of diet. Physicians who subscribe to a leading complementary and alternative medicine journal recommended dietary treatments for asthma more than any other complementary therapy. The second and third most common approaches, "environmental" medicine and nutritional supplements, respectively, have strong components of dietary manipulation. Other recommended treatments include homeopathy, botanical agents, and meditation. Nonphysicians were more likely to recommend homeopathy and acupuncture than physicians.

6. Should patients with asthma take vitamin C supplements?

High doses of ascorbic acid should not be recommended on a routine basis.

Several studies have shown decreased airway hyperreactivity with consumption of large doses, but other studies have found no benefit. More research is required to determine who, if anyone, will benefit from large-dose supplementation of ascorbic acid.

7. Should physicians advise patients to use homeopathy as a treatment for asthma?

No. A Cochrane Collaboration assessment of the data from well-designed trials found only three trials that varied widely in methodology and interventions. Three different remedies were used, two of the studies reported positive results and one reported negative results. The insufficient data and implausible mechanism of action argue against routine recommendation of homeopathy. Additionally, effective treatments are readily available and their use should not be delayed.

8. Describe the relationship between asthma severity and patient self-treatment with herbal remedies, ephedrine, and coffee or black tea.

Self-treatment with one or more of these nonprescription remedies was found in 16% of 601 patients recruited from pulmonary and allergy subspecialty practices. Self-treatment was associated with a higher incidence of asthma-related hospitalization. Possible reasons for this association include a less-than-optimal treatment program, a decreased adherence with prescribed regimens, a delay of appropriate treatment, or, perhaps, a sicker population of patients.

9. What are the theoretical bases for therapy with yoga in the treatment of asthma?

Yoga is an essential part of the practice of Ayurvedic medicine, one of the oldest medical systems in the world. It's utility for prevention and treatment of asthma exacerbation is just now being investigated. Theoretical bases for its efficacy include:
- Stress reduction, with concomitant physical and mental relaxation, diminished muscle tension with more efficient use of the diaphragm and thoracic musculature, and decreased oxygen utilization. These changes all suggest decreased vagal tone and bronchoconstriction, and enhanced bronchodilatation.

• Enhanced adrenocoritcal activity. Unfortunately the early reports of this association have not been further elucidated in the medical literature.
• Improved mechanics of breathing directly related to the breathing exercises and attention to posture.

10. Should supplementation with fish oil be recommended to patients with asthma?
Patients should be advised that increased consumption of fish with high content of omega 3/6 fatty acids may add to a complete asthma care regimen. There are at least two small studies in adults that show promise, although the quantity, type and frequency of optimal essential fatty acid supplementation are unknown. For most patients, substitution of cold water fish for red meat makes good dietary sense whether or not asthma is an active concern.

11. Describe the indirect adverse effects of using "alternative" therapies for asthma.
• Delay of diagnosis. Patients who self-treat or see practitioners who are unable to assess the severity of disease risk delay of approriate treatment and increased requirements for hospitalization. There are documented deaths of patients who rejected conventional therapies in favor of acupuncture, and died due to the severity of untreated disease. Without appropriate anti-inflammatory therapy, patients risk long-term damage to the lungs.
• Inappropriate diagnosis. Not all that wheezes is pure asthma. Persistent or significant symptoms should be evaluated for alternate etiologies such as allergic bronchopulmonary aspergillosis, foreign body, or chronic obstructive pulmonary disease.
• Unrecognized adverse effects. Patients who trust that "natural" medicines are safe may not suspect that their difficulties are due to the chosen remedies. Moreover patients who self-treat have fewer resources for reporting potential adverse outcomes.

12. What is the evidence for chiropractic in the treatment of asthma?
The only relatively well-designed trials of chiropractic for asthma fail to demonstrate benefit. This information and the lack of a plausible mechanism argue against the use of chiropractic for asthma unless evidence to the contrary is presented.

13. Are rotation diets effective therapy for atopic dermatitis in adults?
No. Patients often initiate restrictive diets based on false assumptions or misinformation from practitioners who use unvalidated diagnostic methods (such as "cytotoxic" food testing). Although recent well-designed studies have demonstrated a relationship between certain foods and exacerbation of atopic eczema in a selected, young, pediatric population, dietary intervention should be contemplated only rarely in adults. The social isolation, risk of malnutrition and effort involved in adhering to a restrictive diet are generally far more detrimental than the effects of the disease.

14. What is the evidence for traditional Chinese herbal formulations for the treatment of atopic eczema?
At least six studies have been published recently that used the same standard Chinese herbal formula for atopic eczema. Compared to other complementary therapies

for atopic eczema, the evidence for benefit of the standard formula is relatively good. Two double-blind, placebo-controlled, crossover trials (one with children, one with adults) demonstrated significant improvement with the formula, although one trial had a high dropout rate. A more recent, well-designed study, however, did not support the positive conclusions of these trials.

Whereas conventional pharmaceutic agents usually contain only 1 or 2 active ingredients, the standard Chinese herbal formula contains 10 different botanical agents, each of which contains many active ingredients. Formula content varies slightly with the age and origin of the plants, time of harvest, soil conditions, and a host of other conditions. The challenge of determining the active agents justifies the expectation of solid clinical outcomes data. Nevertheless, a number of studies are underway to assess immunologic responses to the standard formula.

15. What unlabeled pharmaceutic agent is found in Chinese herbal creams prescribed for atopic dermatitis?

Dexamethasone has been found in varying quantities in containers of individually prepared Chinese herbal creams. One study found in it every bottle prescribed for atopic dermatitis. The creams are often applied by patients to large areas of skin, or to sensitive areas, such as the face and flexural areas. As such, patients should be aware the potential adverse effects of these substances.

16. List the essential oils that are associated with new onset eczematous dermatitis.

Lavender

Jasmine

Rosewood

Allergic airborne contact dermatitis from aromatherapy is unusual but increasingly described in the literature.

17. Does the medical literature support acupuncture as a treatment for allergic rhinitis?

Although many studies report positive results using acupuncture to treat allergic rhinitis, their methodologic quality is quite low. Most studies lack effective control groups, and adequate detail is often missing. Evidence-based conclusions are lacking, such that acupuncture cannot yet be recommended as a viable alternative to conventional therapy. Some physicians argue that because allergic rhinitis is generally not life threatening, a course of acupuncture is unlikely to be of harm and may be of benefit in a way that is yet to be elucidated. Studies have shown that patients often use multiple modalities simultaneously to treat chronic medical problems, including the use of acupuncture while taking prescription medication.

18. Which complementary therapies are most frequently used by patients for relief of allergic rhinitis?

Homeopathy

Herbal medicine

Dietary changes and restrictions

Acupuncture

Hypnosis

19. Is acupuncture an effective treatment for urticaria?

Although acupuncture has long been used in Asia to treat acute and chronic urticaria, there are no well-designed trials of its efficacy. There are generally four acupuncture points prescribed for acute symptoms with a 90% cure rate claimed. For chronic urticaria the same points are used, along with other acupuncture techniques, such as cupping, point bleeding, and point injection with thiamine, although the cure rate is only claimed to be about 30 to 50%. Proponents cite evidence of increased circulating levels of cortisol and corticotropin in humans following acupuncture as a possible mechanism.

20. Which common herbal tea should be avoided in patients with allergy to ragweed?

Chamomile should not be consumed by patients with allergy to ragweed, asters, chrysanthemums, and other members of the family Compositae (Asteraceae). Tea prepared with pollen-laden flower heads has caused contact dermatitis, anaphylaxis, and other severe hypersensitivity reactions. Milk thistle is also a member of the Compositae family, and there is evidence for cross-sensitivity with echinacea as well.

21. Name the common contaminants and adulterants of Asian patent medications.
- Ephedrine
- Chlorpheniramine
- Methyltestosterone
- Phenacetin
- Lead, arsenic, and mercury

Approximately one-third of Asian patent medications contain undeclared pharmaceutics or heavy metals. The potential benefits and adverse effects are evident from the list of substances. Unlabeled ephedrine may serve as a weak bronchodilator but it should not be used by patients with hypertension, anxiety, and many other disorders. The sedative properties of chlorpheniramine pose a danger to those who take it unknowingly. Patients should be warned about the pharmacologic effects, both known and hidden, of Asian patent medications.

22. What adverse effects have been related to use of Chinese herbal medicine for atopic dermatitis?

Hepatotoxicity
Dilated cardiomyopathy
Skin atrophy due to unlabeled steroid content of topical agents
The true incidence of toxicity is unknown.

CONTROVERSIES

23. Should homeopathic remedies be used to treat allergic rhinitis?

Background: What is homeopathy? Homeopathy is a system of medical practice founded by Samuel Hahnemann, a German physician who was discouraged by the "heroic" practice of medicine in the late 1700s, which included such treatments

as blood-letting and purging. Homeopathy is based on the belief that substances that cause disease or symptoms in healthy people can treat those same diseases or symptoms when administered in dilute solution to sick people (the principle of "like treats like"). For example, whereas syrup of ipecac normally causes nausea and vomiting, homeopathy uses dilute solutions of ipecac as a treatment for nausea and vomiting. The law of infinitesimals holds that the more dilute the remedy the more potent it is. The most powerful remedies are those diluted even beyond Avogadro's number (6×10^{27}).

During the 1800s, homeopathy became a popular system of practice among American physicians who were happy to have less toxic methods of treating patients. A number of American medical schools taught homeopathy, and many physicians practiced in both systems. The founding of the American Medical Asssociation was due in part to the popularity of homeopathy as a perceived threat to the "regular" physicians. With scientific advancement and critical analysis of medical education early in the twentieth century, homeopathy almost disappeared in the United States. Its reemergence at the end of the century was due to renewed interest in "alternative medicine" generally, and "natural" treatments specifically. However, most practitioners of homeopathy in the United States are no longer licensed physicians. Homeopathy has enjoyed ongoing popularity in Europe, and India has many homeopathic colleges and over 100,000 homeopathic doctors. Importantly, most people assume incorrectly that homeopathy is synonymous with herbal medicine. In reality, homeopathic treatments use a wide variety of animal, mineral, and plant substances.

Homeopathy has been used to treat allergic rhinitis for over 100 years. The evaluation of its efficacy, however, is in its early stages. The challenges of studying homeopathy include the many different remedies prescribed at different doses, the individual nature of prescription to which some practitioners adhere, the difficulty of comparing studies that use different remedies, and the lack of a known mechanism of action, to name a few.

A 1997 meta-analysis of homeopathy included six articles that met methodologic criteria and examined the effects of homeopathy on symptoms of allergic rhinitis. Five of these studies reported positive effects. However, the studies used different substances and tested for different outcomes, and the authors concluded that there was not enough evidence to support the use homeopathic remedies for any single indication. One study demonstrated benefit to the use of the remedy Galphimia glauca for ocular symptoms. Another study showed improved symptoms and decreased antihistamine use compared to placebo in patients who took a homeopathic remedy of mixed grass pollen.

"Homeopathic immunotherapy" is the name given to the practice of "isopathy" for the treatment of allergic rhinitis. Isopathy dictates that the patient be given dilute quantities of the very pollens to which he or she is allergic. Is the solutional "memory" concept of standard homeopathy still considered to be the mechanism of action, or are isopathic solutions of low dilution efficacious in a manner similar to conventional immunotherapy?

For: Proponents argue that homeopathy is a time-tested system of practice that stimulates the body to heal itself. Whereas some practitioners argue that homeopathy cannot be tested in the Western "paradigm," others have made systematic attempts

to do just that. Indeed, several apparently well-designed studies of different remedies for different symptoms of allergic rhinitis have yielded positive results.
Homeopathic remedies are an inexpensive and generally safe alternative to prescription medications.

Against: The proposed mechanism of action of homeopathy (solutions retain a
memory of the diluted substance) makes no sense on the basis of present knowledge
of chemistry and physics. Extraordinary claims require extraordinary proof, which
homeopathy has not yet supplied. Patients may suffer or undergo delay of appropriate
diagnosis by self-treating or not receiving timely medical evaluation and treatment.

BIBLIOGRAPHY

1. Bielory L, Gandhi R: Asthma and vitamin C. Ann Allergy 73:89–96, 1994.
2. Blanc PD, Kuschner WG, Katz PP, Smith S, Yelin EH: Use of herbal products, coffee or black tea,
   and over-the-counter medications as self-treatments among adults with asthma. J Allergy Clin
   Immunol 100:789–791, 1997.
3. Burnham TH (ed): The Review of Natural Products. Facts and Comparisons. St. Louis, 2000
   (monthly updates).
4. Ernst E: Complementary therapies for asthma: What patients use. 35:667–671, 1998.
5. Fung AY, Look PC, Chong LY, But PP, Wong E: A controlled trial of traditional Chinese herbal medicine in Chinese patients with recalcitrant atopic dermatitis. Int J Dermatol 38:387–392, 1999.
6. Hackman RM, Stern JS, Gershwin ME: Complementary/alternative therapies in general medicine:
   Asthma and allergies. In Spencer W, Jacobs J (eds): Complementary/Alternative Medicine: An
   Evidence-Based Approach. St. Louis, CV Mosby, 1999, pp 65–89.
7. Ko R. Adulterants in asian patent medications. N Engl J Med 339:847, 1998.
8. Lewith GT, Watkins AD: Unconventional therapies in asthma: An overview. Allergy 51:761–69,
   1996.
9. Linde K, Clausius N, Ramirez G, et al: Are the clinical effects of homeopathy placebo effects? A
   meta-analysis of placebo-controlled trials. Lancet 350:834–843, 1997.
10. Linde K, Jobst KA: Homeopathy for chronic asthma. Cochrane Database Syst Rev 2:CD000353,
    2000.
11. Shenefelt PD: Hypnosis in dermatology. Arch Dermatol 136:393–399, 2000.
12. Singh V, Wisniewski A, Britton J, Tattersfield A: Effect of yoga breathing exercises (pranayama) on
    airway reactivity in subjects with asthma. Lancet 335:1381–1383, 1990.

20. SYSTEMIC MAST CELL DISEASES

Christopher Chang, M.D., Ph.D.

1. What are mast cells and when were they discovered?

Paul Ehrlich first discovered mast cells in 1877, at the Freiburg University. He named them *mastzellen*, after the Greek term *mastos* for feeding, because he thought that the cytoplasmic granules that he observed were a result of phagocytosis. Mast cells are mononuclear cells that are rarely seen in peripheral blood but that are present in tissue. They are particularly abundant in the connective tissue that surrounds areas of the body that interface with the environment, such as the respiratory tract, gastrointestinal tract, and skin. The function of mast cells remained unknown for many years. Currently, mast cells are thought to be involved in inflammatory and allergic diseases, as well as infectious, parasitic, and neoplastic conditions. Mast cells are present in all mammalian species. Initially, they were thought to be the tissue equivalent of basophils in the peripheral circulation. Recently, they have been well characterized in humans and mice, and have been found to be distinct from basophils.

2. How are mast cells identified?

Under light microscopy, mast cells appear as small round cells present in nasal mucosa, skin, intestinal mucosa, respiratory tract, and conjunctival tissue. Like basophils, the intracellular granules of mast cells stain metachromatically with an aniline dye. The color of the granules, when stained, are violet to reddish purple. This is because of the reaction between the high concentration of highly acidic heparin in the mast cells and basic aniline blue dyes. Mast cells do not stain with hematoxylin-eosin stain. Mast cells can also be identified (a) under electron microscopy, (b) by virtue of specific proteases in their cytoplasmic granules, and (c) by characterization of cell-surface markers specific for mast cells.

3. What is the structure of the mast cell?

Mast cells are usually round but can be spindly or elongated in shape. The diameter of the mast cell ranges from 10 to 20 microns. The nuclei of mast cells are ovoid in shape. The cytoplasm of the mast cell contains many granules. These secretory granules have a unique bilaminar phospholipid membrane. Mast cells also contain lysosomes, which carry oxidative enzymes and acid hydrolases.

4. What is the ontogeny of the mast cell?

Mast cells originate from a pluripotent CD34+ stem cell derived from the bone marrow. When cultured in the presence of IL-3, these stem cells are triggered to produce inordinately high numbers of mast cells. Contrary to earlier beliefs, mast cells and basophils do not share a common lineage. Mast cells complete their final maturation and differentiation in the tissues. There is heterogeneity in the structure and function of mast cells in different tissues, based on microenvironmental stimuli during the differentiation and maturation of mast cells. Mast cell growth factors include the *c-kit* ligand, or stem cell factor (stem cell factor is the high affinity ligand of a *c-kit* proto-oncogene), which is secreted by fibroblasts. Mast cell precursors

cultured with fibroblasts give rise to more mature cell lines as compared with those cultured only with IL-3. When both fibroblasts and IL-3 are present in these cultures, mast cell differentiation increases in synergistic fashion, due to the synergistic activity of stem cell factor and other growth factors, such as granulocyte-macrophage colony-stimulating factor (GM-CSF), IL-3, IL-6, and so on.

5. Describe the different types of mast cells.

In rodents, mast cells are classified as either connective tissue mast cells (CTMC) or mucosal mast cells (MMC). This differentiation is based on the phenotypic and staining characteristics of the mast cell and is not dependent on the histologic location of the mast cell. In humans, there are also two kinds of mast cells: those that secrete the neutral protease tryptase, and those that secrete other enzymes as well, primarily carboxypeptidase, cathepsin G, and chymase. These mast cells are designated as MC_T and MC_{TC} respectively. Both forms of human mast cells contain similar amounts of histamine. The different forms of mast cells are preferentially found in different tissues of the body. For example, MC_T cells are predominantly found in gastrointestinal submucosa, skin and vascular structures. These mast cells appear to be more closely linked with inflammatory disorders or allergic diseases. They are referred to as *immune system-associated mast cells*. They also play a role in host defense and are decreased in immunodeficiency syndromes. Mast cells have been linked to defense against parasitic diseases of the gut as well as involvement in innate host immunity against bacterial invasion. They are increased around areas of TH2-cell activation. MC_{TC} cells are more commonly found in the connective tissue of the lung, upper respiratory tract, and small intestine. These mast cells appear to function more in angiogenesis and tissue remodeling. They are sometimes referred to as the *nonimmune system-associated mast cell.*

6. What cell-surface receptors do mast cells possess?

The primary cell-surface receptor of the mast cell is the high-affinity FcεRI receptor. The FcεRI receptor consists of an a chain, α β chain, and two γ chains. Signal transduction across the cell membrane is regulated by alterations in the carboxyterminal cytoplasmic tail of the β or γ chains.

Other cell-surface receptors include CD43, CD44, CD54, CD68, KIT, and IL4R. Mast cells also possess receptors for IgG, and the receptors for the anaphylatoxins, complements C3a and C5a.

7. What preformed mediators are released by mast cells?

Mast cells release both preformed and newly generated mediators. The clinical effects of mastocytosis syndromes are directly related to the effects of release of both categories of mast cell mediators. The best known of the preformed mast cell mediators is histamine. Histamine is derived from the amino acid histidine and is spontaneously secreted from mast cells at low levels. The amount of histamine contained in a human mast cell is approximately 3 to 8 pg. The biogenic amine, serotonin, is another of the preformed mediators that can have significant inflammatory properties. Heparin is also present in large amounts in mast cells. Effects of heparin include endothelial cell stimulation and kinin pathway activation.

Mast cells also have a high concentration of the neutral proteases (about 60 pg per cell). The neutral protease, tryptase, is present in both human and rodent mast cells. Tryptase is a serine protease present in tetrameric form, with a total molecular weight of 130 kD. There are two pairs of two subunits designated α and β, with variable molecular weights (due to varying degrees of glycosylation) between 31 and 38 kD. Mast cells also contain proteoglycans; chemotactic factors such as eosinophil chemotactic factor (ECF) and neutrophil chemotactic factor (NCF); oxidative enzymes; other biogenic amines; and acid hydrolases, such as β-hexosaminidase and β-glucuronidase, β-D-galactosidase, and arylsulfatase.

8. What is the pathway by which mast cells are activated?

Mast cells are primarily activated as a result of antigen-triggered IgE binding to the high-affinity FcϵRI receptor on the surface of the mast cell, followed by cross-linking. Mast cells also possess the low-affinity IgG receptors FcγRII and FcγRIII. Antigen-IgE interaction leads to cross-linking of FcϵRI molecules on the surface of the mast cell. This leads to activation of tyrosine kinase, which catalyzes phosphorylation of a number of substrates, including phospholipase Cγ1 and the β and γ chains of the FcϵRI receptor, that, in turn, leads to activation of protein kinase and mobilization of intracellular calcium ions, which then leads to phospholipase A2 activation. This results in cleavage of arachidonic acid from the membrane phospholipids. The resulting lysophospholipids are active in fusion of plasma membrane with the secretory granule membrane and leads to extrusion of bioactive mediators such as histamine from the cell (degranulation). Histamine release from mast cells can also be induced by autoantibodies to the IgE FcϵRI receptor in patients with chronic idiopathic urticaria (CIU). Nonimmune-related factors, such as exercise, pressure, trauma, or cold, may also lead to activation of the FcϵRI receptor.

9. How many FcϵRI receptors are on the surface of a mast cell?

There are 10,000 to 1,000,000 FcϵRI receptors on the surface of a mast cell. Aggregation of anywhere from 1 to 15% of these receptors leads to degranulation.

10. What are the biologic effects of histamine?

Histamine is a hormone that exerts its effects on other cells, by binding to cell-surface receptors of both inflammatory and noninflammatory cells. There are two common types of histamine receptors, designated H1 and H2. A third type of histamine receptor, H3, is found on presynaptic nerve endings in both the peripheral and central nervous system. There does not appear to be a significant role for the H3-receptor in allergic or inflammatory conditions. Effects of histamine include gastrointestinal and bronchial smooth muscle contraction; gastric acid secretion; endothelial cell retraction leading to increased vascular permeability; vasodilatation; increased permeability of plasma membranes; stimulation of chemotaxis and infiltration of neutrophils and eosinophils; and stimulation of the release of other neuropeptide mediators. Clinically, this can lead to pruritus; wheezing; a wheal and flare response in the skin or urticarial rash; increased mucus secretion; gastrointestinal cramping; development of gastritis or peptic ulcers; circulatory instability; or even collapse, pulmonary edema, and death. These effects can be present to different degrees. They may be augmented by the presence of other mediators such as the leukotrienes.

11. What is the role of tryptase in acute inflammation and mastocytosis?

Tryptase is present in high concentrations in mast cells but not in other cell types. Because tryptase is not released by basophils, measurement of tryptase levels can be a more specific indicator of mast cell activation and degranulation than histamine. In patients with asthma, anaphylaxis, or systemic mastocytosis, tryptase can be found in bronchoalveolar lavage fluid after an exacerbation. Tryptase has been found to have complement activation activity and can cleave fibrinogen.

12. What are the newly generated mediators derived from mast cells?

In contrast to preformed mediators, mast cells also generate mediators only upon activation by antigen binding to the FcεRI receptor or other stimuli. These mediators include the arachidonic acid metabolites prostaglandin D2 (PGD2), leukotriene C4 (LTC4), and platelet-activating factor (PAF), which is synthesized through the action of lipoxygenase and cyclooxygenase, both of which are present in mast cells. Mast cell degranulation is also an important cytokine-releasing event. Mast cells release proinflammatory and immunomodulatory cytokines including tumor necrosis factor-alpha (TNF-α), the interleukins 1, 2, 3, 4, 5, 6, 8, and 16 (IL-1, IL-2, IL-3, IL-4, IL-5, IL-6, IL-8, IL-16), lymphotoxin, transforming growth factor-β (TGF-β), and endothelin. Some of the interleukins have both proinflammatory and mitogenic activity.

13. What are triggers for degranulation of mast cells?

Many different types of stimuli, which are described in the following list, can trigger mast cell degranulation:

A. Antigen-induced cross-linking of the FcεRI receptor on the surface of the mast cell
B. IgG-autoantibodies to IgE or the FcεRI receptor
C. Physical events
  i.   Cold
  ii.   Heat
  iii. Pressure
  iv.   Water
  v.   UV light
  vi.   Vibration
  vii. Exercise
D. Cellular mediators
  i.   Major basic protein
  ii.   Interleukins such as IL-3
  iii. Stem cell factor
E. Chemicals
  i.   Dextran
  ii.   Compound 40/80
  iii. Phorbol myristate acetate
  iv.   Ionophore A23187
  v.   Protamine sulfate
F. Medications and drugs
  i.   Radiocontrast
  ii.   ACTH

    iii. Doxorubicin
    iv. Daunorubicin
    v. Codeine
    vi. Morphine
    vii. Vancomycin
    viii. Vitamin A
    ix. Polymyxin B
G. Naturally occurring substances
    i. Anaphylatoxins C3a and C5a
    ii. Neuropeptides—substance P
    iii. Venoms

14. What is systemic mastocytosis?

Systemic mastocytosis is a heterogeneous collection of disorders with clinical symptomatology resulting from an increase in mast cells in the tissues. Organ systems involved can include skin, gastrointestinal tract, lung, brain, bone, bone marrow, liver, spleen, and lymph nodes. The disease is classified based on severity of disease and organ system involvement, with category I syndromes being the least severe and category IV being of the highest severity with the poorest prognosis. All of the categories can involve any or all of the above organ systems, but category I disease is generally more indolent and can be managed with pharmaceutic intervention for a long period of time. Category II disease involves and associated hematologic condition such as myeloproliferative or myelodysplastic disease. Category III disease is more aggressive, and Class IV disease carries an associated malignancy of the bone marrow, generally referred to as mast cell leukemia. Mastocytosis can occur at any age, but about 60% of cases develop before the age 2 years, 75% occur before age 15 years, and most other cases occur before age 40 years.

15. How is the diagnosis of systemic mastocytosis syndromes made?

The diagnosis of systemic mastocytosis is primarily made based on clinical history and physical examination. Laboratory evaluation of mastocytosis may include skin biopsy; bone marrow biopsy; measurement of plasma or urine histamine and tryptase, urinary prostaglandin D_2 metabolites, or thromboxane B_2 (of limited value). Radiographic evaluation of mastocytosis may include plain film radiography of skull and skeletal system to identify bone marrow hyperplastic lesions. Gastrointestinal workup including CT scan, plain-film radiography of the abdomen, or upper gastrointestinal series can help to identify hepatic or splenic involvement, gastric ulcers, or, in more severe cases, the presence of ascites. In addition, bone scan and endoscopy may be of diagnostic value. Magnetic resonance imaging (MRI) is a sensitive technique for isolating bone marrow pathology in patients with systemic mastocytosis.

16. What is the frequency of the various organ system involvements in systemic mastocytosis?

The frequency of organ system involvement seen in systemic mastocytosis varies significantly from study to study. With that in mind, some often-quoted frequency rates are:

Organ system	Percentage	Conditions most frequently seen
Skin	90–100%	Urticaria pigmentosa, solitary mastocytomas
Hematologic	28–70%	To various degrees including peripheral blood abnormalities, lytic bone lesions, mast cell leukemia
Gastrointestinal	70%	Peptic ulcer disease, malabsorption, hepatic or splenic involvement
Lymphatic	26%	Peripheral lymphadenopathy

17. What is urticaria pigmentosa?

The skin is the most commonly affected organ system in systemic mastocytosis, followed by the gastrointestinal tract, bone marrow, liver, spleen, and lymph nodes. One of the most common skin presentations of systemic mastocytosis is urticaria pigmentosa. This skin condition was first described by Nettleship in the mid-nineteenth century. Sangster first used the term *urticaria pigmentosa* in 1878. Initially, all the cases were described in patients only a few days to months of age, with spontaneous resolution followed by hyperpigmentation. Urticaria pigmentosa can occur in any age group, but the appearance of urticaria pigmentosa can vary. Urticaria pigmentosa is typically described as tan to red-brown macules appearing on the trunk and spreading outwards. Urticaria pigmentosa tends to spare the palms and soles, and it is generally very pruritic. The pruritus can be exacerbated by environmental changes including heat or friction. In biopsy specimens of urticaria pigmentosa, there are large numbers of mast cells, spanning all of the dermal layers.

18. In addition to urticaria pigmentosa, what are the other skin manifestations of systemic mast cell disease?

The other cutaneous presentations of systemic mast cell disease are a solitary mastocytoma and telangiectasia macularis eruptiva perstans. Approximately 1% of patients with systemic mast cell disease may present with telangiectasia macularis eruptiva perstans. This condition usually occurs in adults, and the appearance is one of numerous telangiectatic macules, primarily on the trunk. Pruritus may vary. Lesions are 3 to 6 mm in diameter. The lesions worsen with trauma.

The mastocytoma is a single nodule; it may be present at birth. It is usually hyperpigmented and present on a distal extremity. There may be associated local pruritus. This is the most common presentation of mastocytosis in children less than 2 years of age.

Any of the above forms of mastocytosis, including urticaria pigmentosa, can appear in a bullous form. Bullous urticaria pigmentosa usually occurs in children less than 3 years of age. Hemorrhagic blister formation and ulceration are characteristics of the lesions. Other organ system involvement is common.

Diffuse cutaneous mast cell disease is another rare presentation in young children. A yellowish-brown or red color, thickening, and lichenification characterize the affected skin.

19. Describe Darier's sign.

In patients with urticaria pigmentosa, scratching of the macular lesion leads to a wheal-and-flare reaction around the original lesion. This is known as Darier's sign.

20. What are skin biopsy findings in urticaria pigmentosa and diffuse cutaneous mastocytosis?

In urticaria pigmentosa, there is an increase in the number of dermal mast cells. Most of the mast cells identified in the skin of these patients are of the MC_{TC} variety. Mast cells primarily infiltrate the upper third of the dermis, but increased numbers can be seen throughout. In patients with systemic involvement, the mast cells may have an atypical morphology. Mast cells may also aggregate perivascularly. The skin biopsy findings in diffuse cutaneous mastocytosis are similar to those of urticaria pigmentosa.

21. List the most common sites of bone marrow lesions in systemic mastocytosis.

In order of decreasing frequency: the long bones, pelvis, ribs, and skull.

22. Is there a genetic component to systemic mastocytosis?

Systemic mastocytosis is generally sporadic, but in some occasions appears to have an autosomal dominant familial pattern. Pediatric onset systemic mastocytosis is more commonly seen in Caucasians. There appears to be a slight male to female predominance.

23. What is the differential diagnosis of urticaria pigmentosa?

Because the skin is the most commonly affected organ system in systemic mastocytosis, the differential diagnosis is often dictated by appearance of the skin. One must consider chronic idiopathic urticaria and angioedema in the differential diagnosis. Other possibilities may be recurrent anaphylaxis and scleroderma. Pheochromocytoma and carcinoid tumor can also present with the same signs of vascular instability that are seen in systemic mastocytosis. These conditions may be ruled in or out by the measurement of urinary catecholamines. In the absence of skin changes, the presence of unexplained flushing, peripheral blood changes, or the presence of visceral organ enlargement may support the diagnosis of mastocytosis. If the diagnosis is suspected, then it is particularly important to obtain a bone marrow biopsy to confirm the diagnosis and characterize the severity, because this plays a role in prognostication.

24. Describe the gastrointestinal manifestations of systemic mastocytosis.

Patients with systemic mastocytosis generally complain of abdominal pain, diarrhea, nausea, and vomiting. Some patients may present with gastric ulcers. Malabsorption can be seen. Liver and spleen involvement can also occur in systemic mastocytosis, although less frequently. Fibrosis of the liver has been observed, and vitamin B12 deficiency has been reported.

25. Define xanthelasmoidea.

Xanthelasmoidea is a term that was used by T. Fox in 1875 to describe the hyperpigmented skin of patients with urticaria pigmentosa. The pigmented skin was described as being smooth, prominent, and firm.

26. What are normal plasma and histamine levels?

The half-life of histamine in blood is only about 20 seconds and measurement of histamine levels as a marker of mast cell activation is not practical. Histamine release

is not solely a function of mast cell activation as histamine is also largely released by basophils. The distribution of histamine levels in asthmatics tends to be skewed toward higher levels, as compared to both nonatopic and atopic nonasthmatic controls. Histamine levels in the latter group range from 1 to 5 nmol/l, while those in asthmatics range from 3 to 14 nmol/l. Histamine levels are increased in asthmatics who are experiencing acute asthma symptoms.

27. How are histamine and tryptase levels measured?

Histamine and tryptase levels can both be measured by immunoassay. Tryptase is measured with the B12 and G5 antibody-based immunoassay. G5 is a mouse monoclonal antibody that recognizes a linear epitope on denatured and inactive tryptase. The active tetramer is not detected by the G5 antibody immunoassay. The sensitivity of the current G5-tryptase assay is 1 ng/mL. The G5-capture monoclonal antibody immunoassay preferentially recognizes the β subunit. In contrast, the B12-capture monoclonal antibody immunoassay detects both the β and α subunits. Of patients with systemic mastocytosis, 50% will have baseline levels of tryptase significantly greater than 1 ng/mL.

28. What is the significance of plasma histamine and tryptase levels?

Unfortunately, because of the short plasma half-life of histamine, there is limited utility in measurement of histamine levels in patients with mastocytosis or anaphylaxis. However, a rise in plasma histamine levels has been observed in patients with severe cold urticaria, with peak levels reached at about 8 minutes after cold stimuli. This corresponds to histamine release observed in skin biopsy specimens. Tryptase has been used in the diagnosis of systemic anaphylaxis because its half-life is somewhat longer (1.5 to 2.5 hours). The mean normal serum or plasma levels for α-tryptase is 4.5 ng/mL. β-Tryptase is normally undetectable. Measurement of serum or plasma tryptase levels can be helpful in determining response to therapy that is directed towards decreasing the degree of mast cell activation. Histamine is released from basophils during blood sampling, so histamine levels are not entirely reflective of mast cell activation.

29. What is the role of mast cells in anaphylaxis?

While not classified as a systemic mastocytosis syndrome, degranulation of mast cells and the resultant release of mediators into the circulation can bring on anaphylaxis. The clinical symptoms of anaphylaxis directly result from the release of histamine, tryptase, and other vasoactive mediators. β-Tryptase is involved in mast cell-dependent systemic anaphylaxis, while α-tryptase is found to be elevated in systemic mastocytosis. Substance P, vasoactive intestinal peptide, and calcitonin gene-related peptide are released during an anaphylactic reaction. Mast cells also release kininogenase. Other mast cell mediators released in anaphylaxis include heparin, prostaglandins D2 and F2a; leukotrienes B4, C4, and D4; platelet-activating factor; lymphokines such as IL-3, IL-5, and TNF; eosinophilic chemotactic factor; neutrophilic chemotactic factor; neutral proteases; major basic protein; and arachidonic acid-stimulating factors.

Anaphylactoid reactions are clinical indistinguishable from anaphylactic events but are not IgE or mast cell mediated. Degranulation of mast cells in anaphylactoid

reactions may be triggered by activation of the FcεRI receptor by nonimmune related stimuli.

30. What is the significance of mast cells in urticaria?

Urticaria is a commonly seen problem. Signs of urticaria include pruritus, vasodilatation, and increased vascular permeability of the superficial dermis. The wheal-and-flare reaction is a hallmark of urticarial lesions. Histamine, prostaglandin D2, the cysteinyl leukotrienes, platelet-activating factor, and bradykinin mediate wheal-and-flare production. Flare production is indicative of increase vasodilatation. In chronic urticaria, it has been found that there is a 10-fold rise in mast cell number in skin biopsy of active urticarial lesions.

31. What are the effects of arachidonic acid metabolites in systemic mastocytosis?

Arachidonic acid is a precursor of a number of newly generated mast cell mediators, including prostaglandin D2, leukotriene C4, and thromboxane A2. Leukotriene C4 is the predominant product of the lipoxygenase pathway. The effects of leukotriene C4 include vasodilation and increased vascular permeability. LTC4 is also an arteriolar constrictor. Mast cells also produce small amounts of LTB4, which plays a role in neutrophil chemotaxis. The effects of PGD2 include increased vasopermeability and vasodilation. PGD2 can also cause pulmonary vasoconstriction and augmentation of basophil histamine release. It is also a neutrophil chemoattractant. This contributes to the skin and gastrointestinal effects seen in mastocytosis. Platelet-activating factor (PAF) can also be released during mast cell activation. In addition to increasing vascular permeability, PAF can also induce neutrophil and eosinophil chemotaxis and activation.

32. Describe the biologic functions of the cytokines released by mast cells.

Cytokines released by mast cells can have proinflammatory, immunomodulatory, and/or mitogenic biologic activity.

IL-1α, IL-1β	Augments histamine release; stimulates IL-10 secretion; increases expression of endothelial cell adhesion molecules, lymphocyte activating factor; stimulates synthesis of IL-2 and IL-2 receptor; stimulates inflammation in allergic diseases
IL-2	Inhibits IL-4 activity
IL-3	Activation, degranulation, and chemotaxis of eosinophils; degranulation of mast cells; activation of monocytes; prolongation of eosinophil survival; induces mast cell proliferation
IL-4	Activates T cells; triggers isotope switching to IgE production; induces IL-6 production by endothelial cells; induces VCAM-1 production
IL-5	Chemotaxis and activation of eosinophils
IL-6	Augments histamine release; inhibits IL-1 and TNF production
IL-8	Chemotaxis of neutrophils; activates neutrophils; inhibits histamine release; induces production of leukotriene B4
IL-10	Inhibits eosinophil survival; inhibits IL-4-induced IgE synthesis, cytokine synthesis inhibitory factor, and mast cell proliferation
IL-13	Plays a role in allergic inflammation; closely related to IL-4 and may share a common receptor

IL-16	Role in inflammatory disorders such as asthma; modulates lymphocyte chemotactic response of CD4+ cells.
TNF-α	Activates a variety of proinflammatory cells, including T-lymphocytes, monocytes, eosinophils, and neutrophils; up-regulates endothelial cell adhesion-molecule expression; stimulates ICAM-1 production
INF-γ	Inhibits IL-4- and IL-13-induced IgE isotope switching
GM-CSF	Prolongs survival of eosinophils; eosinophil, monocyte, and neutrophil activation; autostimulatory mast cell degranulation; eosinophil chemotaxis

33. How is systemic mastocytosis treated?

There is no known cure for systemic mastocytosis. Thus, the treatment of mast cell disorders is focused upon control of symptoms related to the release of mast cell mediators. Avoidance of common physical and chemical triggers is of the utmost importance. Treatment of the effects of histamine, including urticaria and pruritus, gastrointestinal cramps, increase in gastric acid production, and episodes of anaphylaxis are also very important. The treatment of these symptoms requires use of antihistamines. While most of the inflammatory effects of mast cells are mediated through H1-receptor activation, gastrointestinal symptomatology, in particular, may be related to H2 receptors, which are present in high concentration in the acid-secreting parietal cells in the gut. Consequently, both H1 and H2 antagonists may be needed. The availability of second-generation antihistamines, including cetirizine, loratadine, and fexofenadine, has provided advances in the control of the above symptoms because of the absence of sedative side effects and because of their long half-life. For this reason, these agents are preferable to over-the-counter medications such as diphenhydramine. On occasion, an additional short-acting antihistamine such as hydroxyzine, or use of the tricyclic antidepressant doxepin, may be added for severe cases. They can primarily be used at night because of their sedative side effects. Doxepin is known to have very potent H1- and H2-antihistaminic activity. Cyproheptadine has both antihistaminic and antiserotonin activity, and has shown benefit in the treatment of mastocytosis. Addition of an H2-receptor antagonist may be beneficial for the gastrointestinal symptoms. Ranitidine and cimetidine are examples of H2-receptor antagonists.

Control of the clinical effects of the other mast cell mediators poses a more difficult problem, because of the lack of specific blocking agents for the other mediators. As yet, there are no clinical data as to the efficacy of leukotriene receptor antagonists in mast cell disorders. Mast cell-stabilizing agents, such as oral disodium cromoglycate, may be particularly useful in control of gastrointestinal symptoms. The dose is 20 to 40 mg/kg/day in four divided doses. Ketotifen may also be used and may have some benefit in controlling skin symptomatology.

Steroids may be used to control the inflammation resulting from release of mast cell mediators. Methylprednisolone has been used in conjunction with cyclosporin to treat aggressive systemic mastocytosis. High potency topical steroids such as betamethasone dipropionate may be used to treat skin manifestations. There has been some success with the used of psoralen with long-wave ultraviolet radiation done over time. For isolated lesions, local injections of corticosteroids may be affective.

Unfortunately, there is no effective treatment for the more aggressive forms of the disease or for mast cell leukemia. Interferon γ-2b at a dose of 0.5 million units per day has been studied and found to be effective in decreasing lymphadenopathy in retroperitoneal and mesenteric locations. There was also some decrease in the number of mast cells in bone marrow. Although the authors of the study did detect a decrease in urinary excretion of histamine metabolites, there was no effect on serum tryptase levels. There are frequent side effects, including hypothyroidism, thrombocytopenia, and depression, with the use of interferon γ-2b.

In patients with severe liver involvement and ascites, steroids may be beneficial, and the use of a portacaval shunt for management of portal hypertension may occasionally be necessary.

34. What is the prognosis of systemic mastocytosis?

The prognosis is dependent on the category of the disease. In general, the prognosis for category 4 disease is worse than that for category 3 disease, and so on. Those with indolent disease can be managed by pharmaceutic intervention and the disease may even spontaneously regress. In the case of mast cell leukemia, the median survival rate is only 6 months. Bone marrow biopsy can be useful for prognostication. Prognosis of systemic mastocytosis is better in children where the onset is under 10 years of age. Overall, 50% of children with urticaria pigmentosa have spontaneous resolution of the disorder by the second decade of life.

35. What is mast cell leukemia?

Patients with mast cell leukemia have a poor prognosis. The bone marrow of these patients is infiltrated with abnormal mast cells. Mast cells can be seen in the peripheral circulation, sometimes occupying up to 90% of peripheral white blood cells. Mast cell leukemia occurs in less than 2% of all patients with systemic mastocytosis.

36. What are the doses of commonly prescribed H1 and H2 antagonists?

H1 antagonists

Drug	Adult Dose	Pediatric dose	Frequency
First-generation antihistamines			
Diphenhydramine	25–50 mg	1–2 mg/kg	q6h
Hydroxyzine	10–25 mg	0.5 mg/kg	q6–8h
Cyproheptadine	4 mg	n.a.	q.i.d.
Clemastine	1 mg	0.25–1 mg	b.i.d.
Chlorpheniramine maleate	8–12 mg	0.2 mg/kg	b.i.d.
Second-generation antihistamines			
Fexofenadine	180 mg	60 mg (> 6 years)	q.d.
Loratadine	10 mg	5 mg (> 6 years)	Once daily
Cetirizine	10 mg	5 mg (> 2 years)	Once daily

H2 antagonists

Drug	Dose	Pediatric dose	Frequency
Cimetidine	300 mg	20–25 mg/kg	q.i.d.
Ranitidine	150 mg	n.a.	b.i.d.
Famotidine	20 mg	n.a.	b.i.d.
Nizatidine	150 mg	n.a.	b.i.d.

37. Are antihistamines safe for use in pregnancy and lactation?

Most of the first-generation antihistamines are classified as FDA pregnancy category C drugs. Some of the more common ones, including diphenhydramine and chlorpheniramine, are category B. Of the second-generation antihistamines, loratadine and cetirizine are category B, while fenofexadine is category C. Both sedating and nonsedating antihistamines are excreted in breast milk, but only the sedating antihistamines seem to produce side effects, such as sedation or irritability, in the breast-fed infant. The current recommendation, as with most other medications that are normally considered to have a low degree of serious adverse effects, is for these medications to be used only if clearly indicated. Further studies are ongoing.

38. What is the role of mast cell activation in sudden infant death syndrome?

Some cases of sudden infant death syndrome (SIDS) have found postmortem evidence of mast cell activation. This evidence consists of elevated tryptase levels in 50 infants with SIDS as compared to 15 normal controls. This observation allows us to speculate that in some patients with sudden infant death syndrome, anaphylaxis because of mast cell activation may be a cause. Of course, at the present time, this is merely speculative.

BIBLIOGRAPHY

1. Benjamini E, Leskowitz S: Immunology: A Short Course, 2nd ed. New York, Wiley-Liss, 1991.
2. Bier OG, Dias da Silva W, Gotze D, Mota I: Fundamentals of Immunology. New York, Springer-Verlag, 1981.
3. Bierman CW, Pearlman DS. Allergic Diseases from Infancy to Adulthood, 2nd ed. Philadelphia, W.B. Saunders, 1988.
4. Church MK, Holgate ST, Shute JK, Walls AF, Sampson AP: Mast cell-derived mediators. In Middleton E Jr, Ellis EF, Yunginger JW, et al (eds): Allergy, Principles and Practice. St. Louis, Mosby, 1998, pp 146–167.
5. Church MK, Levi-Schaffer F: The human mast cell. J Allergy Clin Immunol 99:155–160, 1997.
6. Galli SJ: New concepts about the mast cell. N Engl J Med 328:257–265, 1993.
7. Hurwitz S: Unclassified disorders. In Clinical Pediatric Dermatology: A Textbook of Skin Disorders of Childhood and Adolescence. Philadelphia, W.B. Saunders, 1993, pp 663–694.
8. Kaposi M: Pathology and Treatment of Diseases of the Skin. New York, William Wood and Company, 1895.
9. Kennard CD: Evaluation and treatment of urticaria. Immunol Allerg Clin North Am 15:785–802, 1995.
10. Kettelhut BV, Metcalfe DD: Pediatric mastocytosis. Ann Allergy 73:197–202, 1994.
11. McNeil HP, Austen KF: Biology of the mast cell. In Frank MM, Austen KR, Claman HN, Unanue ER (eds): Samter's Immunological Diseases, Fifth Edition, Boston, Little, Brown and Company, 1995 pp 185–204.
12. Metcalfe DD: Mastocytosis syndromes. In Middleton E Jr, Ellis EF, Yunginger JW, et al (eds): Allergy, Principles and Practice, 5th ed. St. Louis, Mosby, 1998, pp 1093–1103.
13. Metcalfe DD, Austen KF: Mastocytosis. In Frank MM, Austen KR, Claman HN, Unanue ER (eds): Samter's Immunological Diseases, 5th ed. Boston, Little, Brown and Company, 1995, pp 599–606.
14. Platt MS, Yunginger JW, Sekula-Perlman A, et al: Involvement of mast cells in sudden infant death syndrome. J Allergy Clin Immunol 94:250–256, 1994.
15. Schwartz LB: Laboratory assessment of immediate hypersensitivity and anaphylaxis: Use of tryptase as a marker of mast cell-dependent events. Immunol Allerg Clin North Am 14:339–350, 1994.
16. Venzor J, Baer SC, Huston DP: Urticaria pigmentosa. Immunol Allerg Clin North Am 15:775–784, 1995.

INDEX

Page numbers in **boldface type** indicate complete chapters.

Eosinophils (*cont.*)
degranulation of, 22
eicosanoid synthesis by, 21–22
hypodense, 22
life cycle of, 19
in nonallergic rhinitis with eosinophilia
syndrome (NARES), 64
receptors for, 21
staining of, 59
in vernal keratoconjunctivitis, 131
Eosinophil secretory granules, 21
Eotaxin, in atopic dermatitis, 113–114
Ephedrine
as Asian patent medicine contaminant, 237
as asthma treatment, 233, 234
Epicoccum, 38
Epidemiology, of allergic diseases, 1–3
Epinephrine
as anaphylaxis/anaphylactoid reaction
treatment, 107, 151
in food allergy, 172
in insect sting allergy, 181, 182
as asthma treatment, during pregnancy, 78
interaction with beta-blocking agents, 148
as status asthmaticus treatment, 82–83
Epiphora, 87
Episcleritis, 139
Epitopes, allergenic, 10
Epstein-Barr virus infections, 211, 218
Erythema multiforme, drug-induced, 189, 190
Erythema nodosum, drug-induced, 189
Erythroderma
drug-induced, 189
differentiated from toxic epidermal
necrolysis, 190–191
Omenn's syndrome-related, 219–220
E-selectin, 219
Ethanolamine, 67
Ethylenediamine, 66
Ethylene oxide, anaphylaxis/anaphylactoid
reactions to, 145, 150
Euroglyphus maynei, 39
Europe, allergic disease prevalence in, 3
European Academy of Allergology and Clinical
Immunotherapy, 228, 229
European Commission Respiratory Health Study, 3
Exercise
as anaphylaxis cause, 144
as food-dependent anaphylactic reaction cause,
164–165
Expiratory reserve volume (ERV), 52
Eye examination, 46
Eyelids
allergic conjunctivitis-related edema of, 124
contact dermatitis of, 136–140
involvement in atopic keratoconjunctivitis, 132
Eyes
allergic conjunctivitis-related redness of, 124
contact dermatitis of, 136–140
watery (epiphora), 87

Facial pain
migraine headache-related, 90
sinusitis-related, 86
temporomandibular joint dysfunction-related,
89–90
Facial pressure, sinusitis-related, 86
Facies
adenoid, 70
atopic, 110
Factor D, platelet release of, 26
Family size, large, as atopic disease preventive, 7
Farm environment, as allergic rhinitis preventive,
7
Farmer's lung, 199, 200
Fat, dietary, allergen content of, 169
Fatigue, sinusitis-related, 86, 87
FcεRI receptors, 242, 243, 244
Feather sensitivity
as allergic conjunctivitis cause, 125
in hypersensitivity pneumonitis, 201
Fetal thymus transplantation, as DiGeorge
syndrome treatment, 215
Fever
pharyngoconjunctival, 138–139
sinusitis-related, 86
Fexofenadine (Allegra), 67, 68, 250, 251
Fibrinogen, 26
Fibrosis, pulmonary
allergic bronchopulmonary aspergillosis-
related, 206
hypersensitivity pneumonitis-related, 201, 202,
203, 204
Fire ants, 177–180
control of, 180–181
Fish oil, as asthma therapy, 235
Fixed drug eruptions, 189, 191
Flixonase, 69. *See also* Fluticasone
Flonase, 69. *See also* Fluticasone
Flour, as aeroallergen source, 43
Flowering plants, allergic reactions to, 36–37
Flunisolide (Nasalide, Nasarel), 69, 74, 78
Fluorescence-activated cell sorter (FACS), 55–56
Fluorometholone, as allergic conjunctivitis
treatment, 129
Flush, carcinoid, 146
Fluticasone (Flonase, Flixonase), 69, 74, 78
Food additives and preservatives, as urticaria and
angioedema cause, 97, 101
Food allergens, "hidden," 170–171, 172
Food allergy, **159–174**
airborne protein reactions in, 163–164
as allergic rhinitis risk factor, 7
anaphylaxis/anaphylactoid reaction in, 144–145
as atopic dermatitis trigger, 115
categorization of, 159
cross-reactivity in, 165–166, 170
definition of, 159
diagnosis of, 51, 161–163
unproven methods in, 172–173
fatal reactions in, 164